JOURNAL OF PROSTHODONTICS
ON DENTAL IMPLANTS

JOURNAL OF PROSTHODONTICS ON DENTAL IMPLANTS

Edited by

AVINASH S. BIDRA, BDS, MS, FACP

STEPHEN M. PAREL, DDS, FACP

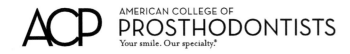

WILEY Blackwell

Cover image [background]: Günay Mutlu/Dental implant model/171225404/Getty Images

Cover design: Wiley

Published by John Wiley & Sons, Inc., Hoboken, New Jersey.
Published simultaneously in Canada.

For general information on our other products and services or for technical support, please contact our Customer Care Department within the United States at (800) 762-2974, outside the United States at (317) 572-3993 or fax (317) 572-4002.

Wiley also publishes its books in a variety of electronic formats. Some content that appears in print may not be available in electronic formats. For more information about Wiley products, visit our web site at www.wiley.com.

Library of Congress Cataloging-in-Publication Data is available.

ISBN: 978-1-119-11536-6

Printed in the United States of America.

10 9 8 7 6 5 4 3 2 1

CONTENTS

Preface   ix

Acknowledgments   xi

American College of Prosthodontists Position Statement on Dental Implants   xiii

PART I   MANAGEMENT OF THE PARTIALLY EDENTULOUS PATIENT

1 **ICK Classification System for Partially Edentulous Arches**   3
Sulieman S. Al-Johany and Carl Andres

2 **A Systematic Approach to Definitive Planning and Designing Single and Multiple Unit Implant Abutments**   10
Sanjay Karunagaran, Sony Markose, Gregory Paprocki, and Russell Wicks

3 **The Digital One-Abutment/One-Time Concept. A Clinical Report**   21
*Florian Beuer, Julian Groesser, Josef Schweiger, Jeremias Hey,
Jan-Frederik Güth, and Michael Stimmelmayr*

4 **Influence of Surgical and Prosthetic Techniques on Marginal Bone Loss around Titanium Implants. Part I: Immediate Loading in Fresh Extraction Sockets**   27
*Antoine N. Berberi, Georges E. Tehini, Ziad F. Noujeim,
Alexandre A. Khairallah, Moustafa N. Abousehlib, and Ziad A. Salameh*

5 **A Prospective Analysis of Immediate Provisionalization of Single Implants**   35
Thomas J. Balshi, Glenn J. Wolfinger, Daniel Wulc, and Stephen F. Balshi

6 **Technique for Removing Cement between a Fixed Prosthesis and Its Substructure**   41
Abdullah S. Alsiyabi and David A. Felton

v

7   **Immediate Loading of Dental Implants in the Esthetic Region Using Computer-Guided Implant Treatment Software and Stereolithographic Models for a Patient with Eating Disorders**   45

Daniel F. Galindo and Caesar C. Butura

8   **A Screwless and Cementless Technique for the Restoration of Single-Tooth Implants: A Retrospective Cohort Study**   52

Rainier A. Urdaneta, Mauro Marincola, Meghan Weed, and Sung-Kiang Chuang

PART II   MANAGEMENT OF THE COMPLETELY EDENTULOUS PATIENT

9   **Evidence-Based Criteria for Differential Treatment Planning of Implant Restorations for the Mandibular Edentulous Patient**   67

Steven J. Sadowsky and Peter W. Hansen

10 **Mandibular Implant Overdenture Treatment: Consensus and Controversy**   77

David R. Burns

11 **Evidence-Based Criteria for Differential Treatment Planning of Implant Restorations for the Maxillary Edentulous Patient**   87

Steven J. Sadowsky, Brian Fitzpatrick, and Donald A. Curtis

12 **Relevant Anatomic and Biomechanical Studies for Implant Possibilities on the Atrophic Maxilla: Critical Appraisal and Literature Review**   103

Paulo Henrique Orlato Rossetti, Wellington Cardoso Bonachela, and Leylha Maria Nunes Rossetti

13 **A Retrospective Analysis of 800 Brånemark System Implants Following the All-on-Four™ Protocol**   114

Thomas J. Balshi, Glenn J. Wolfinger, Robert W. Slauch, and Stephen F. Balshi

14 **Practice-Based Evidence from 29-Year Outcome Analysis of Management of the Edentulous Jaw Using Osseointegrated Dental Implants**   121

Matilda Dhima, Vladimira Paulusova, Christine Lohse, Thomas J. Salinas, and Alan B. Carr

15 **Double Full-Arch Versus Single Full-Arch, Four Implant-Supported Rehabilitations: A Retrospective, 5-Year Cohort Study**   131

Paulo Maló, Miguel De Araújo Nobre, Armando Lopes, and Rolando Rodrigues

16 **The Influence of Rehabilitation Characteristics in the Incidence of Peri-Implant Pathology: A Case-Control Study**   140

Miguel Alexandre de Araújo Nobre and Paulo Maló

17 **Concepts for Designing and Fabricating Metal Implant Frameworks for Hybrid Implant Prostheses**   152

Carl Drago and Kent Howell

18   **Complications and Patient-Centered Outcomes with an Implant-Supported Monolithic Zirconia Fixed Dental Prosthesis: 1 Year Results**   166
     Bryan Limmer, Anne E. Sanders, Glenn Reside, and Lyndon F. Cooper

19   **Prosthetic Improvement of Pronounced Buccally Positioned Zygomatic Implants: A Clinical Report**   177
     Ataís Bacchi, Mateus Bertolini Fernandes dos Santos, Marcele Jardim Pimentel, Mauro Antonio de Arruda Nóbilo, and Rafael Leonardo Xediek Consani

PART III   MANAGEMENT OF PATIENTS WITH MAXILLOFACIAL DEFECTS

20   **Implant-Supported Facial Prostheses Provided by a Maxillofacial Unit in a U.K. Regional Hospital: Longevity and Patient Opinions**   185
     S.M. Hooper, T. Westcott, P.L.L. Evans, A.P. Bocca, and D.C. Jagger

21   **Immediate Obturator Stabilization Using Mini Dental Implants**   192
     Gregory C. Bohle, William W. Mitcherling, John J. Mitcherling, Robert M. Johnson, and George C. Bohle III

22   **Prosthetic Reconstruction of a Patient with an Acquired Nasal Defect Using Extraoral Implants and a CAD/CAM Copy-Milled Bar**   197
     Carolina Vera, Carlos Barrero, William Shockley, Sandra Rothenberger, Glenn Minsley, and Carl Drago

PART IV   IN VITRO STUDIES

23   **Influence of Implant/Abutment Connection on Stress Distribution to Implant-Surrounding Bone: A Finite Element Analysis**   207
     Marcia Hanaoka, Sergio Alexandre Gehrke, Fabio Mardegan, César Roberto Gennari, Silvio Taschieri, Massimo Del Fabbro, and Stefano Corbella

24   **An In Vitro Comparison of Fracture Load of Zirconia Custom Abutments with Internal Connection and Different Angulations and Thickness: Part I**   215
     Abdalah Albosefi, Matthew Finkelman, and Roya Zandparsa

25   **Surface Characteristics and Cell Adhesion: A Comparative Study of Four Commercial Dental Implants**   221
     Ruohong Liu, Tianhua Lei, Vladimir Dusevich, Xiamei Yao, Ying Liu, Mary P. Walker, Yong Wang, and Ling Ye

PART V   GENERAL CONSIDERATIONS

26   **Outcomes of Dental Implants in Osteoporotic Patients. A Literature Review**   237
     Ioanna N. Tsolaki, Phoebus N. Madianos, and John A. Vrotsos

27 **Updated Clinical Considerations for Dental Implant Therapy in Irradiated Head and Neck Cancer Patients**   254

Takako Imai Tanaka, Hsun-Liang Chan, David Ira Tindle, Mark MacEachern, and Tae-Ju Oh

28 **Implant Treatment Record Form**   263

Tony Daher, Charles J. Goodacre, and Steven M. Morgano

Index   267

PREFACE

The *Journal of Prosthodontics* has been the official publication of the American College of Prosthodontists (ACP) for over 20 years. More than 1000 peer-reviewed articles on a wide variety of subjects are now in print, representing a treasure chest of history and valuable information on a myriad of topics of interest to our specialty.

The Board of Directors of the ACP recently began a project to classify and collate articles of significance into a book format, to allow both easier reference and enhanced access to areas of specialty interest for our membership. This specific project is a collection of different types of articles from a number of years, on the multiple applications of osseointegrated implants for the management of partially edentulous and completely edentulous patients as well as patients with maxillofacial defects. There are also articles on in vitro studies and general considerations to round out the readership selections.

The *Journal of Prosthodontics* has played an important role in the dissemination of quality implant research and patient care information, especially in more recent issues. Authors of prominence have begun to select the *Journal* with increasing regularity, as its reputation for quality of content and review process has become more accepted as the industry standard for the specialty.

We hope you enjoy this collection!

AVINASH S. BIDRA, BDS, MS, FACP
STEPHEN M. PAREL, DDS, FACP

ACKNOWLEDGMENTS

The editors are thankful to the authors whose work is collected in this volume; to Ms. Alethea Gerding, Managing Editor of the *Journal of Prosthodontics* since 2003; to Mr. Mark Heiden from the ACP, for his help in coordinating the efforts of everyone involved in this project; to editors-in-chief Dr. Patrick Lloyd (1998–2003) and Dr. David Felton (2003–present), for their tireless efforts on behalf of the *Journal* during the period when these articles were originally published; and to Dr. John Agar, who as President of the American College of Prosthodontists was instrumental in bringing this book to fruition.

AMERICAN COLLEGE OF PROSTHODONTISTS POSITION STATEMENT ON DENTAL IMPLANTS

Placement of dental implants is a procedure, not an American Dental Association (ADA) recognized Dental Specialty. Dental implants like all dental procedures require dental education and training.

Implant therapy is a prosthodontic procedure with a surgical component. Using a dental implant to replace missing teeth is dictated by individual patient needs as determined by their dentist. An implant is a device approved and regulated by the FDA, which can provide support for a single missing tooth, multiple missing teeth, or all teeth in the mouth. The prosthodontic and the surgical part of implant care can each range from straightforward to complex.

A General Dentist who is trained to place and restore implants may be the appropriate practitioner to provide care for straightforward dental implant procedures. This will vary depending on an individual clinician's amount of training and experience. However, the General Dentist should know when care should be referred to a specialist (a Prosthodontist, a Periodontist or an Oral and Maxillofacial Surgeon). Practitioners should not try to provide care beyond their level of competence.

Orthodontists may place and use implants to enable enhanced tooth movement. Some Endodontists may place an implant when a tooth can't be successfully treated using endodontic therapy. Maxillofacial Prosthodontists may place special implants or refer for placement when facial tissues are missing and implants are needed to retain a prosthesis. General Dentists are experienced in restorative procedures, and many have been trained and know requirements for the dental implant restorations they provide.

However, if a patient's implant surgical procedure is complex and beyond the usual practice of a dentist, this part of the care should be referred to a Dental Specialist that is competent in placement of implants. The referring dentist should effectively communicate and provide specific instructions and any necessary surgical guide(s) for appropriate care.

Likewise, the patient should be referred to a Prosthodontic specialist (a Prosthodontist) if the restorative procedure is complex and beyond the usual practice of the General Dentist. Prosthodontists may place implants as part of their patients' reconstruction, but they also may refer with instructions and surgical guides when the implant placement is beyond their level of competence. An example would be referral to an Oral and Maxillofacial Surgeon for more complicated surgical procedures or for patients with serious medical conditions. Referral to a Periodontist would be indicated when a patient exhibits significant periodontal disease that needs to be treated in combination with the implant restorations.

Dentists vary greatly in the procedures they perform and the ones they refer. Procedures that dentists perform should meet the standard of care for that procedure. A dentist should refer to a specialist those procedures they are not experienced and trained to do. Dental Specialists also vary in their level of experience and training relative to the use of dental implants. Therefore, any practitioner's implant knowledge and experience needs to be known by the referring dentist and to the patient regardless of the specialty.

Placement of implants without careful diagnosis and treatment planning should be avoided. The more complex and extensive the care, the more important it is to obtaining a satisfactory outcome for the patient. Implants placed without proper planning can result in an implant being placed with improper position, orientation, or without adequate space for the restoration. This can result in compromise of function, durability, esthetics or any combination of these problems. Implants may even need to be removed to get anticipated results for the patient. In addition to producing a compromised outcome, restoration of improperly placed implants can be expensive and burdensome.

In summary, not all General Dentists and Dental Specialists perform dental implant therapy in their practice. When considering a dental implant, patients should ask what training and credentials a particular dentist has that makes them appropriate to be doing the implant procedure. Just as in medicine, consumers should research their dentist's credentials and training. They should ask the same questions about any dentist(s) they may be referred to for all or part of the implant care. A list of some good questions to ask is below. Patients should check a dentist's web site for information and also check for comments by patients on the web.

(1) How often do you do this procedure?
(2) How many times have you done this procedure?
(3) What has been your training in this procedure? How long was it? (weekend course, lecture, 14–20 weeks CE at a dental school, or years of specialty training at an accredited dental school?)
(4) Where were you taught?

(5) Do you take lifelong learning/Continuing Education credit and if so, when, where, how often and in what area?
(6) What's the success rate for this procedure for me and how long will it last?
(7) How long will the procedure take from beginning until I have my permanent teeth?
(8) Will I have to be without teeth for any period of time?
(9) How much will it cost for the entire treatment from start to completion?
(10) How much will it cost for follow-up maintenance of my restoration?
(11) What are alternative treatment options for this procedure?
(12) What training do you have in these alternative options?
(13) May I get my treatment plan in writing?
(14) How do you feel about me getting a second opinion?

Author
John R. Agar, DDS, MA, FACP

Date
Approved ACP Executive Committee: October 1, 2014
Affirmed ACP Board of Directors: November 4, 2014

PART I

MANAGEMENT OF THE PARTIALLY EDENTULOUS PATIENT

1

ICK CLASSIFICATION SYSTEM FOR PARTIALLY EDENTULOUS ARCHES

SULIEMAN S. AL-JOHANY, BDS, MSD,[1] AND CARL ANDRES, DDS, MSD[2]

[1]Assistant Professor, Department of Prosthetic Dental Sciences, College of Dentistry, King Saud University, Riyadh, Saudi Arabia
[2]Professor and Director, Graduate Prosthodontics, Department of Restorative Dentistry, Indiana University, School of Dentistry, Indianapolis, IN

Keywords
Classification system; dental implants; removable partial denture.

Correspondence
Sulieman S. Al-Johany, College of Dentistry, King Saud University, P.O. Box 60169, Riyadh 11545, Saudi Arabia. E-mail: saljohany@hotmail.com

Previously presented at the Table Clinic Session at the American College of Prosthodontists 2006 Annual Session, Miami, FL.

Accepted May 24, 2007

Published *Journal of Prosthodontics* August 2008; Vol. 17, Issue 6

doi: 10.1111/j.1532-849X.2008.00328.x

ABSTRACT

Several methods of classification of partially edentulous arches have been proposed and are in use. The most familiar classifications are those originally proposed by Kennedy, Cummer, and Bailyn. None of these classification systems include implants, simply because most of them were proposed before implants became widely accepted. At this time, there is no classification system for partially edentulous arches incorporating implants placed or to be placed in the edentulous spaces for a removable partial denture (RPD). This article proposes a simple classification system for partially edentulous arches with implants based on the Kennedy classification system, with modification, to be used for RPDs. It incorporates the number and positions of implants placed or to be placed in the edentulous areas. A different name, Implant-Corrected Kennedy (ICK) Classification System, is given to the new classification system to be differentiated from other partially edentulous arch classification systems.

Partial edentulism is defined as the absence of some but not all the natural teeth in a dental arch.[1] Several methods of classification of partially edentulous arches have been proposed and are in use. It has been estimated that there are over 65,000 possible combinations of teeth and edentulous spaces in opposing arches.[2]

The most familiar classifications are those originally proposed by Kennedy,[3] Cummer,[4] and Bailyn.[5] Costa[6] in 1974 summarized most of the classification systems for partially edentulous arches and the rationale of the classification. These included: (i) the number and position of direct retainers,[4] (ii) the relation of edentulous spaces to abutment teeth,[3] (iii) the type of denture support, that is, tooth-supported, tissue-supported, or a combination,[5,7] (iv) the quality and degree of support a removable partial denture (RPD) receives from the abutment teeth and residual ridge,[8] (v) the number, length, and position of edentulous spaces and the number and position of remaining teeth,[9] (vi) the location and extent of edentulous spaces,[10] (vii) the boundaries of the spaces,[11] and (viii) combinations of these principles.[3,12,13] Classifications have also been proposed by Neurohr,[14] Austin and Lidge,[15] Avant,[16] and others.[6,17] Kennedy's method of classification is probably the most widely accepted classification of partially edentulous arches today.[2,17] None of these classification systems include implants, simply because most were proposed before implants became widely accepted. Recently, Misch and Judy[18] described a classification system depending on the Applegate–Kennedy system, with emphasis on the available bone in the edentulous area for implant placement. Their classification involves four divisions: Divisions A and B when bone is available for implant placement, division C when bone is not available for implant placement, and division D, restricted to cases with severe atrophy of the edentulous area involving basal bone.

Implants with or without attachments can be used to improve the support, stability, and retention of an RPD. The esthetic result of the RPD can be greatly improved by the use of implant attachments, thus eliminating unesthetic clasps. With the use of implants, the options for RPD use have increased, and the high demands of many patients for esthetic prostheses have been satisfied.[19–21]

At this time, there is no classification system for partially edentulous arches incorporating implants placed or to be placed in the edentulous spaces for an RPD.

The purpose of this article is to present a simple classification system for partially edentulous arches with implants based on the Kennedy classification system, with modification, to be used for RPDs.

KENNEDY CLASSIFICATION SYSTEM

The Kennedy method of classification was originally proposed by Dr. Edward Kennedy in 1925.[3] He divided all partially edentulous arches into four basic classes. Edentulous areas other than those determining the basic classes were designated as modification spaces.

> Class I: Bilateral edentulous areas located posterior to the remaining natural teeth,
>
> Class II: A unilateral edentulous area located posterior to the remaining natural teeth,
>
> Class III: A unilateral edentulous area with natural teeth remaining both anterior and posterior to it, and
>
> Class IV: A single, but bilateral (crossing the midline), edentulous area located anterior to the remaining natural teeth.

In 1954, Applegate[12] provided eight rules governing the application of the Kennedy system and proposed a new classification named the Applegate–Kennedy classification system for partially edentulous situations. These rules can be summarized in three general principles.[18] The first principle is that the classification should include only natural teeth involved in the definitive prostheses and follow rather than precede any extractions of teeth that might alter the original classification. The second principle is that the most posterior edentulous area always determines the classification. The third principle is that the edentulous areas other than those determining the classification are referred to as modifications and are designated by their number. The extent of modification is not considered, only the number of additional edentulous areas.

GUIDELINES FOR THE NEW CLASSIFICATION SYSTEM

The new classification system will follow the Kennedy method with the following guidelines:

(1) No edentulous space will be included in the classification if it will be restored with an implant-supported fixed prosthesis.

(2) To avoid confusion, the maxillary arch is drawn as half circle facing up and the mandibular arch as half circle facing down. The drawing will appear as if looking directly at the patient; the right and left quadrants are reversed.

(3) The classification will always begin with the phrase "Implant-Corrected Kennedy (class)," followed by the description of the classification. It can be abbreviated as follows:

   (i) ICK I, for Kennedy class I situations,

   (ii) ICK II, for Kennedy class II situations,

   (iii) ICK III, for Kennedy class III situations, and

   (iv) ICK IV, for Kennedy class IV situations.

(4) The abbreviation "max" for maxillary and "man" for mandibular can precede the classification. The word modification can be abbreviated as "mod."

(5) Roman numerals will be used for the classification, and Arabic numerals will be used for the number of modification spaces and implants.

(6) The tooth number using the American Dental Association (ADA) system is used to give the number and exact position of the implant in the arch. (*Note*: other tooth numbering systems such as Fédération Dentaire Internationale [FDI] can be used, as can the tooth name. The ADA system was used by the authors because of familiarity).

(7) The classification of any situation will be according to the following order: main classification first, then the number of modification spaces, followed by the number of implants in parentheses according to their position in the arch preceded by the number sign (#).

(8) The classification can be used either after implant placement to describe any situation of RPD with implants, or before implant placement to indicate the number and position of future implants with an RPD.

(9) A different name, ICK Classification System, is given to this classification system to be differentiated from other partially edentulous arch classification systems.

THE PROPOSED ICK CLASSIFICATION SYSTEM FOR PARTIALLY EDENTULOUS ARCHES

Examples for Kennedy Class I Situations

For Kennedy class I situations, Figures 1.1–1.3 show the classification if no modification spaces exist. The full text can be used, or preferably the abbreviation (Fig 1.1).

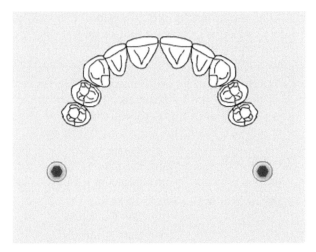

FIGURE 1.1 Maxillary implant-corrected Kennedy class I (#2, 15) or ICK I (#2, 15).

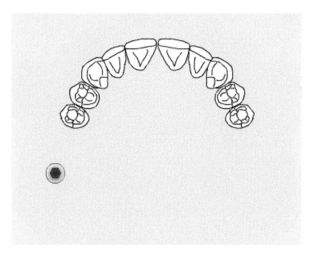

FIGURE 1.2 ICK I (#2).

If only one implant is placed in one of the two edentulous areas, it will be indicated between parentheses. This will mean that no implants were placed or to be placed in the other edentulous area (Fig 1.2).

The main classification, followed by the number of modification spaces, will be placed first, followed by the position (number) of the implants in the edentulous areas in parenthesis arranged according to the tooth numbering system used.

The arrangement of the implants will be from right to left in the maxillary arch and from left to right in the mandibular arch, following the arrangement of the tooth numbering system (Fig 1.3).

Figures 1.4–1.6 show the classification with modification spaces. Figure 1.4 shows the situation if only one modification space exists, and Figure 1.5 if two modification spaces exist.

If only one of the modification spaces or one of the main edentulous spaces has implants, it will be the same as in Figure 1.5.

When more than two modification spaces exist, it will be as shown in Figure 1.6.

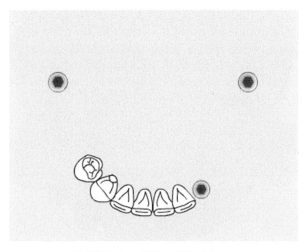

FIGURE 1.3 ICK I (#18, 22, 31).

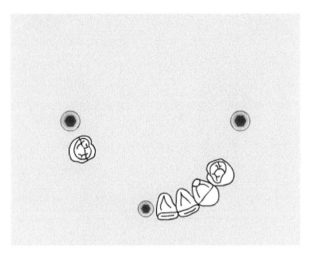

FIGURE 1.4   ICK I mod 1 (#19, 25, 30).

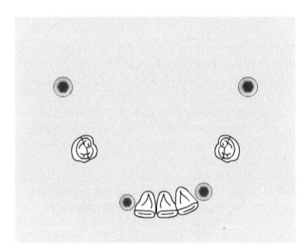

FIGURE 1.5   ICK I mod 2 (#18, 22, 26, 31).

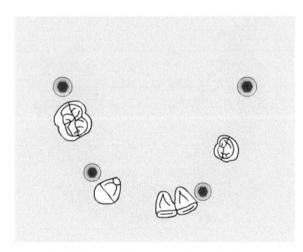

FIGURE 1.6   ICK I mod 3 (#18, 22, 28, 31).

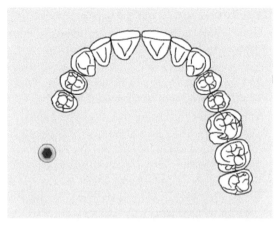

FIGURE 1.7   ICK II (#2).

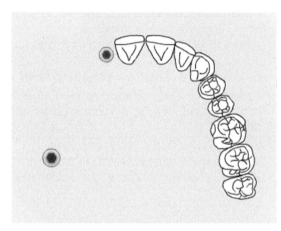

FIGURE 1.8   ICK II (#2, 7).

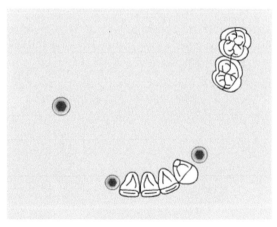

FIGURE 1.9   ICK II mod 1 (#21, 26, 30).

Examples for Kennedy Class II Situations

Figures 1.7 and 1.8 show the implant-corrected classification (ICK) for Kennedy class II situations without any modification spaces; Figures 1.9 and 1.10 show the same, but with modification spaces.

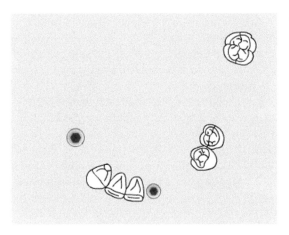

FIGURE 1.10   ICK II mod 2 (#24, 29).

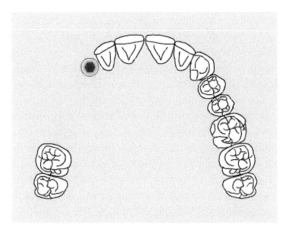

FIGURE 1.11   ICK III (#6).

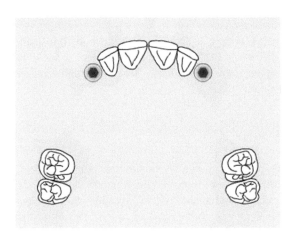

FIGURE 1.12   ICK III mod 1 (#6, 11).

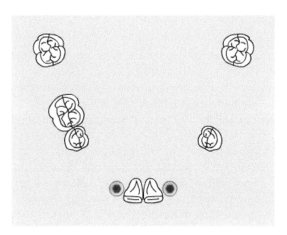

FIGURE 1.13   ICK III mod 3 (#23, 26).

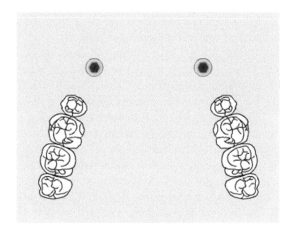

FIGURE 1.14   ICK IV (#6, 11).

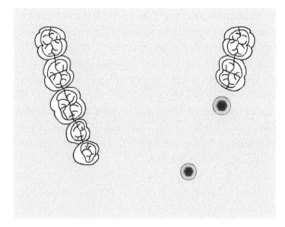

FIGURE 1.15   ICK IV (#19, 22).

Examples for Kennedy Class III Situations

Figure 1.11 shows the implant-corrected classification for Kennedy class III without modification spaces; Figures 1.12 and 1.13 show the same, but with modification spaces.

Examples for Kennedy Class IV Situations

Figures 1.14 and 1.15 show the implant-corrected classification for Kennedy class IV situations.

DISCUSSION

One requirement of a classification of partially edentulous arches is that it provides immediate visualization of the edentulous situation and the proposed treatment planning and design.

The proposed classification can be used before or after implant placement. The original Kennedy classification can be used to describe the situation without implants, and then the implant-corrected classification can be used to describe the situation with implants. It means that the classification can be used either retrospectively to describe an existing situation, or prospectively for future planning. For example, in a Kennedy class I situation with two implants already placed in the area of teeth #2 and 15, this system can be used to describe the existing situation as shown in Figure 1.1, retrospectively. If the same situation has no implants placed, but implants were planned to be placed in the area of teeth #1 and 15, this system can be used prospectively to describe the future situation and help in treatment planning.

Any edentulous space to be restored with an implant-supported fixed prosthesis will not be included in the classification as mentioned earlier in the guidelines. A description of the types of the removable and/or fixed prosthesis can be mentioned following the classification. The implant size, length, and system can also be included.

Misch and Judy[18] classification can be used for the edentulous area regarding the available bone for implant placement, as follows: divisions A and B for edentulous areas with bone available for implant placement, division C when bone is insufficient for implant placement, and division D when the edentulous area is severely atrophied involving basal bone. The authors did not use this in the classification to avoid complexity. It can be mentioned after the classification, if desired.

For dental schools using Kennedy's classification system for the classification of partially edentulous arches, this new classification system can be included to make the original classification broader to incorporate implants with RPDs. This can be done by explaining the original Kennedy classification first, then after the students become familiar with the original classification, the new implant-corrected classification can be introduced. Emphasis should be made about using the new classification system only when implants are incorporated with an RPD, not to be confused with the original classification without implants.

The guidelines of the new classification system can be summarized or compacted for teaching purposes. The examples provided with drawings showing the use of this new classification in different Kennedy classification classes should be helpful in explaining the use of this new classification for educational purposes.

The recently developed Prosthodontic Classification System, or Prosthodontic Diagnostic Index (PDI) for complete edentulism,[22] partial edentulism,[1] and completely dentate patients,[23] has gained more interest among educational centers and clinicians. Implants are involved in the classification for complete edentulism. If the condition requires a simple implant procedure, it will be classified as class III. If the condition requires complex implant procedures with bone graft, it will be class IV.

For partial edentulism, the residual ridge will be classified according to the complete edentulism classification. For example, if the residual ridge is classified as class III according to the complete edentulism classification, the condition will be class III, if no other factors make it class IV, and so on.

The authors suggest that this new classification be used with the PDI for partial edentulism according to the following: if the implant-corrected classification (ICK) of the condition involves the placement of two or fewer implants, the condition will be considered as simple and placed as class III (implants-simple) in the PDI. If the condition involves placement of more than two implants, with or without bone graft, it will be considered as complex and placed as class IV (implants-complex) in the PDI.

The presented classification is simple, but needs practice for familiarization. A software program (Dental Flash, Attachments International, San Mateo, CA) can be used to assist in drawing and designing any classification, and printing the design cleanly. This is very helpful for students and residents.

A widely used classification (Kennedy) is followed with modification for implant location and number. The classification is simple and easy to visualize, it can be done by observing the diagnostic casts or radiograph (e.g., Panorex), and assists in proposed treatment planning and design. The system provides ease in communication with the laboratory and assists professional communication regarding the different situations of partially edentulous arches with implants for RPDs.

The classification will be difficult for individuals who are unfamiliar with the Kennedy classification. Information is provided about the location and the number of the implants, but not the quality of the bone. Refinement and revision may be required.

SUMMARY

A classification system for partially edentulous arches with implants has been proposed. The Kennedy classification was used with modification. It incorporates the number and positions of implants placed or to be placed. A different name, ICK Classification System, is given to the new classification system to be differentiated from other partially edentulous arch classification systems.

ACKNOWLEDGMENTS

The authors thank Drs. Amir Saad and Mounir Iskandar, residents in the Graduate Prosthodontics Program, Indiana

University, for their help in using the software that produced the figures.

REFERENCES

1. McGarry TJ, Nimmo A, Skiba JF, et al: Classification system for partial edentulism. *J Prosthodont* 2002;11:181–193.
2. McGivney GP, Castleberry DJ: *McCracken's Removable Partial Prosthodontics* (ed 9). St. Louis, MO, Mosby, 1995, p. 17.
3. Kennedy E: Partial denture construction. *Dent Items Interest* 1928;1:3–8.
4. Cummer W: Partial denture service. In Anthony LP (ed): *American Textbook of Prosthetic Dentistry*. Philadelphia, PA, Lea & Febiger, 1942, pp. 339–452.
5. Bailyn M: Tissue support in partial denture construction. *Dent Cosmos* 1928;70:988–997.
6. Costa E: A simplified system for identifying partially edentulous dental arches. *J Prosthet Dent* 1974;32:639–645.
7. Beckett L: The influence of saddle construction on the design of partial removable restoration. *J Prosthet Dent* 1953;3:506–516.
8. Skinner C: A classification of removable partial dentures based upon the principles of anatomy and physiology. *J Prosthet Dent* 1959;9:240–246.
9. Mauk E: Classifications of mutilated dental arches requiring treatment by removable partial dentures. *J Am Dent Assoc* 1942;29:2121–2131.
10. Godfrey RJ: A classification of removable partial dentures. *J Am Coll Dent* 1951;18:4–13.
11. Friedman J: The ABC classification of partial denture segments. *J Prosthet Dent* 1953;3:517–524.
12. Applegate O: *Essentials of Removable Partial Prostheses* (ed 1). Philadelphia, PA, Saunders, 1954, pp. 4–9.
13. Terkla L, Laney W: *Partial Dentures* (ed 3). St. Louis, MO, Mosby, 1963, pp. 40–50.
14. Neurohr F: *Partial Dentures: A System of Functional Restoration* (ed 1). Philadelphia, PA, Lea & Febiger, 1939, pp. 120–137.
15. Austin K, Lidge E: *Partial Dentures: A Practical Textbook* (ed 1). St. Louis, MO, Mosby, 1957, pp. 17–21.
16. Avant WE: A universal classification for removable partial denture situations. *J Prosthet Dent* 1966;16:533–539.
17. Miller EL: Systems for classifying partially dentulous arches. *J Prosthet Dent* 1970;24:25–40.
18. Misch CE, Judy KW: Classification of partially edentulous arches for implant dentistry. *Int J Oral Implantol* 1987;4:7–13.
19. Jenkins G: *Precision Attachments: A Link to Successful Restorative Treatment* (ed 1). London, Quintessence, 1999, pp. 91–125.
20. Kuzmanovic DV, Payne AG, Purton DG: Distal implants to modify the Kennedy classification of a removable partial denture: a clinical report. *J Prosthet Dent* 2004;92:8–11.
21. Chee WW: Treatment planning: implant-supported partial overdentures. *J Calif Dent Assoc* 2005;33:313–316.
22. McGarry TJ, Nimmo A, Skiba JF, et al: Classification system for complete edentulism. *J Prosthodont* 1999;8:27–39.
23. McGarry TJ, Nimmo A, Skiba JF, et al: Classification system for the completely dentate patient. *J Prosthodont* 2004;13:73–82.

2

A SYSTEMATIC APPROACH TO DEFINITIVE PLANNING AND DESIGNING SINGLE AND MULTIPLE UNIT IMPLANT ABUTMENTS

Sanjay Karunagaran, bds, dds, msd,[1] Sony Markose, bds, dds, msd,[2,3] Gregory Paprocki, dds,[4] and Russell Wicks, dds, ms[5]

[1]Graduate Prosthodontic Resident, Advanced Education Program in Prosthodontics, Department of Prosthodontics, University of Tennessee Health Science Center, Memphis, TN
[2]Private Practice, Carrolton, TX
[3]Formerly, Assistant Director and Assistant Professor, Advanced Education Program in General Dentistry, Baylor College of Dentistry, Dallas, TX
[4]Director, Maxillofacial Prosthodontics, Memphis Veterans Affairs Medical Center, Memphis, TN
[5]Chairman and Professor, Department of Prosthodontics, University of Tennessee Health Science Center, Memphis, TN

Keywords
Implant dentistry; implant-supported abutment; abutment selection; prosthesis; restoration.

Correspondence
Sanjay Karunagaran, University of Tennessee Health Science Center – Prosthodontics, 875 Union Ave., Memphis, TN 38163. E-mail: skaruaga@uthsc.edu

The authors deny any conflicts of interest.

Accepted November 3, 2013

Published *Journal of Prosthodontics* December 2014; Vol. 23, Issue 8

doi: 10.1111/jopr.12161

ABSTRACT

With an increase in the availability of implant restorative components, the selection of an appropriate implant abutment for a given clinical situation has become more challenging. This article describes a systematic protocol to help the practitioner more thoughtfully select abutments for single and multiple unit fixed implant prostheses. The article examines the evaluation, planning, design, and fabrication processes for the definitive restoration. It includes an assessment of a variety of factors, namely restorative space, soft and hard tissues, the location of the implant platform, the type of platform connection, platform switching indications, tissue collar heights, emergence profile, implant angulation, and finally the design and esthetic options for the final implant abutment.

TABLE 2.1   **Assessment Criteria for Abutment Design**

Criteria	Implication for Abutment Selection
Determine restorative space available	Abutment height must not exceed the space available for the restoration
Evaluate the soft and hard tissue for possible grafting requirements	Placement of a bone graft may be required to correct vertical and horizontal defects prior to placement in order to achieve a more proportional and esthetic final abutment restoration
Determine implant platform location	Abutment margins should be supragingival in nonesthetic zones and slightly subgingival in the esthetic zone. Locate depth of soft tissue when deciding on the collar design (bone level, tissue level) with or without a transmucosal abutment
Choose engaging/nonengaging connection	Decide on the type of connection based on the type of restoration (single-unit, multi-unit)
Determine choice to platform switch	Decide on platform width based on adjacent teeth/implants and available or grafted bone
Determine existing tissue collar height	Bone sound the tissue to determine tissue thickness
Plan to customize emergence profile	Depending on the soft-tissue profile at the restorative stage, prefabricated or customized abutments can be made
Plan to correct implant angulation	If unavoidable, the abutment must counter an implant angulation to allow the restoration to emerge in the correct position relative to adjacent teeth
Plan for esthetic abutment	Ceramic/zirconia abutment may improve the esthetics

The dental implant has become a cornerstone in the current practice of restorative dentistry. The predictability of implant-supported restorations as a treatment modality has been sustained by a considerable amount of research. The continued development of implant surfaces, surgical protocols, and prosthetic components have enhanced the planning, placement, and restoration of missing dentitions.[1] An abutment is a component between the implant and the restoration, usually retained to the implant by a screw. The abutment provides retention, support, stability, and an optimal position for the definitive restoration.

Implant dentistry may be technically considered a prosthodontic procedure with a surgical component and, as such, it should be restoratively derived. The protocol for abutment selection should therefore begin with an understanding of the factors controlling prosthetic outcomes. The prosthetic selection process can be divided into planning phases. Related criteria and decision-making processes have been suggested.[2,3] Additional factors also requiring consideration include: (1) the proposed need for retrievability, (2) the passivity of fit of the prosthesis, (3) the occlusal scheme to be established, (4) predicting and planning for failure, and (5) the cost limitations and expectations of the patient.[3,4]

As part of the initial diagnostic assessment, the clinician should: (1) establish well-extended and articulated diagnostic casts. (2) Perform a diagnostic wax-up of the intended definitive restoration, reflecting its 3D size and exact location. (3) Begin to consider a protocol for rehabilitation, in the order outlined in Table 2.1 and described in detail below.

RESTORATIVE SPACE EVALUATION

Examine the distance from the crest of the alveolar ridge or the implant platform to the proposed occlusal plane in the posterior region and the incisal edge in the anterior region.[5]

Restorative space has been classified by the American College of Prosthodontists as follows: Class 1: 15 mm or greater; Class 2: 12 to 14 mm; Class 3: 9 to 11 mm; Class 4: Less than 9 mm.[6] An excessive crown height space is considered to be a distance greater than 15 mm.[7] These distances outline the restorative boundary of the definitive prosthesis and provide the clinician with the ability to decide between a screw- or cement-retained, fixed or removable prosthesis. The ideal space for a fixed prosthesis is suggested to be between 8 and 12 mm.[7]

The choice of fixed restoration is dependent on the preference of the clinician, and equal success has been accomplished when using either cemented or screw-retained prosthetics. The tissue may respond more favorably to a screw- vs. a cement-retained restoration, due to potential extrusion of the luting media on cementation.[8] Screw-retained restorations have disadvantages, including a higher cost of fabrication, and difficulty in optimally positioning the access opening in the design of the occlusion. As a result, some clinicians may prefer to use traditional crown and bridge protocols and use cemented restorations for prosthetic convenience.

A cementable restoration requires 8 to 10 mm of clearance from the implant platform to the opposing dentition. Clinicians should note that variations in the location of these restorations when considering anterior or posterior regions of the mouth may pose their own set of restorative space requirements. The dimensions requiring consideration for the abutment design should incorporate the 3-mm occlusogingival distance necessary for creating the ideal emergence profile, 2 mm for the ideal porcelain thickness, and 3 to 5 mm for the abutment to generate the retention, stability, and support needed for the definitive prosthesis. If 8 to 10 mm is not readily available, the dentist may choose to eliminate the abutment altogether, and retain the prosthesis directly into the body of the implant as a screw-retained restoration. Alternatively, if only the minimum of 3 mm for the construction of the abutment is available, the clinician may choose to modify the cementation method of the definitive restoration.

If between 3 and 4 mm of restorative space exists between the implant platform and the proposed occlusal plane, screw retention is most often chosen to accommodate the restorative space deficiencies. If 5 to 7 mm of restorative space exists, screw retention may be used. Additionally a cement-retained restoration (abutment-supported) may also be chosen if the implant has not been placed in its ideal location, to accommodate awkward screw access openings. Finally, if more than 8 mm of restorative space exists, the choice of either a cement- or screw-retained (abutment-supported) prosthesis may be possible.[7] The clinician should plan and consider the required restorative space prior to implant surgery and not consider it as an afterthought following implant placement.

Interocclusal distances exceeding 15 mm may be a concern when considering fixed restorations, as ideal tooth proportions can be challenging to accomplish and can often be avoided and corrected if an examination of the soft and hard tissue is accomplished concurrently with an assessment of restorative space.[7] Available intraoral restorative space may be estimated using a vacuum-formed shell of the diagnostic wax-up and a periodontal probe.

SOFT AND HARD TISSUE EVALUATION

An assessment of the supporting tissues is critical in implant treatment planning. In most instances, the proposed implant site presents itself with deficiencies due to trauma, tooth loss, or periodontal disease. This loss in architecture translates to both hard and soft tissue deficiencies. The position of the definitive restoration therefore has to be assessed in relation to these existing deficiencies. This is accomplished both clinically and radiographically.

Vertical, horizontal, and combined ridge defects should be examined and classified relative to the planned restorative position,[9] in addition to the quality and quantity of bone (Fig 2.1). These sites may require corrective grafting procedures or implant site development to have the implant platform placed in an ideal position for the definitive restoration. Careful planning will allow the implant restoration to have a good esthetic result and enable the definitive prosthesis to be placed in conformity with the body of the implant, thereby preventing any angulation and offset load issues.[10]

IMPLANT PLATFORM LOCATION AND EVALUATION

Incorrect implant placement can lead to both esthetic and prosthetic complications. Positional complications may result from an incorrect placement of the implant platform

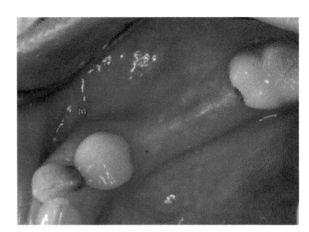

FIGURE 2.1 Alveolar ridge defects.

in mesiodistal, apicocoronal, or buccolingual directions. Positional requirements should be addressed at the soft and hard tissue evaluation phase, and if changes cannot be made by grafting, a custom abutment may be incorporated.

Mesiodistal positional errors should not exceed 3 mm from the intended prosthetic position, to prevent unreasonable esthetic and functional challenges.[11] Figure 2.2 illustrates a less than ideal placement in this direction. In these instances, it is often difficult to obtain a fixture level impression of both implants at the same time, as the impression copings have no space to be placed next to each other. In such instances, departures from recommended impression protocols may present restorative complications. It might even become necessary to leave one of the implants unrestored if an anatomical, cleansable, and esthetic result cannot be obtained.

Apico-coronal positional errors should not lead to exposure of the metal collar and implant platform. Figure 2.3 illustrates an incorrect apico-coronal position that had to be corrected prosthetically. In such situations, crown height becomes excessive, producing an unesthetic result. In most instances, a gingival porcelain collar is often required,

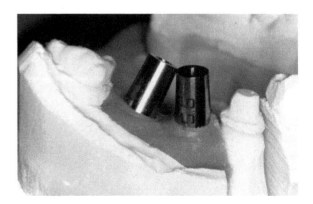

FIGURE 2.2 Incorrect mesiodistal placements.

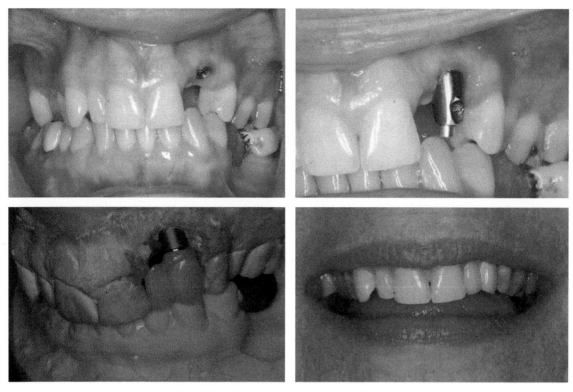

FIGURE 2.3   Incorrect apico-coronal placement.

and a customized abutment will need to be constructed. The definitive prosthesis can then be cemented into place or tapped into the custom abutment if screw retention is preferred. As previously mentioned, an assessment of grafting requirements should be considered in advance so as to avoid the need for such prosthetic corrections.

Buccolingual positional errors should not result in a ridge lap design in the definitive prosthesis, as this invariably makes oral hygiene almost impossible for the patient.[12] Placement should also not be directed buccally, as recession of facial tissue will often ensue. Figure 2.4 illustrates an incorrect buccolingual placement that had to be corrected

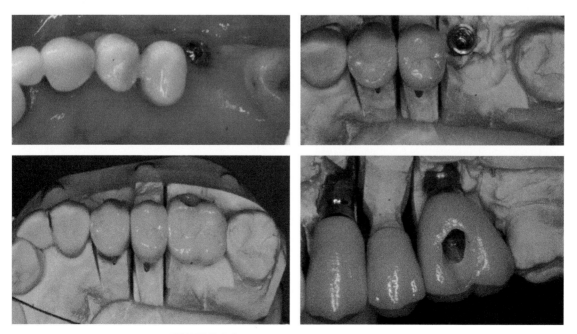

FIGURE 2.4   Incorrect buccolingual placement.

prosthetically. In this instance, the access hole for the restoration emerges from the buccal surface of the first molar, as an intervening abutment could not be used, a result of a desire to keep the prosthesis retrievable. In this instance, a ridge lap design was unavoidable.

INTERNAL ENGAGING/NONENGAGING CONNECTION EVALUATION

The term "engaging" is an antirotational component that prevents the turning of the abutment at the implant interface, thereby preserving the integrity of the preload on the abutment screw interface. The type of prosthetic connection is established (Fig 2.5) in conjunction with the type of implant platform to be used, whether it be at the bone level or the tissue level. Interfaces are divided into internal and external connections.[13] Both connections have been successfully used in the past; however, authors have suggested that under high occlusal loads the external connection abutments have been subject to greater micromovement, causing abutment joint instability associated with screw loosening.[14]

A resulting new preference of design has evolved favoring the internal connection; however, with the variation in manufacturers and the multitude of designs available, differences in performance between varieties of internal connections have been described.[15] These variations will require consideration during the selection process. Authors have outlined some factors for choosing a particular connection that may influence the success of the definitive prosthesis.[16]

These factors help the clinician control the design of the implant/abutment interface to establish stability and longevity in the implant prosthesis. Substantial evidence suggests that eliminating misfit in the prosthesis and engaging the antirotational features while applying adequate preload on the abutment screw significantly reduces mechanical

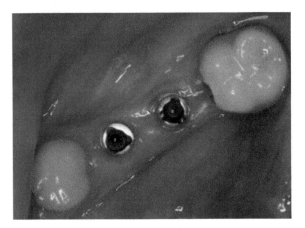

FIGURE 2.5   Platform connection, inter-implant, and inter-tooth distance.

complications and screw loosening.[17,18] Selection of compatible components between manufacturers should always be considered with care and caution.

The depth of penetration of the abutment within the fixture of the implant should be known. In the past, screw loosening and difficulty with seating restorations were attributed to the short lateral wall heights of external indexed implant systems, which on average had 0.8 mm index heights.[19] The newer more commonly used internal engaging connection systems have wall heights for lateral wall engagement on average of 2.4 mm, which provides a biomechanical advantage.[19] The intimacy of fit between the walls of the abutment and the internal surface of the implant fixture has become important, as these internally indexed abutments may be a challenge to seat accurately, especially when using multiple abutments. To overcome this problem, nonengaging implant connections are being used.

In a recent study of cantilevered prostheses, the presence and position of engaging components was shown to have a significant effect on the amount of axial force and the number of cycles it took to see prosthesis failure resulting in screw fracture and separation.[19] The authors concluded that using an engaging abutment in a screw-retained fixed cantilevered fixed dental prosthesis (FDP) provided a mechanical advantage.

The dimensions of the abutment screw should also be noted, as well as the type of thread design and the type of driver interface present (whether it is square, hexed, or unigrip), as these will influence individual torqueing protocols. Screw preload and torque protocols vary for the specific implant and the manufacturer.

Three types of connection methods are available to the clinician to connect and retain the abutment to the implant platform. One method involves a screw in addition to the antirotational interface (Astra, Nobel Biocare, Zurich, Switzerland). The other involves a tapered conical interference fit or Morse Taper (Bicon Implant, Boston, MA). Finally, the last mode of connection involves a combination of the above two systems (Ankylos, Straumann, Basel, Switzerland). When using the screw type of connection, mechanical complications such as screw loosening when occlusal loads exceed the preload were observed.[20] When tapered-fit connections are used, abutment loosening seems to be less of a concern.[21]

PLATFORM SWITCH EVALUATION

The implant platform is the area or the interface at which the implant and the abutment come together. Platform diameters can vary and can range from 3 to 6 mm depending on the implant system used. All platforms are divided into groups: narrow (3 mm), regular (4 mm), and wide (5–6 mm). The width of the implant platform chosen is often indicated by the width of the tooth being restored.

The size of the edentulous space will also dictate the potential width of the proposed implant platform. Authors have shown that a minimum space of 1.5 mm is required mesiodistally between an implant and a tooth to maintain both the soft tissue and the architecture of the bone. When placing an implant adjacent to another implant, a greater distance has been recommended, with a minimum space of 3 mm.[22]

The term "platform switching" is a concept first described in 1991 when Implant Innovations introduced its wide diameter implants, but they failed to develop an abutment to restore their implants. They therefore recommended using smaller standard diameter abutments and healing abutments as a substitute for their restorative protocol. They noticed that when these "platform-switched" components were used, there was a smaller change in crestal bone height around the implants than when restored in the conventional fashion.[23] Since this discovery, implant manufacturers have tried to establish their own systems of platform switched implants.

Platform switching is a treatment philosophy, and a recent systematic review concluded that platform switching appears to be a promising tool in the preservation of peri-implant bone, but more research is needed to validate its application.[24] Several confounding variables will need to be standardized in existing studies to reach a definitive conclusion.

TISSUE COLLAR HEIGHT EVALUATION

A measurement of the soft tissue sulcular depth from the surface of the implant platform to the free gingival margin should be reflected in the design of the abutment. This depth can be determined 6 to 8 weeks following stage 2 surgery.[1] Assessment of gingival tissue thickness should begin prior to surgical placement. The need to determine if a restoration will connect straight to the implant or if an intermediary transmucosal abutment is preferred will depend on the amount of tissue present and the availability of an adaptable manufactured abutment collar height.

Abutment collar heights can affect the design of the final abutment restoration. Abutment marginal placement should ideally follow the anatomy of the gingival margin as it rises

and falls past the interdental col areas. Abutment margins on the buccal and mesial should be placed at or 1 mm below the gingival margin based on the site and location of the restoration. Palatal and distal abutment margins may be placed at the gingival crest or 0.5 mm below the crest based on operator preference, as nonesthetic sites. This helps account for and controls any gingival recessional changes that may occur over time. If a cemented restoration is chosen, cement clean-up is easier to accomplish if abutment margins are placed within 1 mm of the gingival crest. Studies have shown that margins placed more below the gingiva can pose a problem to cement removal. A recent study has indicated that 80% of peri-implant disease was a result of the bacterial colonization of the extruded cement.[25] An exactingly detailed custom abutment may be fabricated using gold, titanium nitride, or zirconia to ideally locate and esthetically enhance the restorative margin.

An implant may have a shallow tissue crevice and still be in a position that is apical in relation to the adjacent teeth. This happens in situations where vertical resorption has occurred prior to implant placement and the implants are placed into these sites without the correct site development protocols, causing an uneven gingival topography (Fig 2.6). If this restoration is within the esthetic zone it may produce an esthetic compromise in soft tissue and gingival architecture. The site may require removal of the implant and grafting to correct the hard and soft tissue deficiency. If this is not possible, pink porcelain can be used to mask the defect[10] (Figs 2.3 and 2.6).

When soft tissue depth ranges from 1 to 3 mm, stock prefabricated abutments may generally be used.[26] Tissue depths greater than 4 mm or presenting unusual gingival contours may, however, benefit from customized cast or milled computer-aided design/computer-aided manufacture (CAD/CAM) abutments.[26]

CAD/CAM abutment designs now allow control of marginal placement based on operator- and patient-specific needs. These margins are designed from a scan of the implant site, either directly in the patient's oral cavity or from an impression of the master cast, and the abutments can then be virtually designed and fabricated. Abutment margins may be placed by a variety of methods; some systems use

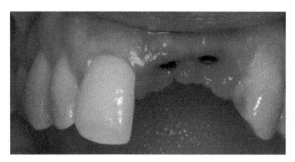
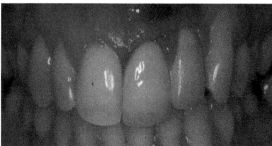

FIGURE 2.6 Gingival porcelain.

subgingival depths by measuring the soft tissue from the gingival crest to the proposed abutment margin at the implant platform. Alternatively, the margin may be designed as close to the implant/abutment interface as possible or by using the neighboring teeth as a guide to its final placement.

EMERGENCE PROFILE EVALUATION

The emergence of an implant restoration is dependent on implant location in three-dimensional space and the width of the implant platform. Anatomically, teeth are ovoid in cross section at the level of the cementoenamel junction (CEJ).[27] Alternatively, implants have circular platforms, and this poses difficulties for the dentist in creating a natural tooth profile as it emerges from the soft tissue. Ideally, the placement of the implant platform should be established 3 mm below the CEJ of the adjacent teeth to provide the distance required to establish the correct emergence of the restoration out of its socket. If this can be established with relative ease, then a prefabricated abutment may be used to construct the definitive prosthesis. If soft tissue depths exceed 3 mm, then customization may become necessary to follow the existing gingival topography. The need for customized abutment may also be beneficial in more challenging situations, especially where anterior restorations are being planned in patients with excessive gingival displays and esthetic challenges.[28]

Keratinized tissues can be customized by a variety of methods, some of which are illustrated in Figure 2.7. The emergence profile may be modified either by a direct or an indirect technique prior to definitive abutment selection. Direct techniques involve customization intraorally, while the indirect technique involves customization within the laboratory setting. When using the indirect technique, authors have contoured the emergence profile on the master cast by shaping the gingival profile in stone or sculpting a gingival substitute after the implant level impression has been made.[29] The disadvantage of using this method is that the technician has no indication of the biotype of the tissue or its tolerance to the contours of the final restoration. If the emergence profile is overcontoured, the tension created may result in trauma to the soft tissue, causing soft tissue recession and hard tissue resorption. In addition, if the tissue is undercontoured, tissue collapse can occur, leaving an unacceptable esthetic result.[30] Figures 2.5 and 2.7 illustrate how the emergence profile can be sculpted by a direct technique.

Implant manufacturers have developed CAD/CAM patient-specific abutments, to optimize function, esthetics, and simplicity. Zirconia abutments are being used and possess favorable esthetic qualities and are available in a variety of shades. These abutments are being virtually designed to correspond to the shape of natural teeth and to the height and width of the healing tissue gingival collar. The ability to customize this space to a variety of dimensions can be chosen

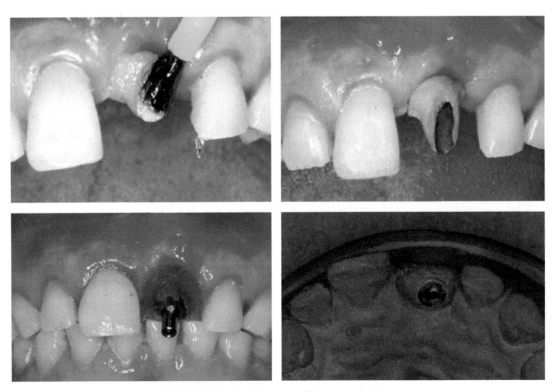

FIGURE 2.7   Emergency profile customization.

by the operator based on the level of soft tissue compression desired to complement the specific emergence profile.

IMPLANT ANGULATION EVALUATION

Improper alignment of implants compromises both esthetics and function due to the unfavorable positioning of the screw access opening. Ideal access openings should be centrally placed (Fig 2.8). As mentioned previously, offset angulation problems should be avoided, and the restorative site must be assessed in mesiodistal, buccolingual, and apicocoronal directions. Figures 2.2–2.4 illustrate some of the problems associated with an incorrect placement as well as the prosthetic corrections required to compensate for faulty surgical placements. One of the major prosthetic problems in correcting such nonoptimal implant placements is screw loosening, which frequently ranges from 2% to 45%.[31]

Prosthetic preangulated abutments are available to correct such problems[32] and are available in a variety of angulations that can range from 15° to 35° depending on the implant manufacturer chosen. The dentist may prefer to fabricate a custom abutment to produce a more ideal abutment design, thereby providing more control in the position of the definitive restoration. Angulations less than 15° are slight and may usually be corrected by modification of straight standard prefabricated abutments. Angulations between 15° and 20° may require the use of angle correcting prefabricated abutments, while an angulation discrepancy greater than 20° will usually require a custom abutment.

Studies have suggested that angulated abutments result in increased strain and stress along the implant and bone interface.[33,34] It was shown that when 15° and 25° angulated abutments are used compared with straight abutments, compressive strain increased fourfold with strain gauge measurements, whereas photoelastic methods showed an 11% increase in fringe order at the implant/bone interface. It is now accepted that angulated abutments result in increased stress on the implant and the adjacent bone, but these stresses are within physiological limits.[35] In addition, the use of angulated abutments has not decreased the survival rate of implants or prostheses in comparison with those of straight abutments, nor has this increase resulted in an increase in bone loss.[35]

Implant angulation issues require additional restorative distances from the implant's prosthetic platform to the free gingival margin. The dentist requires this distance to transition from the small-diameter, circular shape of the implant platform to the final shape of the tooth being restored.[35] Larger distances can often be beneficial in creating a transition from the implant platform to the free gingival margin in situations where implants were incorrectly placed. Custom abutments are often preferred in these situations.

IMPLANT ABUTMENT—ESTHETICS AND FUNCTION

An ideal abutment should be durable and able to undergo functional loads without a risk of deformation and fracture. Within the anterior region, the abutment should ideally be tooth colored and allow soft tissue coloration. In sites of thin gingival biotypes, the implant abutment can often show through at the cervical extent of the tissue surface, producing an unesthetic result. In such instances, three options are available in abutment design. The operator may choose to use a zirconium abutment, a titanium nitride coated abutment, or a titanium abutment with pink gingival porcelain to mask the color show through the gingiva. Titanium abutments are the standard, but there is now a growing trend for titanium-reinforced zirconia abutments and zirconium or alumina abutments, which are often the choice if restorations are planned within the anterior esthetic zone to produce more satisfactory results; however, all-ceramic abutments are brittle and susceptible to fracture in thin sections, and careful examination and design of the prosthetic abutment is required.[36] An alternative to the all-ceramic abutment is the traditional porcelain fused to metal gold cast-to abutment. In situations of lost gingival profile, gingival contours can be recreated in the definitive restoration (Fig 2.6). The uses of CAD/CAM abutments have their benefits, namely increased accuracy or precision of fit, durability, and simplicity of construction.[37]

With the advent of computer-generated technology in the 1980s, many manufacturers have now incorporated CAD/CAM technology into the production of their implant abutments. Traditional prosthodontic techniques used the lost-wax technique and relied on the processes of impression materials, gypsum products, waxing crowns, investing, and casting with alloys at high temperatures. The accuracy of this process is limited by the expansion and contraction of the

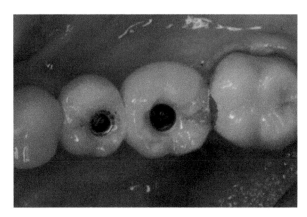

FIGURE 2.8   Ideal implant location to access hole.

materials at each stage. CAD/CAM production involves the steps of scanning, CAD modeling, and CAM production.

All implant manufacturers offer ceramic abutments that are available in either a prefabricated or a customizable form. The current materials of preference are densely sintered high purity alumina (Al_2O_3) and yttria-stabilized tetragonal zirconia poly-crystal ceramics. Zirconia has been shown to possess superior properties due to the stabilizing effect of yttria that allows the zirconia to be processed in a metastable tetragonal crystalline structure at room temperature. This tetragonal phase that is stable at room temperature allows transformation into the monoclinic form under stress, preventing crack propagation, a process called transformation toughening.[38]

Alumina abutments are composed of 99.5% pure alumina ceramic.[39] This abutment provides a more esthetic abutment when compared to the more whitish zirconia. Alumina abutments are also easier to prepare but are not as resistant to fracture as their zirconia counterparts.[40] A study showed the masticatory loading after fixation of various zirconia, alumina, and titanium abutments and their restoration and adhesive cementation of metal crowns. The median fracture loads for the zirconia, alumina, and titanium abutments were 294 N, 239 N, and 324 N, respectively. The authors

1. **PERFORM TRIAL TOOTH WAX-UP**

2. **DETERMINE RESTORATIVE SPACE AVAILABLE**

8-10 MM: CEMENT-RETAINED   5-7 MM: CEMENT- OR SCREW-RETAINED   < 4 MM: SCREW-RETAINED

3. **EVALUATE SOFT AND HARD TISSUE**

SOFT TISSUE GRAFT REQUIRED	SOFT TISSUE GRAFT NOT REQUIRED
HARD TISSUE GRAFT REQUIRED	HARD TISSUE GRAFT NOT REQUIRED
COMBINATION GRAFT REQUIRED	COMBINATION GRAFT NOT REQUIRED
BONE LEVEL IMPLANT REQUIRED	TISSUE LEVEL IMPLANT REQUIRED

4. **DETERMINE IMPLANT PLATFORM LOCATION**

MESIODISTAL POSITION   BUCCOLINGUAL POSITION   APICOCORONAL POSITION

5. **DETERMINE NEED FOR IMPLANT ENGAGING/ NON ENGAGING CONNECTION**

EXTERNAL CONNECTION   INTERNAL CONNECTION

6. **DETERMINE NEED TO PLATFORM SWITCH**

NARROW PLATFORM- INCISOR, CANINE   REGULAR PLATFORM-PREMOLAR   WIDE PLATFORM-MOLAR

7. **DETERMINE EXISTING TISSUE COLLAR HEIGHT**

1-4 MM: PREFABRICATED ABUTMENT   >4 MM: CUSTOMIZED ABUTMENT

8. **PLAN TO CUSTOMIZE EMERGENCE PROFILE**

3 MM: PREFABICATED ABUTMENT   >4 MM: CUSTOMIZED ABUTMENT

9. **PLAN TO CORRECT ANY IMPLANT ANGULATION**

<15°: (STANDARD PREFABRICATED ABUTMENT)   15°-20°: (ANGLE CORRECT PREFABRICATED ABUTMENT)
>20°: CUSTOMIZE CAST OR CAD/CAM ABUTMENT

10. **CONSIDER INDIVIDUAL ABUTMENT REQUIREMENTS**

ANTERIOR RESTORATION (Zr)   POSTERIOR RESTORATION (Ti-reinforced Zr, Ti, Ti Nitride, Alloys)

FIGURE 2.9 Flow chart (single and multiple units).

concluded that titanium-reinforced zirconia abutments were comparable to metal abutments and can therefore be used as an alternative in the anterior region.[40]

When considering the definitive restoration, studies have shown that the highest fracture resistance value was found with a titanium and alumina crown combination, whereas the smallest fracture resistance was found with an alumina abutment and a zirconia crown. They concluded that all abutment and crown combinations have the potential to withstand occlusal loads in the anterior region. For the posterior region, the routine use of zirconia abutments still must be validated.[41,42] Zirconia abutments benefit from the process of customization, as this will ensure maximal bulk in the final prosthesis to aid with durability. More recently, clinicians are using titanium nitride abutments, which are gold colored and have quite impressive esthetics through ceramic restorations as they impart a warm natural hue through the crown and gingiva.

CONCLUSION

Abutment selection is an important step in the process of creating the ideal restorative prosthesis. This article presents some of the factors and protocols needed for consideration in making this definitive restoration possible. Figure 2.9 presents a flow chart summarizing these factors. The treatment, however, remains the same and will invariably involve correct treatment planning, decision making, and finally sequencing of treatment to ensure a successful end result.

REFERENCES

1. Giglio GD: Abutment selection in implant-supported fixed prosthodontics. *Int J Periodontics Restorative Dent* 1999;19:233–241.

2. Drago CJ: Two new clinical/laboratory protocols for CAD/CAM implant restorations. *J Am Dent Assoc* 2006;137:794–800.

3. Wicks RA: A systematic approach to definitive planning for osseointegrated implant prostheses. *J Prosthodont* 1994;3:237–242.

4. Lee A, Okayasu K, Wang HL: Screw- versus cement-retained implant restorations: current concepts. *Implant Dent* 2010;19:8–15.

5. Misch CE, Goodacre CJ, Finley JM, et al: Consensus conference panel report: crown-height space guidelines for implant dentistry-part 1. *Implant Dent* 2005;14:312–318.

6. McGarry TJ, Nimmo A, Skiba JF, et al: Classification system for complete edentulism. The American College of Prosthodontics. *J Prosthodont* 1999;8:27–39.

7. Misch CE, Goodacre CJ, Finley JM, et al: Consensus conference panel report: crown-height space guidelines for implant dentistry-part 2. *Implant Dent* 2006;15:113–121.

8. Wadhwani CP, Pineyro AF: Implant cementation: clinical problems and solutions. *Dent Today* 2012;31:56, 58, 60–62; quiz 63, 54.

9. Seibert JS: Ridge augmentation to enhance esthetics in fixed prosthetic treatment. *Compendium* 1991;12:548, 550, 552 passim.

10. Cavallaro JS, Greenstein G: Prosthodontic complications related to non-optimal dental implant placement. In Froum JS (ed): *Dental Implant Complications. Etiology, Prevention and Treatment.* Hoboken, NJ, Wiley-Blackwell, 2010, p. 156.

11. Chen ST, Bruser D: Esthetic complications due to implant malpositions: etiology, prevention, and treatment. In Froum JS (ed): *Dental Implant Complications. Etiology, Prevention and Treatment.* Hoboken, NJ, Wiley-Blackwell, 2010, p. 134.

12. Goodacre C, Kattadiyil MT: Prosthodontic-related dental implant complications: etiology, prevention, and treatment. In Froum JS (ed): *Dental Implant Complications. Etiology, Prevention and Treatment.* Hoboken, NJ, Wiley-Blackwell, 2010, p. 172.

13. Finger IM, Castellon P, Block M, et al: The evolution of external and internal implant/abutment connections. *Pract Proced Aesthet Dent* 2003;15:625–632; quiz 634.

14. Jemt T, Laney WR, Harris D, et al: Osseointegrated implants for single tooth replacement: a 1-year report from a multicenter prospective study. *Int J Oral Maxillofac Implants* 1991;6:29–36.

15. Steinebrunner L, Wolfart S, Ludwig K, et al: Implant-abutment interface design affects fatigue and fracture strength of implants. *Clin Oral Implants Res* 2008;19:1276–1284.

16. Gracis S, Michalakis K, Vigolo P, et al: Internal vs. external connections for abutments/reconstructions: a systematic review. *Clin Oral Implants Res* 2012;23 Suppl 6:202–216.

17. Martin WC, Woody RD, Miller BH, et al: Implant abutment screw rotations and preloads for four different screw materials and surfaces. *J Prosthet Dent* 2001;86:24–32.

18. Piermatti J, Yousef H, Luke A, et al: An in vitro analysis of implant screw torque loss with external hex and internal connection implant systems. *Implant Dent* 2006;15:427–435.

19. Dogus SM, Kurtz KS, Watanabe I, et al: Effect of engaging abutment position in implant-borne, screw-retained three-unit fixed cantilevered prostheses. *J Prosthodont* 2011;20:348–354.

20. Schwarz MS: Mechanical complications of dental implants. *Clin Oral Implants Res* 2000;11 Suppl 1:156–158.

21. Morgan KM, Chapman RJ: Retrospective analysis of an implant system. *Compend Contin Educ Dent* 1999;20:609–614, 616–623 passim; quiz 626.

22. Tarnow DP, Cho SC, Wallace SS: The effect of inter-implant distance on the height of inter-implant bone crest. *J Periodontol* 2000;71:546–549.

23. Lazzara RJ, Porter SS: Platform switching: a new concept in implant dentistry for controlling postrestorative crestal bone levels. *Int J Periodontics Restorative Dent* 2006;26:9–17.

24. Annibali S, Bignozzi I, Cristalli MP, et al: Peri-implant marginal bone level: a systematic review and meta-analysis of studies comparing platform switching versus conventionally restored implants. *J Clin Periodontol* 2012;39:1097–1113.

25. Wilson TG, Jr.: The positive relationship between excess cement and peri-implant disease: a prospective clinical endoscopic study. *J Periodontol* 2009;80:1388–1392.

26. Drago CJ, Lazzara RJ: Guidelines for implant abutment selection for partially edentulous patients. *Compend Contin Educ Dent* 2010;31:14–20, 23–24, 26–27; quiz 28, 44.

27. Goodacre CJ, Campagni WV, Aquilino SA: Tooth preparations for complete crowns: an art form based on scientific principles. *J Prosthet Dent* 2001;85:363–376.

28. Bidra AS, Agar JR, Parel SM: Management of patients with excessive gingival display for maxillary complete arch fixed implant-supported prostheses. *J Prosthet Dent* 2012; 108:324–331.

29. Macintosh DC, Sutherland M: Method for developing an optimal emergence profile using heat-polymerized provisional restorations for single-tooth implant-supported restorations. *J Prosthet Dent* 2004;91:289–292.

30. Alani A, Corson M: Soft tissue manipulation for single implant restorations. *Br Dent J* 2011;211:411–416.

31. Goodacre CJ, Kan JY, Rungcharassaeng K: Clinical complications of osseointegrated implants. *J Prosthet Dent* 1999; 81:537–552.

32. Priest G: Virtual-designed and computer-milled implant abutments. *J Oral Maxillofac Surg* 2005;63(9 Suppl 2): 22–32.

33. Brosh T, Pilo R, Sudai D: The influence of abutment angulation on strains and stresses along the implant/bone interface: comparison between two experimental techniques. *J Prosthet Dent* 1998;79:328–334.

34. Clelland NL, Gilat A: The effect of abutment angulation on stress transfer for an implant. *J Prosthodont* 1992;1:24–28.

35. Cavallaro J, Jr., Greenstein G: Angled implant abutments: a practical application of available knowledge. *J Am Dent Assoc* 2011;142:150–158.

36. Aboushelib MN, Salameh Z: Zirconia implant abutment fracture: clinical case reports and precautions for use. *Int J Prosthodont* 2009;22:616–619.

37. Abduo J, Lyons K: Rationale for the use of CAD/CAM technology in implant prosthodontics. *Int J Dent* 2013; 2013:768121. doi: 10.1155/2013/768121. Epub 2013 Apr 16.

38. Maerten A, Zaslansky P, Mochales C, et al: Characterizing the transformation near indents and cracks in clinically used dental yttria-stabilized zirconium oxide constructs. *Dent Mater* 2013;29:241–251.

39. Andersson M, Oden A: A new all-ceramic crown. A dense-sintered, high-purity alumina coping with porcelain. *Acta Odontol Scand* 1993;51:59–64.

40. Kohal RJ, Att W, Bächle M, Butz F: Ceramic abutments and ceramic oral implants. An update. *Periodontol 2000* 2008; 47:224–243.

41. Att W, Kurun S, Gerds T, et al: Fracture resistance of single-tooth implant-supported all-ceramic restorations after exposure to the artificial mouth. *J Oral Rehabil* 2006;33: 380–386.

42. Att W, Kurun S, Gerds T, et al: Fracture resistance of single-tooth implant-supported all-ceramic restorations: an in vitro study. *J Prosthet Dent* 2006;95:111–116.

3

THE DIGITAL ONE-ABUTMENT/ONE-TIME CONCEPT. A CLINICAL REPORT

Florian Beuer, prof. dr. med. dent.,[1] Julian Groesser,[1] Josef Schweiger, cdt,[1] Jeremias Hey, dr med dent, msc,[2] Jan-Frederik Güth, priv doz dr med dent,[2] and Michael Stimmelmayr, priv doz dr med dent[1]

[1]Department of Prosthodontics, Munich Dental School, Munich, Germany
[2]Department of Prosthodontics, Martin Luther University, Halle, Germany

Keywords

Dental implant; digital dentistry; one-abutment one-time; computer aided impressions; single-tooth implant; implant prosthodontics.

Correspondence

Florian Beuer, Department of Prosthodontics, Munich Dental School, Goethestr. 70, 80336 Munich, Germany.
E-mail: florian.beuer@med.uni-muenchen.de

Presented at the American College of Prosthodontists Annual Session, October 12, 2013; Las Vegas, NV.

The authors deny any conflicts of interest.

Accepted June 10, 2014

Published in *Journal of Prosthodontics*, online January 5, 2015

doi: 10.1111/jopr.12256

ABSTRACT

The digital fabrication of dental restorations on implants has become a standard procedure during the last decade. Avoiding changing abutments during prosthetic treatment has been shown to be superior to the traditional protocol. The presented concept for implant-supported single crowns describes a digital approach without a physical model from implant placement to final delivery in two appointments. A 54-year-old man was provided with a single-tooth implant on his left mandibular first molar. Before wound closure, the implant position was captured digitally with an intraoral scanning device. After bone healing at the time of second-stage surgery the final screw-retained crown fabricated without a physical model was inserted. Soft tissue healing took place at the definitive restoration, avoiding abutment changes or changes of the healing cap. These led to stable soft tissues with a minimum of surgery. The benefits of digital fabrication and the unique way to scan the implant right after placement give an additional value that would not be achieved by analog techniques. In addition to financial benefits it represents a biologically advantageous, one-abutment/one-time approach with customized screw-retained, full-contour crowns or cemented crowns on custom abutments.

Over the last several decades, implant-supported restorations have significantly changed prosthetic treatment concepts and proven their clinical reliability.[1–4] In particular, single implants help avoid sacrificing natural tooth structure when fixed dental prostheses (FDPs) supported from adjacent teeth can be avoided; however, to achieve clinical long-term success, several clinical considerations have to be taken into account, of which the soft tissue conditions around the implant can be considered one of the most important.[5]

The established interface during soft tissue healing between the peri-implant mucosa and the implant/abutment consists of an epithelium and a connective tissue component.[6] Berglundh et al reported a length of approximately 2 mm for the junctional epithelium and a height of 1 to 2 mm for the connective tissue zone, resulting in a total transmucosal attachment of 3 to 4 mm.[7] Several technical factors might possibly influence the condition of this critical peri-implant mucosa. These factors include the material of the abutment, the veneering material, the fit of the abutment, or a platform switch.[8–10]

In contrast, some clinical procedures are known to influence the soft tissue around dental implants. Frequent probing at dental implants during the soft-tissue healing period has been shown to increase the pocket probing depths and markedly disrupt the epithelial and connective tissue attachment.[11] Additionally, an elevation of a full flap (periosteum) leads to a substantial loss of hard tissues and, therefore, influences the soft tissue behavior.[12–14] Furthermore, the prosthetic treatment concept was reported to influence the stability of the soft tissues. Repeated abutment change was associated with a disruption of the mucosal seal and an increase of the dimension of the transmucosal barrier and an increase of bone remodeling in an animal study.[15] As such, from a histological point of view, abutments should not be changed once they have been placed.[16] In this context, interesting concepts (e.g., the "one-abutment/one-time concept") have already been described. Against a control group using provisional abutments, the "one-abutment/one-time" group showed significantly less bone loss at the 18-month and 3-year recalls after implant placement.[17]

Today, the computer-aided design (CAD)/computer aided manufacturing (CAM) of implant abutments has become a new standard for customized abutments.[18–20] However, using digital technology for fabrication of dental restorations requires the digitalization of the oral situation. This can be done either by direct digitalization, using an intraoral scanning device, or by indirect digitalization of a plaster model in the dental laboratory.[21] Because of the multiple potential sources of error during the conventional way, including conventional impression, plaster model, and indirect digitalization, the direct digitalization using an intraoral scanner seems to be the most logical way to access the digital workflow and CAD/CAM.[22–24] As a whole, the digital workflow offers the possibility to facilitate the daily procedures and offers new, innovative treatment strategies that provide advantages for dentists, dental technicians, and patients.[25–28]

Against this background, this report introduces the Munich Implant Concept (MIC), describing the treatment of a patient with an implant-supported, full-contour crown within two appointments without any physical model, using intraoral scanning and CAD/CAM technology.

CLINICAL REPORT

Anamnesis and Preoperative Procedure

A generally healthy 54-year-old male patient was referred to the Department of Prosthodontics at Munich Dental School with a missing mandibulary left first molar (FDI position 36, Fig 3.1). After discussion of the alternative treatments, the patient decided to have a single-tooth implant and gave his informed consent. As he lived 2000 km from the clinic, the number of appointments necessary until delivery needed to be limited to a minimum. A cone-beam computed tomography (CBCT) of the site was made to receive 3D information

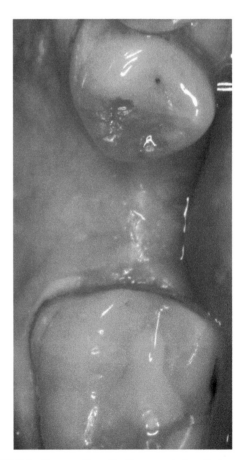

FIGURE 3.1 Preoperative situation: a missing first mandibular molar (FDI position 36).

about the soft and hard tissues (CS 9300; Carestream Dental, Rochester, NY) at the desired implant position.

Appointment 1: Implant Surgery and Scanning

The intraoral situation was digitized using an intraoral scanning device (Intrascan; Zfx, Dachau, Germany) to receive a dataset of the clinical situation. This scan involved the mandible (gap and adjacent teeth), the maxilla, and a vestibular scan for bite registration.

The patient was instructed to take antibiotics (Amoxicillin, 1.000 mg t.i.d.) and 400 mg of Ibuprofen 1 hour before surgery to prevent inflammation and swelling. Ibuprofen was continued for 2 days. Immediately before surgery, the patient rinsed his mouth with a 0.2% chlorhexidine solution for 3 minutes.[29] A crestal incision in region 36 was followed by sulcular incisions at both neighboring teeth without relieving incisions. A full-thickness flap was elevated, and all inflammatory and granulation tissue was debrided with a curette. For a tension-free wound closure, the periosteum was slit at the basal of the flap, right at beginning of the surgery. An implant (length 11 mm, diameter 4.3 mm, Camlog Screwline; Camlog Biotechnologies, Basel, Switzerland) was placed at the planned position according to the manufacturer's protocol (Fig 3.2).

After placement, a scan body (3shape, Copenhagen, Denmark) was screwed to the primary stable implant to enable the direct digitalization of the implant position (Fig 3.3). The precise fit of the scan body could be controlled easily, and the scan was conducted within the "gingiva-extra" scan mode. During scanning, it was of paramount importance to also scan the adjacent teeth to enable a superimposition of the scan body dataset with the situation scan, which was conducted before surgery.

After scanning, the scan body was removed, a covering screw was placed, and the wound was closed with a deep horizontal mattress (Prolene 5.0; Ethicon, Johnson & Johnson Medical, Norderstedt, Germany) and interrupted sutures (Prolene 6.0; Ethicon). A control X-ray was made for forensic reasons, and the patient was instructed on adequate

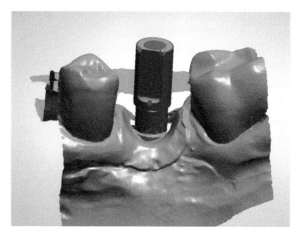

FIGURE 3.3 Screen shot of the virtual model in the CAD program (Dental Designer; 3shape).

care for the next several days. Wound healing was uneventful. The sutures were removed 8 days after implant placement. Subsequently, the scan data was exported in standard tessellation language (STL) format and transferred to the dental laboratory of the Department of Prosthodontics of Martin Luther University, Halle, Germany, where the crown was manufactured during the healing period.

Laboratory

The scan data were imported into a CAD-Software (Dental Designer; 3shape) to design the final restoration (Fig 3.4). The bottom line of the presented concept is to prevent changes of abutments or healing caps. Therefore, two restoration options are possible: (1) a final screw-retained crown; (2) a final custom abutment made from zirconia or titanium with a provisional crown. In this case, the restorative team decided to deliver a screw-retained full-contour crown made from lithium disilicate (IPS e.max CAD; Ivoclar Vivadent, Schaan, Liechtenstein), which was stained and glazed.[30] The finalized crown was adhesively bonded (Multilink Implant; Ivoclar Vivadent) to a Ti insert (Fig 3.5) in accordance with the manufacturer's recommendations.[31,32]

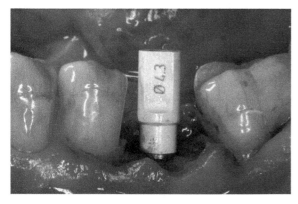

FIGURE 3.2 Situation during implant placement: scanning post mounted to the implant.

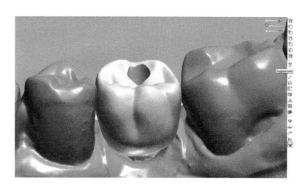

FIGURE 3.4 Screen shot of the CAD design (Dental Designer) of a screw-retained crown.

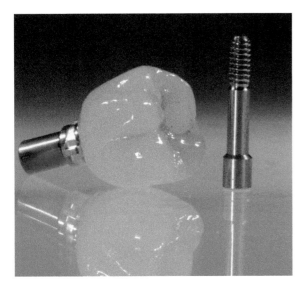

FIGURE 3.5 Screw-retained crown fabricated in full contour from lithium disilicate (e.max CAD, Ivoclar Vivadent) bonded to a titanium insert.

Appointment 2: Re-entry and Delivery

After 12 weeks of healing, second-stage surgery was performed, and the final crown was inserted. Therefore, only a mucosal flap was necessary, and the periosteum remained on the bone (Fig 3.6). The covering screw was removed. The

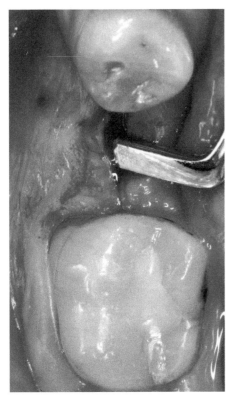

FIGURE 3.6 Second-stage surgery: raising a mucosal flap and undermining the buccal soft tissue.

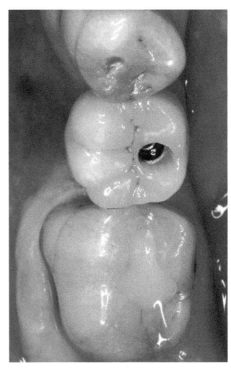

FIGURE 3.7 Second-stage surgery: placement of screw-retained final crown.

implant was rinsed with isotonic sodium chloride solution and dried. The screw-retained crown was tried in, and occlusal and proximal contacts were checked and adapted. The crown was polished in the dental laboratory according to the manufacturer's recommendations and was cleaned in an ultrasonic bath. Before placing, the restoration was disinfected in 0.2% chlorhexidine solution. The crown was placed, and the screw was fixed with a torque moment of 20 N cm (Fig 3.7). The soft tissue was adapted to the crown with two papilla sutures (Prolene 6.0). Sutures were removed after uneventful healing after 6 days.

DISCUSSION

Today, the CAD/CAM-supported fabrication of abutments and implant-supported restorations can be considered as the new standard.[33,34] In consideration of the industrial quality of the applied materials and the almost unlimited design opportunities regarding the emergence profile, the dimensions and angulation of the restorations have to be considered as the major advantage of this digital procedure. In addition to the higher mechanical stability that can be achieved by CAD/CAM-fabricated restorations,[30] concepts that offer additional value to patients and practitioners mean further advantages of digital implant-supported prosthodontics.

Regarding the MIC, the fabrication of the restoration during the (closed) healing-phase of the implant rationalizes the treatment procedure. The accuracy of the transfer of the implant position by an intraoral scan seems to be sufficient for single-tooth implants.[35] Also, the adjacent teeth and antagonists are directly digitized, which facilitates the transfer of the situation to the dental laboratory. The scanning device allows the export of STL data, which allows importing the data in all major CAD programs. Based on the authors' experience, physical models are not necessary for that kind of single-tooth restoration.

The question of screw retention or cementation is controversial; however, the presented concept allows both protocols. The primary objective of omitting detaching of the epithelium from the abutment or healing cap can easily be followed when a screw-retained restoration is placed. The gingival line represents no esthetic limitation, as abutment and crown are one part, made from a tooth-colored material (e.g., lithium disilicate). If a cemented approach is used, the part in direct contact with the soft tissue must be final. Abutments fabricated from zirconia or titanium are treatment options of choice. If a cemented restoration is used, the gingiva line becomes more important, as visible Ti, in particular, might be an esthetic drawback. Therefore, provisional crowns are cemented on the final abutments at the time of re-entry. After soft tissue consolidation, the preparation margin of the abutment can be adjusted without removing the abutment in the patient's mouth. An additional (conventional or digital) impression is made for the fabrication of the final crown.

After placement of the restoration at the time of uncovering the implant, the healing of the soft tissue takes place at the definitive restoration instead of at a healing abutment. Consequently, the emergence profile heals immediately toward an optimal shape. In contrast, standard healing abutments exhibit a round profile, which means that the cross section of the emergence profile has to be modified from round-shaped toward root-shaped before placement of the definitive restoration. This is achieved by repeated change of interim prostheses or continuously individualized healing abutments to apply gentle pressure on the emergence profile.[36] However, too much high pressure might cause a change of the mucosa that can lead to a loss of attached gingiva and recessions.[37]

Additionally, the immediate placement of the definitive restoration enables the formation of a long junctional epithelium between the restoration and soft tissues that should not be separated again.[6,16,38,39] This sealing between the oral environment and the alveolar bone is an important factor for the long-term success of implant-supported restorations.[9,38,40] In consideration of these findings, less peri-implant inflammation can be expected when the junctional epithelium is not detached and injured; however, this has to be proven in animal experiments and clinical studies.

Observed from the economic standpoint, the concept offers clear advantages for dentists and patients. On one hand, the concept saves treatment time, yet the healing period does not have to be abbreviated. On the other hand, the MIC concept offers saving potential regarding additional implant parts, as there is no need for transfer posts and healing abutments.

A screw-retained full contour crown from lithium disilicate on a Ti insert seems to be the best restorative approach for the presented concept based on today's knowledge. Even in cases where the soft-tissue level might heal more apically from the planned level, there will be no esthetic or functional disadvantages due to the continuous color and form of the restoration.

CONCLUSION

The Munich Implant Concept offers economical and biological advantages for practitioners and patients, and the ongoing integration of the digital workflow offers the potential for further enhancements and simplifications.

REFERENCES

1. Akca K, Uysal S, Cehreli MC: Implant-tooth-supported fixed partial prostheses: correlations between in vivo occlusal bite forces and marginal bone reactions. *Clin Oral Implants Res* 2006;17:331–336.

2. Buser D, Mericske-Stern R, Bernard JP, et al: Long-term evaluation of non-submerged ITI implants. Part 1: 8-year life table analysis of a prospective multi-center study with 2359 implants. *Clin Oral Implants Res* 1997;8:161–172.

3. Kopp KC, Koslow AH, Abdo OS: Predictable implant placement with a diagnostic/surgical template and advanced radiographic imaging. *J Prosthet Dent* 2003;89:611–615.

4. Krennmair G, Krainhofner M, Waldenberger O, et al: Dental implants as strategic supplementary abutments for implant-tooth-supported telescopic crown-retained maxillary dentures: a retrospective follow-up study for up to 9 years. *Int J Prosthodont* 2007;20:617–622.

5. Happe A, Stimmelmayr M, Schlee M, et al: Surgical management of peri-implant soft tissue color mismatch caused by shine-through effects of restorative materials: one-year follow-up. *Int J Periodont Rest* 2013;33:81–88.

6. Zucchelli G, Mazzotti C, Mounssif I, et al: A novel surgical-prosthetic approach for soft tissue dehiscence coverage around single implant. *Clin Oral Implants Res* 2013;24:957–962.

7. Berglundh T, Lindhe J, Ericsson I, et al: The soft tissue barrier at implants and teeth. *Clin Oral Implants Res* 1991;2:81–90.

8. Rodriguez AM, Rosenstiel SF: Esthetic considerations related to bone and soft tissue maintenance and development around dental implants: report of the Committee on Research in Fixed Prosthodontics of the American Academy of Fixed Prosthodontics. *J Prosthet Dent* 2012;108:259–267.

9. Esposito M, Maghaireh H, Grusovin MG, et al: Soft tissue management for dental implants: what are the most effective techniques? A Cochrane systematic review. *Eur J Oral Implantol* 2012;5:221–238.

10. Schwarz F, Alcoforado G, Nelson K, et al: Impact of implant-abutment connection, positioning of the machined collar/microgap, and platform switching on crestal bone level changes. Camlog Foundation Consensus Report. *Clin Oral Implants Res* 2014;25:1301–1303.

11. Schwarz F, Mihatovic I, Ferrari D, et al: Influence of frequent clinical probing during the healing phase on healthy peri-implant soft tissue formed at different titanium implant surfaces: a histomorphometrical study in dogs. *J Clin Periodontol* 2010;37:551–562.

12. Araujo MG, Lindhe J: Ridge alterations following tooth extraction with and without flap elevation: an experimental study in the dog. *Clin Oral Implants Res* 2009;20:545–549.

13. Greenstein G, Cavallaro J, Tarnow D: Confronting controversial issues in dental implant therapy, part 2. *Dent Today* 2013;32:80, 82, 84–86; quiz 87.

14. Greenstein G, Cavallaro J, Tarnow D: Confronting controversial issues in dental implant therapy, part I. *Dent Today* 2013;32:36, 38–40; quiz 41.

15. Rodriguez X, Vela X, Mendez V, et al: The effect of abutment dis/reconnections on peri-implant bone resorption: a radiologic study of platform-switched and non-platform-switched implants placed in animals. *Clin Oral Implants Res* 2013;24:305–311.

16. Becker K, Mihatovic I, Golubovic V, et al: Impact of abutment material and dis-/re-connection on soft and hard tissue changes at implants with platform-switching. *J Clin Periodontol* 2012;39:774–780.

17. Canullo L, Bignozzi I, Cocchetto R, et al: Immediate positioning of a definitive abutment versus repeated abutment replacements in post-extractive implants: 3-year follow-up of a randomised multicentre clinical trial. *Eur J Oral Implantol* 2010;3:285–296.

18. Borges T, Lima T, Carvalho A, et al: The influence of customized abutments and custom metal abutments on the presence of the interproximal papilla at implants inserted in single-unit gaps: a 1-year prospective clinical study. *Clin Oral Implants Res* 2014;25:1222–1227.

19. Parpaiola A, Norton MR, Cecchinato D, et al: Virtual abutment design: a concept for delivery of CAD/CAM customized abutments – report of a retrospective cohort. *Int J Periodont Rest* 2013;33:51–58.

20. Canullo L: Clinical outcome study of customized zirconia abutments for single-implant restorations. *Int J Prosthodont* 2007;20:489–493.

21. DIN 13995:2010–02. Dentistry – Terminology of process chain for CAD/CAM-systems. 2010.

22. Christensen GJ: The challenge to conventional impressions. *J Am Dent Assoc* 2008;139:347–349.

23. Christensen GJ: The state of fixed prosthodontic impressions: room for improvement. *J Am Dent Assoc* 2005; 136:343–346.

24. Christensen GJ: Laboratories want better impressions. *J Am Dent Assoc* 2007;138:527–529.

25. Stapleton BM, Lin WS, Ntounis A, et al: Application of digital diagnostic impression, virtual planning, and computer-guided implant surgery for a CAD/CAM-fabricated, implant-supported fixed dental prosthesis: a clinical report. *J Prosthet Dent* 2014;112:402–408.

26. Kurtzman GM, Dompkowski DE: Using digital impressions and CAD/CAM in implant dentistry. *Dent Today* 2014;33:114, 116–117.

27. Kim C, Kim JY, Lim YJ: Use of CAD/CAM to fabricate duplicate abutments for retrofitting an existing implant prosthesis: a clinical report. *J Prosthet Dent* 2014; 112:429–433.

28. Kapos T, Evans C: CAD/CAM technology for implant abutments, crowns, and superstructures. *Int J Oral Max Implants* 2014;29 (Suppl): 117–136.

29. Stimmelmayr M, Stangl M, Edelhoff D, et al: Clinical prospective study of a modified technique to extend the keratinized gingiva around implants in combination with ridge augmentation: one-year results. *Int J Oral Max Implants* 2011;26:1094–1101.

30. Guess PC, Zavanelli RA, Silva NR, et al: Monolithic CAD/CAM lithium disilicate versus veneered Y-TZP crowns: comparison of failure modes and reliability after fatigue. *Int J Prosthodont* 2010;23:434–442.

31. Stimmelmayr M, Edelhoff D, Guth JF, et al: Wear at the titanium-titanium and the titanium-zirconia implant-abutment interface: a comparative in vitro study. *Dent Mater* 2012;28:1215–1220.

32. Stimmelmayr M, Sagerer S, Erdelt K, et al: In vitro fatigue and fracture strength testing of one-piece zirconia implant abutments and zirconia implant abutments connected to titanium cores. *Int J Oral Max Implants* 2013;28:488–493.

33. Beuer F, Schweiger J, Edelhoff D, et al: Reconstruction of esthetics with a digital approach. *Int J Periodont Rest* 2011;31:185–193.

34. Beuer F, Schweiger J, Edelhoff D: Digital dentistry: an overview of recent developments for CAD/CAM generated restorations. *Br Dent J* 2008;204:505–511.

35. Syrek A, Reich G, Ranftl D, et al: Clinical evaluation of all-ceramic crowns fabricated from intraoral digital impressions based on the principle of active wavefront sampling. *J Dent* 2010;38:553–559.

36. Khoury F, Happe A: Soft tissue management in oral implantology: a review of surgical techniques for shaping an esthetic and functional peri-implant soft tissue structure. *Quintessence Int* 2000;31:483–499.

37. Stimmelmayr M, Allen EP, Reichert TE, et al: Use of a combination epithelized-subepithelial connective tissue graft for closure and soft tissue augmentation of an extraction site following ridge preservation or implant placement: description of a technique. *Int J Periodont Rest* 2010;30:375–381.

38. Cochran DL, Mau LP, Higginbottom FL, et al: Soft and hard tissue histologic dimensions around dental implants in the canine restored with smaller-diameter abutments: a paradigm shift in peri-implant biology. *Int J Oral Max Implants* 2013;28:494–502.

39. Welander M, Abrahamsson I, Berglundh T: The mucosal barrier at implant abutments of different materials. *Clin Oral Implants Res* 2008;19:635–641.

40. Cutrim ES, Peruzzo DC, Benatti B: Evaluation of soft tissues around single tooth implants in the anterior maxilla restored with cemented and screw-retained crowns. *J Oral Implantol* 2012;38:700–705.

4

INFLUENCE OF SURGICAL AND PROSTHETIC TECHNIQUES ON MARGINAL BONE LOSS AROUND TITANIUM IMPLANTS. PART I: IMMEDIATE LOADING IN FRESH EXTRACTION SOCKETS

ANTOINE N. BERBERI, BDS, MSC, PHD,[1] GEORGES E. TEHINI, DDS, MSC,[2] ZIAD F. NOUJEIM, DDS, CES,[3] ALEXANDRE A. KHAIRALLAH, BDS, DESS,[4] MOUSTAFA N. ABOUSEHLIB, DDS, MSC, PHD,[5,6] AND ZIAD A. SALAMEH, DDS, MSC, PHD[3]

[1]Department of Oral and Maxillofacial Surgery, School of Dentistry, Lebanese University, Beirut, Lebanon
[2]Department of Prosthodontics, School of Dentistry, Lebanese University, Beirut, Lebanon
[3]Research Department, School of Dentistry, Lebanese University, Beirut, Lebanon
[4]Department of Radiology, School of Dentistry, Lebanese University, Beirut, Lebanon
[5]Department of Materials Science, ACTA, Amsterdam, The Netherlands
[6]Faculty of Dentistry, Department of Materials Science, Alexandria University, Alexandria, Egypt

Keywords
Marginal bone loss; immediate loading; radiological evaluation; titanium implant.

Correspondence
Moustafa N. Aboushelib, ACTA – Material Science, Louwesweg 1 Amsterdam 1066 EA, The Netherlands.
E-mail: info@aboushelib.org, bluemarline_1@yahoo.com

This work received support from a reintegration grant (Grant number 489) provided by the Science and Technology Department Fund.

The authors deny any conflicts of interest.

Accepted October 22, 2013

Published in *Journal of Prosthodontics* October 2014; Vol. 23, Issue 7

doi: 10.1111/jopr.12153

ABSTRACT

Purpose: Delayed placement of implant abutments has been associated with peri-implant marginal bone loss; however, long-term results obtained by modifying surgical and prosthetic techniques after implant placement are still lacking. This study aimed to evaluate the marginal bone loss around titanium implants placed in fresh extraction sockets using two loading protocols after a 5-year follow-up period.

Material and Methods: A total of 36 patients received 40 titanium implants (Astra Tech) intended for single-tooth replacement. Implants were immediately placed into fresh extraction sockets using either a one-stage (immediate loading by placing an interim prosthesis into functional occlusion) or a two-stage prosthetic loading protocol (insertion of abutments after 8 weeks of healing time). Marginal bone levels relative to the implant reference point were evaluated at four time intervals using intraoral radiographs: at time of implant placement, and 1, 3, and 5 years after implant placement. Measurements were obtained from mesial and distal surfaces of each implant ($\alpha = 0.05$).

Results: One-stage immediate implant placement into fresh extraction sockets resulted in a significant reduction in marginal bone loss ($p < 0.002$) compared to the traditional two-stage technique. Whereas mesial surfaces remained stable for the 5-year observation period, significant marginal bone loss was observed on distal surfaces of implants after cementation of interim prostheses ($p < 0.007$) and after 12 months ($p < 0.034$).

Conclusions: Within the limitations of this study, immediate loading of implants placed into fresh extraction sockets reduced marginal bone loss and did not compromise the success rate of the restorations.

Radiological assessment of bone quality and quantity around dental implants is one of the most important evaluation criteria in long-term follow-up studies; however, with regard to marginal bone loss (MBL), most reports present only mean values, while frequency distributions of the data have rarely been described. Only a few long-term studies have addressed this issue from the patient level.[1–9]

Several criteria have been proposed for the evaluation of the success of dental implants. A commonly used criterion was suggested by Albrektsson et al[10] and was further revised in 1993.[11] According to the authors,[12] a successful dental implant should sustain less than 1.5 mm of bone loss during the first year in function and less than 0.2 mm annually thereafter. In 1999, Wennström and Palmer[13] suggested a modification of the radiological criteria used to assess MBL. They suggested that a maximum bone loss of 2 mm could be accepted over a 5-year period after functional loading of the restoration.

The peri-implant tissue or biological width is composed of connective tissue coated by layers of epithelial cells that attach to the implant surface, forming the junctional epithelium.

Biologic width should be physiologically and dimensionally stable before and after loading.[14,15] Dynamic changes can be observed over time regarding the dimensions of gingival sulcus, junctional epithelium, and connective tissue.[16–20]

Achieving optimal peri-implant mucosal dimension is a challenging procedure, and maintaining it over time can be an equally demanding task.[21,22] In fact, peri-implant mucosal architecture implicates the position of the gingival zenith and the interproximal tissue volume (papillae). It is also well accepted that peri-implant soft tissue preservation is related to many anatomical and clinical parameters,[23–27] and that following implant, abutment, or crown placement, peri-implant soft tissue changes may include papillary regrowth, among other changes.[15,19,20] Presence and maintenance of papillae is primarily related to the bone level at the adjacent tooth,[15,22,28] and bone preservation is a key factor for the esthetic outcome.[29,30]

MBL can be influenced by several surgical and prosthetic factors, such as immediate insertion of implants in fresh extraction sockets, the time of fixation of the implant superstructures, and the time of functional loading.[31–33] Previous studies[9,34–38] have reported a possible association between increase in the MBL and the removal of cover screws,

placement of healing abutments, and subsequent manipulations of the abutment. This prosthetic handling is a potential compromising factor for the stability of the subcrestal biological area. In 2006, Lazzara and Porter[39] reported that "the removal and reconnection of the abutment created a soft tissue wound with subsequent bone re-sorption due to the attempt made by the soft tissue to establish a proper biologic dimension of the mucosal barrier attachment to a stable implant surface."[38]

Several studies have reported inconclusive evidence regarding the advantages or disadvantages of immediate versus delayed implant placement.[39,40] The correlation between the timing of implant placement and tooth extraction has been evaluated and has been reported not to be crucial for implant survival or MBL.[41,42] Some investigations[43–45] have compared bone level changes for immediately loaded versus conventionally loaded implants and have not reported any differences in MBL levels. The results of recent studies have shown that insertion of abutments at the time of implant placement resulted in a significant reduction in MBL.[38,43–47]

Unfortunately, sound guidelines regarding the interaction of these variables are not yet available in the dental literature, especially over long-term observation periods. The aim of this retrospective study was to evaluate the influence of two prosthetic techniques on MBL around titanium implants placed into maxillary fresh extraction sockets over a 5-year period. The null hypothesis was that more MBL would not be observed around immediately loaded implants compared to the delayed loading technique.

MATERIALS AND METHODS

This study included 36 patients (21 men and 15 women, mean age 31 years) who required single implant placement in anterior maxillae. Ethics Committee approval (School of Dentistry, Lebanese University, Beirut, Lebanon) was obtained for all patients.

Patient Selection Criteria

Patients in need of bone grafts or bone regeneration, medically compromised patients (corticosteroid therapy, uncontrolled diabetes, bisphosphonate therapy, immunocompromised cases), smokers, and patients with periodontal disease were excluded from the study. The selected cases included 20 central incisors, 13 lateral incisors, 1 canine, and 6 premolars; all were treated by the same oral surgeon ($n = 40$). Study casts, diagnostic waxing, and surgical guides were prepared for all patients. Provisional crowns were prepared for implants when sufficient initial primary stability was observed (20 N/cm).[48,49]

Surgical Phase

The diseased teeth were extracted, and full-thickness muco-periosteal flaps were raised for direct exposure of the surgical fields. Titanium implants (Astra Tech Implant system; Dentsply Implants, Mölndal, Sweden) were inserted into the prepared sites using successive drill sizes and were counter-sunk to levels approximately 2 mm apical to the cemento–enamel junctions of the adjacent teeth. This process resulted in implant collars 1 mm below the crest of the ridge for greater primary stability and optimal esthetics. Bone chips collected during drilling were packed to fill the gaps between the defects and the inserted implants. Implants with initial primary stability of 20 N/cm or more were immediately restored; implants placed with less than 20 N/cm of insertion torque were restored with a delayed loading protocol. Initial stability was evaluated during insertion of the implants in the prepared sockets with a torque-controlled low-speed handpiece. The torque (N/cm) values were visualized on the surgical motor (Aseptico Inc., Woodinville, WA). A manual torque control (Astra Tech Implant system) was used to confirm initial stability by engaging it in the removal position; force was stopped once the indicator passed the required level (20 N/cm).

Immediate Loading Protocol (One Stage)

Definitive abutments (Ti Design or Zir Design; Astra Tech Implant system) were prepared outside the mouth for use intraorally, and abutment screws were tightened with finger pressure. No further preparation of the abutments was required. Interim prostheses were fabricated and adjusted in the mouth with demonstrable contact (holding shimstock) in the maximum intercuspal position. No eccentric contacts were permitted. Temporary cement (Temp-Bond; Kerr USA, Romulus, MI) was used to cement the acrylic resin interim prostheses (Pro-Temp Garant III; 3M ESPE America, Norristown, PA). Excess cement was removed, and the flaps were closed around the cemented restorations by means of interrupted sutures (Vicryl 4–0; Johnson & Johnson Medical Ltd., Wokingham, UK).

Delayed Loading Protocol (Two Stages)

Implants that did not achieve 20 N/cm of insertion torque were covered using flathead cover screws. After 8 weeks of healing time, a tissue punch and small crestal incisions were used to expose the cover screws, and the previously described prosthetic protocol was applied. Abutment screws were tightened with a torque controller, according to the manufacturer's recommendations (20 N/cm for 3.5 and 4 S abutments; 25 N/cm for ST abutments). Provisional crowns were prepared as for the immediate loading group and cemented with occlusal contacts until the delivery of the definitive restorations. Definitive crowns (Empress 2; Ivoclar Vivadent, Schaan, Liechtenstein) were cemented with glass ionomer cement (Ketac-Cem; 3M ESPE America). Patients were instructed to rinse three times daily (0.12% digluconate chlorhexidine, for 3 minutes after each meal over a 2-week period) and to maintain proper oral hygiene.

Radiological Evaluation

Standardized periapical radiographs were obtained using a long-cone paralleling technique, with the central beam perpendicular to the alveolar crest (XCP holder Rinn; Dentsply International, York, PA). Each X-ray holder was individualized with an occlusal record to standardize the procedure between visits for each patient. Radiographs were obtained at the time of implant placement, after 8 weeks, then at 1, 3, and 5 years of function. All radiographs were processed according to time/temperature guidelines (processing solutions were maintained at 20°C and an immersion time of 4 minutes).

A digital camera (Kodak EOS camera equipped with 1:1 100 mm macro lens; Kodak, Rochester, NY) was used to convert the images into digital formats (JPEG format). Measurements were obtained with the aid of image-processing software (DBSWIN 5; DÜRR DENTAL AG, Bietigheim-Bissingen, Germany) and were used to calculate the vertical distance between the bone level and the implant shoulder (calibrated 10× magnifications). Marginal bone level relative to the implant reference point (implant shoulder) was measured on mesial and distal surfaces of the implants (Fig 4.1). Two calibrated examiners performed all measurements, which were recorded in millimeters.

Statistical Analysis

Interexaminer correlation analysis was performed to calibrate the accuracy of the measuring procedure. One- and two-way ANOVA were performed to detect significant changes in the marginal bone level at every time interval ($\alpha = 0.05$). Measurements were obtained on the mesial and distal surfaces of each implant. Pairwise comparisons were performed using Bonferroni's post hoc test. Analyses were performed using computer software (SPSS, version 18.0; SPSS Inc., Chicago, IL).

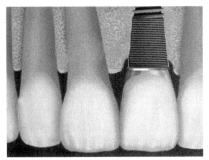

A

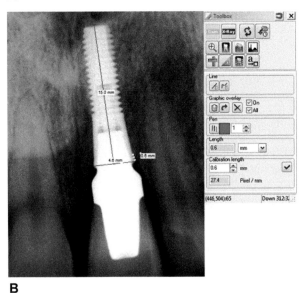

B

FIGURE 4.1 Measurement technique: (A) Mesial and distal marginal bone loss (MBL) calculated as the vertical distance between the crestal bone level and the implant neck; (B) software calculation of the MBL.

RESULTS

Interexaminer correlation analysis revealed a nonsignificant error margin for all of the measurements obtained ($p < 0.11$). Statistical analysis showed that immediate placement of interim prostheses in occlusion as described resulted in a significant reduction in MBL ($F = 21.5, p < 0.002$), compared to the two-stage technique, where abutments were inserted 8 weeks following implant placement. This finding was observed at all time intervals (Figs 4.2 and 4.3). Significant MBL was observed on the distal surfaces of the implants after cementation of provisional crowns ($F = 8, p < 0.007$) and at 1 year ($p < 0.034$), compared to the mesial surfaces, which remained stable over the 5-year observation period (Table 4.1).

DISCUSSION

All 40 implants were successfully integrated at the time of definitive crown cementation. No failures were recorded over the 5-year evaluation period. Complications included fracture of three provisional crowns, two in the immediate group and one on the delayed group, during the healing period. Minor incisal porcelain chipping of four crowns occurred after 1 year, and two crowns were replaced for esthetic reasons. The patients reported no crown or abutment loosening.

Data analysis revealed that the majority of MBL was observed during the second observation period, 8 weeks after insertion of implants. Almost 85% of the total MBL observed after 5 years occurred during the first 8-week period following implant placement, after which the rate of bone loss remained relatively constant (0.01 to 0.02 mm/year). This could be related to the early loss of the bundle bone of the buccal aspect.[26] After the 8-week healing period, the formation of soft tissue attachment, which protects peri-implant crestal bone from oral cavity products, was observed. This tissue is important for initial healing, osseointegration maintenance, and long-term implant behavior.[15,19–21]

Significantly lower MBL associated with immediately loaded implants inserted into fresh extraction sockets was observed when compared to the delayed loading technique. Thus, the suggested hypothesis that greater MBL would be observed in immediately loaded implants was rejected.

During the one-stage surgery, the concept of immediate placement of definitive abutments and insertion of immediate interim prostheses appeared to protect the blood clot and to prevent interruption of the early mineralization of marginal bone.[31] This was in contrast with several studies that reported no differences in MBL between immediate and delayed loading of dental implants.[33,41–45] This phenomenon was more obvious in fresh extraction sockets, which demonstrated early MBL during the first 8 weeks, after which a constant marginal bone height was observed over 5 years.[9,36,37]

Evaluation of the MBL in extraction sites was also related to discrepancies between the socket walls and the final drilling dimensions. Filling the extraction sockets with bone chips resulted in preservation of the marginal buccal wall during the observation period of this study. The MBL values reported in this study were lower compared to other studies with similar observation periods.[30,43–47] Another concern for the immediate loading group was the predictability of peri-implant mucosal healing, based on positive adaptation to the implant–abutment complex. The rapid and reproducible reformation of peri-implant mucosa within the gingival embrasures can be attributed to minimal MBL, immediate delivery of the interim prostheses, and absence of abutment manipulation during the healing period.

Two-phase surgical procedures have been associated with continuous MBL of between 0.01 and 0.02 mm/year, which could be in part related to the additional surgical procedure. During the removal of cover screws and tightening of implant abutments, greater stress is delivered to the initially

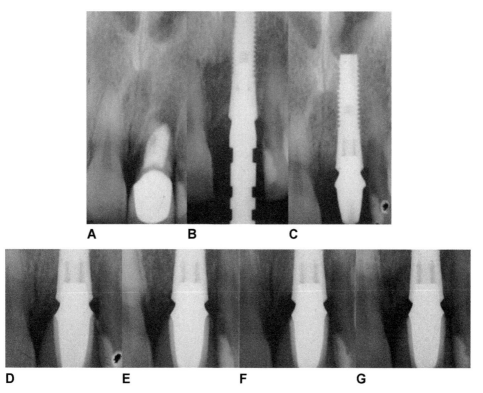

FIGURE 4.2 Digital intraoral radiographs of implants placed into fresh extraction sockets with immediate loading (one-stage technique) at different observation times. (A) Preoperative; (B) on the day of surgical placement of the implant; (C) placement of the abutment and provisional crown; (D) 8 weeks after definitive crown cementation; (E) after 1 year; (F) after 3 years; (G) after 5 years.

mineralizing marginal bone; this manipulation could interfere with the healing process and thus result in increased MBL.[19,34,35] Moreover, the amount of initial MBL during the first 8 weeks was significantly greater (more than twofold), compared to immediately loaded implants inserted into fresh extraction sockets. Vascular ischemia associated with flap reflection for second-stage surgery has been implicated as a potential source of MBL.[18] Significant changes did occur

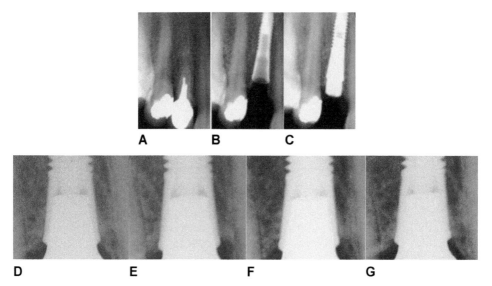

FIGURE 4.3 Digital intraoral radiographs of implants placed into fresh extraction sockets with delayed loading (two-stage technique): (A) preoperative; (B) implant placement; (C) healing abutment placement; (D) 8 weeks after definitive crown cementation; (E) after 1 year; (F) after 3 years; (G) after 5 years.

TABLE 4.1   Marginal Bone Loss (mm) at Different Time Intervals

Technique	Observation Interval	Distal	Mesial	Average
One-stage	8 weeks	0.189 ± 0.270	0.039 ± 0.104	0.114 ± 0.135
	1 year	0.261 ± 0.243	0.217 ± 0.233	0.239 ± 0.158
	3 years	0.247 ± 0.270	0.220 ± 0.221	0.233 ± 0.182
	5 years	0.200 ± 0.271	0.160 ± 0.241	0.180 ± 0.183
Two-stage	8 weeks	0.300 ± 0.283	0.160 ± 0.230	0.230 ± 0.244
	1 year	0.400 ± 0.071	0.340 ± 0.241	0.370 ± 0.144
	3 years	0.420 ± 0.084	0.300 ± 0.200	0.360 ± 0.089
	5 years	0.450 ± 0.071	0.300 ± 0.141	0.375 ± 0.106

MBL was significantly greater for the two-stage technique at all time intervals ($F = 14$, $p < 0.005$). For every group, there was no significant difference in MBL between the second and third observation periods or between the fourth and fifth observation periods.

within the soft tissue compartments, such that sulcus depth and connective tissue contact dimensions decreased while the length of epithelium barrier increased.[24] The formation and maturation of the soft tissue around implants in fresh extraction sockets were higher than in healed sockets.[19]

Other reports have shown that simple procedures, such as removing healing screws, are associated with an increase in MBL.[35,36] Thus, prevention of further disturbance of the implant bone–soft tissue interface favored early placement of definitive implant abutments.[37] In some cases, if reflection of a flap is required, greater bone loss is expected due to the interruption of the blood supply reaching the bone crest. The results of these studies warrant the immediate placement of implant abutments when primary stability was achieved, to reduce MBL.[34–36,47]

The difference in MBL values between mesial and distal surfaces was observed statistically; however, this difference was too small to have any clinical relevance (maximum difference of 0.2 mm at all observation intervals). This difference could be related to anatomical features, such as incisive fissures and interdental septa, or due to the direction of stress around the implant neck.[23,32] Periodic follow-up radiographs are required to detect the early stages of MBL and peri-implantitis.

An interesting observation was the remodeling of peri-implant marginal bone around the implant collars, in association with healthy gingival margins and sulcular depths. In an environment with active biomechanical stimulation, several factors should be considered to preserve marginal bone for adequate protection and support of soft tissue, careful and regular oral hygiene, and for proper placement of implant abutments.

CONCLUSIONS

Within the limitations of this study, less MBL was associated with immediately loaded implants inserted into fresh extraction sockets.

REFERENCES

1. Lekholm U, Gunne J, Henry P, et al: Survival of the Brånemark implant in partially edentulous jaws: a 10-year prospective multicenter study. *Int J Oral Maxillofac Implants* 1999; 14:639–645.

2. Ekelund J-A, Lindquist LW, Carlsson GE, et al: Implant treatment in the edentulous mandible: a prospective study on Brånemark system implants over more than 20 years. *Int J Prosthodont* 2003;16:602–608.

3. Jemt T, Johansson J: Implant treatment in the edentulous maxillae: a 15-year follow-up study on 76 consecutive patients provided with fixed prostheses. *Clin Implant Dent Relat Res* 2006;8:61–69.

4. Roos-Jansåker A, Lindahl C, Renvert H, et al: Nine to fourteen-year follow-up of implant treatment. Part II: presence of peri-implant lesions. *J Clin Periodontol* 2006;33:290–295.

5. Örtorp A, Jemt T: Clinical experiences with laser-welded titanium frameworks supported by implants in the edentulous mandible: a 10-year follow-up study. *Clin Implant Dent Relat Res* 2006;8:198–209.

6. Örtorp A, Jemt T: Laser-welded titanium frameworks supported by implants in the partially edentulous mandible: a 10-year comparative study. *Clin Implant Dent Relat Res* 2008;10:128–139.

7. Wennström J, Ekestubbe A, Gröndahl K, et al: Oral rehabilitation with implant-supported fixed partial dentures in periodontitis-susceptible subjects: a 5-year prospective study. *J Clin Periodontol* 2004;31:713–724.

8. Fransson C, Lekholm U, Jemt T, et al: Prevalence of subjects with progressive bone loss at implants. *Clin Oral Implants Res* 2005;16:440–446.

9. Albrektsson T, Zarb GA, Worthington P, et al: The long-term efficacy of currently used dental implants: a review and proposed criteria of success. *Int J Oral Maxillofac Implants* 1986;1:11–25.

10. Albrektsson T, Zarb GA: Current interpretations of the osseointegrated response: clinical significance. *Int J Prosthodont* 1993;6:95–105.

11. Albrektsson T, Isidor F: Consensus report of session IV. In Lang NP, Karring T (eds): *Proceedings of the 1st European*

Workshop on Periodontology. London, Quintessence, 1993, pp. 365–369.

12. Wennström J, Palmer R: Consensus reports session 3: clinical trials. In Lang NP, Karring T, Lindhe J (eds): *Proceedings of the 3rd European Workshop on Periodontology. Implant Dentistry.* Berlin, Quintessence, 1999.

13. Cochran DL, Hermann JS, Schenk RK, et al: Biologic width around titanium implants. A histometric analysis of the implanto-gingival junction around unloaded and loaded non-submerged implants in the canine mandible. *J Periodontol* 1997;68:186–198.

14. Henriksson K, Jemt T: Measurements of soft tissue volume in association with single-implant restorations: a 1-year comparative study after abutment connection surgery. *Clin Impl Dent Relat Res* 2004;6:181–189.

15. Abrahamsson I, Berglundh T, Lindhe J: The mucosal barrier following abutment dis/reconnection. An experimental study in dogs. *J Clin Periodontol* 1997;24:568–572.

16. Hermann JS, Buser D, Schenk RK, et al: Biologic width around titanium implants. A physiologically formed and stable dimension over time. *Clin Oral Impl Res* 2000;11:1–11.

17. Buser D, Martin W, Belser U: Surgical considerations with regard to single-tooth replacements in the esthetic zone. In Buser D, Belser U, Wismeijer D (eds): *ITI Treatment Guide, Vol 1. Implant Therapy in the Esthetic Zone: Single-Tooth Replacements.* Berlin, Quintessenz, 2007, pp. 26–37.

18. Vignoletti F, de Sanctis M, Berglundh T, et al: Early healing of implants placed into fresh extraction sockets: an experimental study in the beagle dog. III: soft tissue findings. *J Clin Periodontol* 2009;36:1059–1066.

19. Blanco J, Carral C, Linares A, et al: Soft tissue dimensions in flapless immediate implants with and without immediate loading: an experimental study in the beagle dog. *Clin Oral Impl Res* 2012;23:70–75.

20. Phillips K, Kois JC: Aesthetic peri-implant site development. The restorative connection. *Dent Clin North Am* 1988; 42:57–70.

21. Kan JY, Rungcharassaeng K, Umezu K, et al: Dimensions of peri-implant mucosa: an evaluation of maxillary anterior single implants in humans. *J Periodontol* 2003;74:557–562.

22. Cardaropoli G, Lekholm U, Wennstrom JL: Tissue alterations at implant-supported single-tooth replacements: a 1-year prospective clinical study. *Clin Oral Impl Res* 2006;17: 165–171.

23. Cooper LF, Ellner S, Moriarty J, et al: Three-year evaluation of single-tooth implants restored 3 weeks after 1-stage surgery. *Int J Oral Maxillofac Implants* 2007;22:791–800.

24. Woelfel JB, Scheid RC: *Dental Anatomy. Its Relevance to Dentistry.* Philadelphia, Lippincott, Williams and Wilkins, 2002, 100 p.

25. Araujo MG, Sukekava F, Wennstrom JL, et al: Ridge alterations following implant placement in fresh extraction sockets: an experimental study in the dog. *J Clin Periodontol* 2005;32:645–652.

26. Cooper LF: Objective criteria: guiding and evaluating dental implant esthetics. *J Esthet Restor Dent* 2008;20:195–205.

27. Choquet V, Hermans M, Adriaenssens P, et al: Clinical and radiographic evaluation of the papilla level adjacent to single-tooth dental implants. A retrospective study in the maxillary anterior region. *J Periodontol* 2001;72:1364–1371.

28. Palmer RM, Farkondeh N, Palmer PJ, et al: Astra Tech single tooth implants: an audit of patient satisfaction and soft tissue form. *J Clin Periodontol* 2007;34:633–638.

29. Degidi M, Piattelli A, Carinci F: Immediate loaded dental implants: comparison between fixtures inserted in postextractive and healed bone sites. *J Craniofac Surg* 2007;18: 965–971.

30. Crespi R, Capparè P, Gherlone E, et al: Immediate occlusal loading of implants placed in fresh sockets after tooth extraction. *Int J Oral Maxillofac Implants* 2007;22:955–962.

31. Donati M, Botticelli D, La Scala V, et al: Effect of immediate functional loading on osseointegration of implants used for single tooth replacement. A human histological study. *Clin Oral Implants Res* 2013;24:738–745.

32. Abrahamsson I, Berglundh T, Sekino S, et al: Tissue reactions to abutment shift: an experimental study in dogs. *Clin Implant Dent* 2003;2:82–90.

33. Rodriguez X, Vela X, Mendez V, et al: The effect of abutment dis/reconnections on peri-implant bone resorption: a radiologic study of platform-switched and non-platform-switched implants placed in animals. *Clin Oral Impl Res* 2013;24: 305–311.

34. Pikner SS, Gröndahl K, Jemt T, et al: Marginal bone loss at implants: a retrospective, long-term follow-up of turned Brånemark System implants. *Clin Implant Dent Relat Res* 2009;11:11–23.

35. Pikner SS, Gröndahl K: Radiographic analyses of "advanced" marginal bone loss around Brånemark dental implants. *Clin Implant Dent Relat Res* 2009;11:120–133.

36. Van Assche N, Collaert B, Coucke W, et al: Correlation between early perforation of cover screws and marginal bone loss: a retrospective study. *J Clin Periodontol* 2008; 35:76–79.

37. Degidi M, Nardi D, Piattelli A: One abutment at one time: non-removal of an immediate abutment and its effect on bone healing around subcrestal tapered implants. *Clin Oral Implants Res* 2011;22:1303–1307.

38. Lazzara RJ, Porter SS: Platform switching: a new concept in implants dentistry for controlling postrestorative crestal bone levels. *Int J Periodontics Restorative Dent* 2006;26:9–17.

39. Esposito M, Grusovin MG, Polyzos IP, et al: Timing of implant placement after tooth extraction: immediate, immediate-delayed or delayed implants? A Cochrane systematic review. *Eur J Oral Implantol* 2010;3:189–205.

40. Sennerby L, Gottlow J: Clinical outcomes of immediate/early loading of dental implants. A literature review of recent controlled prospective clinical studies. *Aust Dent J* 2008;53 (Suppl 1): S82–S88.

41. Ormianer Z, Piek D, Livne S, et al: Retrospective clinical evaluation of tapered implants: 10-year follow-up of delayed and immediate placement of maxillary implants. *Implant Dent* 2012;21:350–356.

42. Ostman PO, Hellman M, Albrektsson T, et al: Direct loading of Nobel Direct and Nobel Perfect one-piece implants: a 1-year prospective clinical and radiographic study. *Clin Oral Implants Res* 2007;18:409–418.

43. Testori T, Del Fabbro M, Capelli M, et al: Immediate occlusal loading and tilted implants for the rehabilitation of the atrophic edentulous maxilla: 1-year interim results of a multicenter prospective study. *Clin Oral Implants Res* 2008;19:227–232.

44. Collaert B, De Bruyn H: Immediate functional loading of TiOblast dental implants in full-arch edentulous maxillae: a 3-year prospective study. *Clin Oral Implants Res* 2008;19: 1254–1260.

45. Boronat A, Peñarrocha M, Carrillo C, et al: Marginal bone loss in dental implants subjected to early loading (6 to 8 weeks postplacement) with a retrospective short-term follow-up. *J Oral Maxillofac Surg* 2008;66:246–250.

46. De Bruyn H, Raes F, Cooper LF, et al: Three-years clinical outcome of immediate provisionalization of single Osseospeed implants in extraction sockets and healed ridges. *Clin Oral Implants Res* 2012;24:217–223.

47. Bergkvist G, Nilner K, Sahlholm S, et al: Immediate loading of implants in the edentulous maxilla: use of an interim fixed prosthesis followed by a permanent fixed prosthesis: a 32-month prospective radiological and clinical study. *Clin Implant Dent Relat Res* 2009;11:1–10.

48. Norton M: A short-term clinical evaluation of immediately restored maxillary TiOblast single-tooth implants. *Int J Oral Maxillofac Implants* 2004;19:274–281.

49. Donati M, La Scala V, Billi M, et al: Immediate functional loading of implants in single tooth replacement: a prospective clinical multicenter study. *Clin Oral Impl Res* 2008; 19:740–748.

5

A PROSPECTIVE ANALYSIS OF IMMEDIATE PROVISIONALIZATION OF SINGLE IMPLANTS

Thomas J. Balshi, DDS, FACP, Glenn J. Wolfinger, DDS, FACP, Daniel Wulc, and Stephen F. Balshi, MBE

Institute for Facial Esthetics, Prosthodontics Intermedica Dental Center, Fort Washington, PA

Keywords
Dental implant; single-tooth implant; immediate provisionalization; Teeth in a Day protocol; osseointegration.

Correspondence
Stephen F. Balshi, Prosthodontics Intermedica—Research, 467 Pennsylvania Ave., Ste 201, Fort Washington, PA 19436. E-mail: balshi2@aol.com

Accepted March 1, 2010

Published in *Journal of Prosthodontics* January 2011; Vol. 20, Issue 1

doi: 10.1111/j.1532-849X.2010.00659.x

ABSTRACT

Purpose: The purpose of this prospective study was to evaluate the viability of immediately provisionalized single-tooth implants.

Materials and Methods: One hundred forty patients (86 female, 54 male) with a mean age at implant placement of 45 years (range, 15–88 years) needing single-tooth replacement, were treated between July 1999 and December 2004. Single-tooth implants were placed and provisionalized the day of the surgery. All implants were manufactured by Nobel Biocare (Yorba Linda, CA) and had multiple diameters and configurations. The majority of the implants used in this study had oxidized titanium surfaces. The contours of the restorations were designed to mimic the original teeth and root forms. The morphology of the restorations provides support of the labial gingiva.

Results: Over 5.5 years, 164 implants were placed and immediately provisionalized. Sixty-four implants were placed immediately post extraction. Seven implants failed, yielding an overall survival rate of 95.73%.

Conclusion: The application of an immediate provisionalization protocol to a single implant can be successful if the proper precautions are taken in achieving passive occlusion.

Excellent long-term results have been achieved with the conventional two-stage implant protocol with delayed loading.[1] Healing periods may be a result of clinical assumptions[2] and appropriate to question as a requisite to osseointegration in all situations. Healing periods for dental implants can impose hardships on patients for many reasons, most obviously inconvenience, discomfort, and embarrassment of removable prostheses. An alternative protocol, known as immediate loading, delivers a prosthesis immediately following implant placement and eliminates many of the aforementioned hardships. Immediate loading features direct occlusal loading and enjoys high success rates.[3] Evidence supports immediate loading if micromotion can be controlled below the threshold that could interfere with osseointegration.[4–6] This technique, however, is susceptible to certain complications, including overload, as exceeding threshold forces of 100 μm can lead to fibrous encapsulation.[7] A third option, known as immediate provisionalization, is becoming a commonplace therapeutic procedure for partially edentulous and dentate patients wishing to replace missing teeth.[8–10] Research illustrates that this technique enjoys high survival rates, varying between 82 and 100%.[11–13] One method of achieving this includes placing sufficient numbers of threaded implants into high-quality bone and connecting them with a rigid restoration.

Immediate loading of multiple implants is significantly different than single, unsplinted implants. Functional loads on a single-tooth implant restoration are applied to the one implant and not spread through a rigid connection to multiple implants. Common clinical practice is for the interim prosthesis placed on the single implant to be fabricated in a manner that eliminates direct occlusal loading.[14,15] After the implant has osseointegrated, the definitive prosthesis can be put into normal function. The purpose of this prospective study was to evaluate the long-term viability of these immediately provisionalized single implants. A secondary purpose of this study was to assess the success rates of varying implant types and surfaces. Past research illustrates that oxidized-titanium-surfaced implants had higher survival rates.[16,17]

MATERIALS AND METHODS

Patients

One hundred forty patients (86 female, 54 male), with a mean age at placement of 45 years (range 15–88 years), needing single-tooth replacement were treated between July 1999 and December 2004 (Fig 5.1). Inclusion criteria were based on current stable medical condition and ability to undergo dental implant surgery. Exclusion criteria were limited to patients with metabolic bone disease or an unstable systemic condition, such as uncontrolled diabetes, untreated hypothyroidism, or a malignancy in mid-treatment. All patients were treated in a

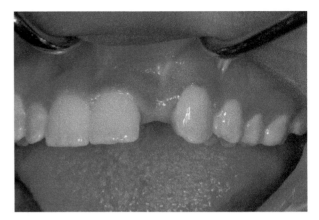

FIGURE 5.1   Retracted facial view of missing maxillary left lateral incisor.

private-practice setting (Prosthodontics Intermedica, Institute for Facial Esthetics, Fort Washington, PA).

Surgical Procedure

Local anesthesia was administered as follows: Marcaine 1:200,000 (Cooke-Waite, Abbott Laboratories, North Chicago, IL) and Lignospan 1:100,000 (Septodont, Inc., New Castle, DE). When teeth were present they were carefully removed using thin elevators to dissect the periodontal ligament and allow atraumatic removal of the tooth from the socket while maintaining all available bone surrounding the area. Clinical palpation and lateral cephalometric radiographs assisted in positioning the drills used to create the implant osteotomy site. Profuse saline irrigation is used throughout the drilling procedure. In the esthetic zone, the osteotomy is designed to orient the receptor site toward the palatal aspect of the socket to create an implant angulation similar to that of the natural root but extending far beyond the apex into the premaxillary basal bone. All immediate implants were placed with an insertion torque of at least 45 N cm using the Nobel-Pharma DEC 100 drill machine (Nobel Biocare, Yorba Linda, CA). Following preparation of the sockets in the esthetic zone, an implant was placed with the shoulder 4 mm below the crest of the gingiva on the labial aspect. A bone guide was often installed and the accompanying trephine was used to remove peripheral bone from the proximal surfaces of the sockets. Typically on external hexed Brånemark implants, a 1-mm CeraOne abutment was installed (Nobel Biocare).

Teeth in a Day Prosthetic Procedures

With the abutment in place, a methyl methacrylate custom coping was fitted over the abutment. A prefabricated acrylic resin crown was carefully connected to the plastic coping with a soft mix of acrylic resin. Once the acrylic resin polymerized to the coping, the crown was removed from the abutment, and an abutment analogue was installed in the coping to preserve

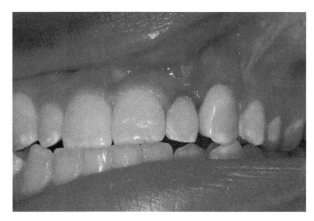

FIGURE 5.2 Delivery of Nobel Perfect implant provisional crown for immediate provisionalization.

the integrity of the acrylic resin margins during the refinishing of the acrylic resin restoration. Small amounts of acrylic resin were added to any voids or thin areas that required reinforcement. Once set, the occlusion was adjusted to eliminate contact in all centric and excursive movements, and final contouring/polishing was accomplished.

Clinical treatment continues during this laboratory phase. If required, autogenous bone obtained from the osteotomy site is used to fill voids between the socket wall and the implant surface.

Cementation of the acrylic resin crown is accomplished with carboxylate cement (Duralon, ESPE America Inc., Norristown, PA). Only the thinnest amount of cement was required as to avoid the extrusion of excess into the cervicular area of the fresh extraction site. The contours of this restoration were designed to mimic the original tooth and root form, sealing the socket and maintaining clot formation subgingivally. The morphology of the restoration provides support of the labial gingiva (Fig 5.2).

No sutures were required when sculpting the restoration in this fashion. This incisionless, sutureless procedure provides an exceptionally fast recovery with very little, if any, postoperative discomfort. Standard protocol for medications following implant surgery was given to patients along with postoperative instructions cautioning premature function on the individual implant.

For many patients, the definitive impression can be made at the time of this one-stage procedure, just prior to cementation of the crown. Cases with gingival swelling due to extensive presurgical periodontal and endodontic pathology are often unsuitable for impression at stage one. Those patients return 4 months after the procedure for the final impression, followed a few days later by delivery of the porcelain-fused-to-gold implant-supported crown. Periapical radiographs were taken on the day of implant placement, definitive prosthesis delivery, and annually. These radiographs had the same angulation through the use of a Rinn Long cone radiographic holder to position the film.

RESULTS

A total of 164 single-tooth implants were placed and provisionalized the day of surgery following the protocol as described above. The implant sites include the maxillary premolar, canine, lateral, central, and molar, as well as the mandibular premolar, canine, and incisor. There was only one single-tooth implant molar restoration in this study because the clinician authors prefer the use of two implants for a molar;[18] therefore, limited data are present for that area. Sixty-four of the 164 implants were placed in fresh extraction sites, two were immediate replacements for failed implants, and the remaining 98 sites were into healed ridges. At the time of implant placement, the bone quality was determined clinically by the surgeon[19] according to the anatomic and bone density criteria established by Lekholm and Zarb.[20]

The implants were various Nobel Biocare implants with differing diameters and configurations. The majority (151) of the implants used in this study had oxidized titanium surfaces (TiUnite, Nobel Biocare USA); the remaining 13 implants had a machine surface. While 7.7% of machine surface-type implants failed, only 4.0% of TiU surface implants failed. One hundred fifteen implants were regular platform, 39 were wide platform, and 10 were narrow platform (Table 5.1). Diameters were predominately 4 and 5 mm with implant lengths distributed primarily between 13 and 18 mm. The teeth most often treated in this study were the maxillary lateral incisors (Table 5.2). Bone quality was primarily type III (59.15%) versus type II (29.88%) and type IV (10.98%) with no type I cases (Table 5.3). Nine patients were smokers, receiving 12 total implants. Seventy-nine autogenous bone grafts were placed.

Of the 164 implants placed with immediate provisionalization seven implants failed, yielding an overall survival rate of 95.73%. Among the complications noted at failure was soft tissue encapsulation, fracture of buccal bone, infection, a decrease in bone quality, and pain. Of the seven failures, four were in the maxillary premolar area, two in the mandibular incisor region, and one in the mandibular premolar region. Three of the failures were type III bone, three were type IV, and one was type II. Four failures were implants placed into immediate extraction sites (6.25%). Twenty percent of Ebon type implants failed, 3.3% of MKIII, and 7.8% of MKIV; there were no failures for MK II, Nobel Perfect, and Brånemark standard type implants (Table 5.4). Two failures had autogenous bone grafts at the time of placement. Six of the failures had TiUnite surfaces (3.97%); one machined surface implant failed (7.69%). None of the failures were associated with smokers, and one occurred in a diabetic patient, otherwise medical conditions were unremarkable. No occlusal adjustments were necessary, and no provisional crowns became loose.

TABLE 5.1 **Implant Distribution Frequency**

Quantity	Diameter	Length	Type	Surface	Platform
1	4	15	Ebon	Machine	RP
4	5	13	Ebon	Machine	WP
1	5	10	MK II	Machine	WP
3	4	13	MK III	TiU	RP
9	4	15	MK III	TiU	RP
3	4	18	MK III	TiU	RP
1	5	13	MK III	TiU	WP
6	3.75	15	MK III	TiU	RP
8	3.75	18	MK III	TiU	RP
7	4	10	MK IV	TiU	RP
12	4	13	MK IV	TiU	RP
21	4	15	MK IV	TiU	RP
18	4	18	MK IV	TiU	RP
5	5	13	MK IV	TiU	WP
1	3.75	18	MK IV	TiU	RP
2	3.5	13	Nobel Perfect	TiU	NP
8	3.5	16	Nobel Perfect	TiU	NP
2	4	13	Nobel Perfect	TiU	RP
1	4.3	10	Nobel Perfect	TiU	RP
3	4.3	13	Nobel Perfect	TiU	RP
14	4.3	16	Nobel Perfect	TiU	RP
1	5	10	Nobel Perfect	TiU	WP
4	5	13	Nobel Perfect	TiU	WP
22	5	16	Nobel Perfect	TiU	WP
3	3.75	15	Standard	Machine	RP
1	3.75	18	Standard	Machine	RP
2	4	18	Standard	Machine	RP
1	5	12	Standard	Machine	WP
Total implant population =	164				

Regular platform (RP), narrow platform (NP), wide platform (WP).

DISCUSSION

Kupeyan and May[4] and Wöhrle[5] reported on a series of 10 and 14 immediately restored implants, respectively, in the maxillary anterior region. Kupeyan and May performed their study in healed ridges with machined titanium implants while Wöhrle reported on roughened implants in immediate extraction sites. All implants in both studies clinically integrated, remaining stable for the observation periods of 6 months to 3 years.

Hui et al[11] did a comparison study of two groups of patients with 24 implants, immediate placement of implants in 11 extraction sites and immediate placement and restoration in 13 extraction sites in the maxillary anterior region. Heavy smokers and patients with a history of bruxism were excluded. Machined-surface implants 13 to 18 mm long were placed with torque values of 40 to 50 N cm attempting to achieve bicortical anchorage. Interim prostheses were placed out of contact in all excursive movements the day of surgery. No implants were lost, and no complications were encountered.

Glauser et al[12] placed 127 implants (76 maxillary, 51 mandibular) in 41 patients, including smokers. Patients with bruxism and imperfect alveolar ridges were not excluded. Restorations were usually placed the day of surgery and were fabricated in centric occlusal contact without excursive contact. After 1 year, results indicated that 22 implants were lost in 13 patients, including 7 maxillary implants in one patient, for a survival rate of 82.7%. Thirty-four percent of 41 implants in the maxillary posterior area failed, while only 9% of the other 86 implants in all other areas failed. Patients with parafunctional habits (22 implants) had failure more often (41%) than nonbruxers (105 implants, 12%).

Following up on their earlier work, Malo et al[13] coordinated a multicenter study with 116 machined-surface implants with various diameters and configurations placed in 76 patients. Implants were placed in the esthetic zone using underpreparation of the apical aspect of the osteotomies to increase initial stability and increasing insertion torque to greater than 30 N cm for all implants. Twenty-four patients in

TABLE 5.2 **Implant Survival Rates by Location and Implant Length**

Tooth Position	Total	Length						Failures
		10 mm	12 mm	13 mm	15 mm	16 mm	18 mm	
Max premolar	37	6		14	5	12	1	4
Max canine	10				3	2	3	
Max lateral	54			9	15	13	17	
Max central	34			4	10	11	10	
Max molar	1	1						
Mand premolar	18	3	1	9	4	1		1
Mand canine	4				1	1	2	
Mand incisors	6				4	1	1	2
Totals	164	10	1	36	42	41	34	7
Failures	7	2	0	1	4	0	0	
Survival rate	95.73%	80.00%	100.00%	97.22%	90.48%	100.00%	100.00%	

TABLE 5.3   **Implant Survival Rates by Location and Bone Quality**

Tooth Position	Total	Bone Quality				Fail	% Survival
		I	II	III	IV		
Max premolar	37		3	28	6	4	89.18%
Max canine	10		5	5			100.00%
Max lateral	54		14	30	10		100.00%
Max central	34		15	19			100.00%
Max molar	1			1			100.00%
Mand premolar	18		6	10	2	1	94.44%
Mand canine	4		3	1			100.00%
Mand incisors	6		3	3		2	66.70%
Totals	164	0	49	97	18	7	95.73%
% of cases		0.00%	29.88%	59.15%	10.98%		
Failures	7		1	3	3		
Survival rate		n/a	97.95%	96.91%	83.33%		

TABLE 5.4   **Implant Failure Rate by Type**

Type	Ebon	MK II	MK III	MK IV	NblPrfct	Standard	
Cases	5	1	30	64	57	7	164
% of total cases	3.0%	0.6%	18.3%	39.0%	34.8%	4.3%	
Failures	1		1	5			7
Fail rate	20.0%	0.0%	3.3%	7.8%	0.0%	0.0%	4.3%

this group smoked more than 10 cigarettes per day. The authors reported a 96.5% (112 of 116) success rate for integration and 100% (22 of 22) integration in fresh extraction sockets.

These studies show promise for immediate provisionalization of single-tooth implants with a success range from 82% to 100%. In this study, the survival rate was 95.7% during the observation period. Schnitman et al[6] reported on factors affecting the outcome of immediately loaded implants as high primary stability, implant to cortical bone contact percentage, cortical bone density, and control of micromotion during the healing process. Brunski[7] suggests the threshold of forces critical to successful integration is 100 μm, and exceeding this level leads to fibrous encapsulation.

This report shows a trend of higher failure rates in immediate provisionalization of single-tooth implants as the bone quality decreases; however, the sample size of implants placed in Type IV bone is limited, and therefore no definitive conclusion can be made from the bone quality figures. This data does illustrate that successful osseointegration can occur in all bone types with a single-tooth implant immediately provisionalized.

Of the implant designs used in this study, the Nobel Perfect implant had the best success rate. All 57 Nobel Perfect implants achieved successful osseointegration. The oxidized Ti surface (TiUnite) implants in this study yielded a 96.03% survival rate, a greater percentage than the implants

with a machined surface (92.31%). These results support the results from previous reports.[16,17] In regards to implant location, the only implants that failed in the maxillary arch were in the premolar areas. This suggests the possibility of micromotion/overload created by larger forces found in the area of the premolar. In the mandible, there was one failure in the area of the premolars and two failures in the area of the incisors.

The implants in this study were placed consecutively as single teeth and immediately provisionalized. Without the confounding variable of operator judgment, the results should be reproducible by attention to detailed replication of technique and materials.

CONCLUSION

Immediate provisionalization protocols have proven to be a successful treatment option for the edentulous and partially edentulous patient. Although loading forces are different from an edentulous arch to a partially edentulous or single-tooth restoration, the application of provisionalization to a single implant can be successful if the proper precautions are taken in achieving passive occlusion. The data from this study supports this treatment option by reporting a 95.73% survival rate for a population of 164 immediately provisionalized single-tooth implants.

ACKNOWLEDGMENTS

The authors would like to thank the staff at Prosthodontics Intermedica for their kind and very gentle treatment of the patients; Robert Winkelman and the staff of Fort Washington Dental Lab for laboratory support; and Christine Raines for image preparation.

REFERENCES

1. Adell R, Lekholm U, Rockler B, et al: A 15-year study of osseointegrated implants in the treatment of the edentulous jaw. *Int J Oral Surg* 1981;10:387–416.

2. Brånemark PI, Hansson BO, Adell R, et al: Osseointegrated implants in the treatment of the edentulous jaw. Experience from a 10-year period. *Scand J Plast Reconstr Surg Suppl* 1977;16:1–132.

3. Glauser R, Ruhstaller P, Windisch S, et al: Immediate occlusal loading of Brånemark System TiUnite implants placed predominantly in soft bone: 4-year results of a prospective clinical study. *Clin Implant Dent Relat Res* 2005;7(Suppl 1):S52–S59.

4. Kupeyan HK, May KB: Implant and provisional crown placement: a one-stage protocol. *Implant Dent* 1998;7:213–217.

5. Wöhrle PS: Single-tooth replacement in the aesthetic zone with immediate provisionalization: fourteen consecutive case reports. *Pract Periodontics Aesthet Dent* 1998;10:1107–1114.

6. Schnitman PA, Rubenstein JE, Whorle PS, et al: Implants for partial edentulism. *J Dent Educ* 1988;52:725–736.

7. Brunski JB: Avoid pitfalls of overloading and micromotion of intraosseous implants. *Dent Implantol Update* 1993;4:77–81.

8. Brunski JB: In vivo bone response to biomechanical loading at the bone/dental implant interface. *Adv Dent Res* 1999;13:99–119.

9. Cameron HU, Pilliar RM, MacNab I: The effect of movement on the bonding of porous metal to bone. *J Biomed Mater Res* 1973;7:301–311.

10. Szmukler-Moncler S, Piattelli A, Favero GA, et al: Considerations preliminary to the application of early and immediate loading protocols in dental implantology. *Clin Oral Implants Res* 2000;11:12–25.

11. Hui E, Chow J, Li D, et al: Immediate provisional for single-tooth implant replacement with Brånemark System: preliminary report. *Clin Implant Dent Relat Res* 2001;3:79–86.

12. Glauser R, Rée A, Lundgren A, et al: Immediate occlusal loading of Brånemark implants applied in various jawbone regions: a prospective, 1-year clinical study. *Clin Implant Dent Relat Res* 2001;3:204–213.

13. Malo P, Friberg B, Polizzi G, et al: Immediate and early function of Brånemark System implants placed in the esthetic zone: a 1-year prospective clinical multicenter study. *Clin Implant Dent Relat Res* 2003;5(Suppl 1):37–46.

14. Ericsson I, Nilson H, Nilner K, et al: Immediate provisional for single-tooth implant replacement with Brånemark System: preliminary report. *Clin Implant Dent Relat Res* 2001;3:79–86.

15. Misch CE, Hahn J, Judy KW, et al: Immediate Function Consensus Conference. Workshop guidelines on immediate loading in implant dentistry. November 7, 2003. *J Oral Implantol* 2004;30:283–288. Review.

16. Glauser R, Lundgren AK, Gottlow J, et al: Immediate occlusal loading of Brånemark TiUnite implants placed predominantly in soft bone: 1-year results of a prospective clinical study. *Clin Implant Dent Relat Res* 2003;5(Suppl 1):47–56.

17. Balshi SF, Wolfinger GJ, Balshi TJ: Analysis of 164 titanium oxide-surface implants in completely edentulous arches for fixed prosthesis anchorage using the pterygomaxillary region. *Int J Oral Maxillofac Implants* 2005;20:946–952.

18. Balshi TJ, Wolfinger GJ: Two-implant-supported single molar replacement: interdental space requirements and comparison to alternative options. *Int J Periodontics Restorative Dent* 1997;17:426–435.

19. Johansson P, Strid K: Assessment of bone quality from cutting resistance during implant surgery. *Int J Oral Maxillofac Implants* 1994;9:279–288.

20. Lekholm U, Zarb G: Patient selection and preparation. In Brånemark P-I, Zarb G, Albrektsson T (eds): *Tissue-Integrated Prostheses: Osseointegration in Clinical Density.* Chicago, Quintessence, 1985, pp. 199–220.

6

TECHNIQUE FOR REMOVING CEMENT BETWEEN A FIXED PROSTHESIS AND ITS SUBSTRUCTURE

ABDULLAH S. ALSIYABI, BDS, MS, FFD RCSI, MRACDS,[1] AND DAVID A. FELTON, DDS, MS, FACP[2]

[1]Head of Prosthodontics Department, Military Dental Services, Royal Army of Oman, Sultanate of Oman, formerly Graduate Prosthodontics Resident, UNC School of Dentistry, Chapel Hill, NC

[2]Professor, Department of Prosthodontics, UNC School of Dentistry, Chapel Hill, NC

Keywords

Loose screw-retained implant prosthesis; debonded cast dowel-core crowns or dowel-core restorations; adhesive luting cements; cement-retained prostheses.

Correspondence

Abdullah Alsiyabi, Military Dental Center, Royal Army of Oman, P.O. Box 1097, Postal Code 132, Alkoudh, Wilayat Alseeb, Sultanate of Oman. E-mail: nibras97@omantel.net.om

Accepted February 11, 2008

Published in *Journal of Prosthodontics* April 2009; Vol. 18, Issue 3

doi: 10.1111/j.1532-849X.2008.00397.x

ABSTRACT

Failed restorations diagnosed with salvageable and subsequently reusable metal substructures that demand their separation can be clinically challenging to undertake without the risk of damaging either the super- or substructures. This article describes a technique to safely separate them from each other in order for the respective substructure to be reused in the fabrication of a newly reconstructed restoration and for the existing restoration to be reused as a provisional where appropriately indicated.

Many present-day implant systems have screw-retained abutments onto which restorations can be cemented. There are situations when a patient presents with an otherwise clinically successful, cement-retained fixed prosthesis that needs to be separated from its respective metallic substructure. This is most often the case when an implant abutment screw loosening has occurred under a cemented restoration due to inadequate torque, or when a cast dowel and core-retained restoration has developed an incipient recurrent caries between the preparation finish line and the prosthetic margin. In both cases, there may or may not be an indication for the fabrication of a new restoration. Some of the traditional methods used to separate cemented retainers from their respective metallic abutments are to physically pull them apart or to use an ultrasonic vibration device to disturb the cement interface.[1] The technique described here is a more "predictable" practical procedure with the least damaging effect on the restoration or its respective substructure. One of the main advantages of this procedure is that the retrieved prosthesis and its metallic substructure can be salvaged and subsequently reused either definitively or provisionally. The technique described below is illustrated through its application in two cases with different clinical presentations.

TECHNIQUE

Clinical Scenario Case 1

1. A patient presents with a loose, implant-retained fixed partial denture (FPD) cemented on screw-retained abutments. An intraoral radiograph is made as a preoperative guide. Upon examination, clinical findings are that the abutments screws are loose and require retightening.

2. The entry to each screw head is carefully gained through access channels prepared from the palatal aspect, using a high-speed diamond bur to cut through porcelain to maintain its integrity and then multifluted carbide burs (SS White, Lakewood, NJ) to cut through the metal substructure (Fig 6.1).

3. The width of the screw-access channels are kept slightly larger than the screw head diameter for unimpeded straight-line access to each screw head.

4. The screw heads are exposed after the screw access channel filling material is removed.

5. Using the appropriate implant system screwdriver, the abutment screws are removed through the access channels, and the FPD is retrieved with its cemented abutments (Fig 6.2).

6. In this particular situation, the fabrication of a new FPD is planned for two reasons. One, the screw access chamber is overenlarged following

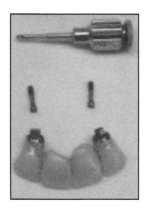

FIGURE 6.2 Ceramometal implant-retained FPD with its associated abutments is retrieved from the implants.

preparation while trying to gain direct straight-line access for the screwdriver to the screw head. With the concern that this channel will weaken the porcelain structural integrity and establish unstable occlusal contact[2] that may compromise the long-term prognosis of the prosthesis, a new FPD is advisable. Second, a new prosthesis is warranted due to the patient's insistence for a cement-retained prosthesis without the esthetic compromise of the filled screw access holes.

7. After disinfection, the retrieved FPD with its associated abutments is placed in the ceramic furnace tray on a fibrous firing support pad (Vita Zahnfabrik, Bad Sackingen, Germany).

8. The ceramic furnace (Programat P80, Ivoclar, Vita Zahnfabrik) is programmed using the following schedule:

   (1) Firing at 650°C (or equivalent) as the high temperature,

   (2) No vacuum used,

   (3) One minute preheat time,

   (4) One minute holding time at the maximum temperature,

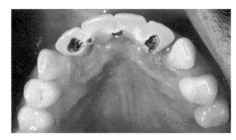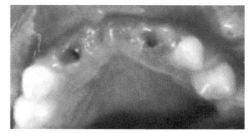

FIGURE 6.1 Screw access channels are prepared from the palatal aspect to retrieve the prosthesis and its respective substructures.

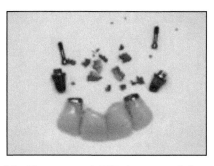

FIGURE 6.3 The cemented FPD is separated from its screw-retained implant abutments through cement disintegration.

(5) Allow to cool on firing tray at room temperature. This firing sequence resulted in the disintegration of the cement layer, leaving the abutment detached from the prosthesis (Fig 6.3).

9. The retrieved abutments' supramarginal areas are carefully air-abraded with 50 μm medium grit lead-free soda particles of glass beads (Perlablast micro, Bego, Bremen, Germany) at 2 bar air pressure to remove the superficial passive postfiring titanium oxide layer, to remove remnants of the old cement, and to increase the surface area necessary to optimize cement adhesion. This mechanical (nonacid) treatment is recommended for base-metal castings instead of pickling (chemical) treatment.[3] With the use of glass bead particles, there is no metal loss, because the surface is compacted rather than abraded. This will maintain the integrity of the machined precision friction-fit of the manufactured plastic or metal coping used in the fabrication of the permanent restoration. The final cleaning step is done by immersing the abutments in a container of distilled water and either cleaned ultrasonically (BioSonic UC100, Coltene Whaledent AG,

Altstatten, Switzerland) or steam cleaned (Impulse, Jacger, Weinsheim, Germany) for 10 to 15 minutes.[4]

10. The abutments are tightened to their recommended torque value of 35 N cm.

11. An impression is made for the fabrication of the new FPD in the conventional manner.

12. The retrieved FPD is cleaned before it is recemented with interim cement as a provisional prosthesis. Screw access channels are sealed with Fermit (Ivoclar North America, Amherst, NY).

Clinical Scenario Case 2

1. The patient presented for his recare visit with a finding of early stage recurrent caries along the finish line of a first molar crown.

2. Bite-wing radiographic analysis revealed a root canal-treated tooth with a cast dowel and core foundation and loss of restoration marginal integrity with natural tooth due to caries.

3. An attempt to remove the crown alone without disturbing its cast dowel and core system was unsuccessful. In this particular case, among other etiological factors, this could be due to intraradicular cement insufficiency, cement adhesion bond failure between the dowel and core system with the root dentine, or poor cementation technique. Inadequate dowel/core system design (e.g., short tapered post) is ruled out.

4. The same laboratory procedure described above (step 8) is used to carefully separate the dowel/core system from its restoration after disinfection (Fig 6.4).

5. The cast dowel and core is air-abraded with 50 μm aluminum oxide particles at 1 to 2 bar air pressure. It is then chemically treated (cleaned) by immersion in nonfuming hot pickling agent (Jet Pak, JF Jelenko,

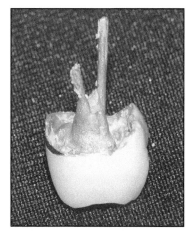
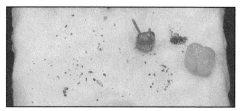

FIGURE 6.4 Retrieved PFM crown with custom cast dowel and core still cemented. The right picture shows the crown separated from its cast dowel-core substructure through cement disintegration.

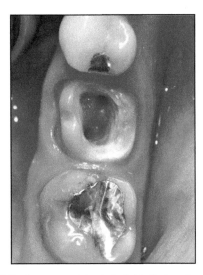

FIGURE 6.5 Lower root-treated right first molar preparation following recurrent caries removal, remargination, and dowel space clean-up.

Armonk, NY) in an ultrasonic bath for several minutes.[5]

6. The existing custom-made cast dowel and core system is recemented after the root canal system is conservatively filled, irrigated, and cleaned of the old residual cement.

7. Following caries removal and remargination, the prepared tooth is impressed for the fabrication of a new crown (Fig 6.5).

8. The existing crown is finally luted with interim cement (Tempbond NE, Kerr, West Collins Orange, CA) and used as a provisional after it has been cleaned and relined intraorally. Due to the near-precise fit of the existing PFM crown used as provisional, and to not disturb the cemented cast dowel and core, the Tempbond NE modifier has been added to the base before it is mixed with the accelerator to make the crown easier to remove thereafter.

In the alternative procedure, if following residual cement removal and canal clean-up, the retrieved cast dowel/core is deemed to be mildly loosely fitting within the caries-free canals (i.e., with suboptimal snug fit), it can be air-abraded, ultrasonically cleaned, and oxidized if it is made of metal base alloy or either silane coupling agent bonded to its surface using special equipment (Silicoater, Kulzer, Irvine, CA) or tin-electroplated if made of noble metal alloy[6] in preparation for adhesive resin bonding. Additionally, the radicular dentine to be conditioned before the cast dowel and core can be bonded using the appropriate etchants and adhesive resin luting cement, which provide significantly higher retentive tensile bond strength[7,8] due to the fact that adhesive cement is an active resin that chemically bonds not only to the restoration but also to the tooth structure preparation, even if designed with suboptimal or less-than-ideal retentive features.[9]

Following the cement disintegration firing cycle, contamination to the ceramic furnace can be overcome by purging it in the manner recommended by the manufacturer. Firing below the auto-glaze temperature of the porcelain minimizes any pyro thermomechanical detrimental effects on the restoration, such as vitrification.

SUMMARY

This technique has several advantages. It enables the clinician to separate the cemented prosthesis from its respective substructure in a practical, simple, and predictable way whenever indicated. It is a chairside, time-saving procedure that can be carried out in the dental laboratory once the restoration components' assembly is safely retrieved. As per clinical judgment, the separated components can be reused either provisionally (interim prostheses) or permanently (the abutments and custom-cast dowel and core system) without a remake. This in turn renders it a cost-effective procedure.

REFERENCES

1. Rosenstiel SF, Land MF, Fujimoto J: Restoration of the endodontically treated tooth. In Rosenstiel SF, Land MF, Fujimoto J (eds): *Contemporary Fixed Prosthodontics* (ed 4). St. Louis, MO, Mosby, 2006, pp. 372–373.

2. Chee W, Felton DA, Johnson PF, et al: Cemented versus screw-retained implant prostheses: which is better? *Int J Oral Maxillofac Implants* 1999;14:137–141.

3. Shillingburg HT Jr, Hobo S, Whitsett LD, et al: Investing and casting. In Shillingburg HT Jr, Hobo S, Whitsett LD, et al (eds): *Fundamentals of Fixed Prosthodontics* (ed 3). Chicago, IL, Quintessence, 1997, p. 382.

4. Naylor WP: *Introduction to Metal Ceramic Technology* (ed 1). Chicago, IL, Quintessence, 1999, pp. 88–89.

5. Shillingburg HT Jr, Hobo S, Whitsett LD, et al: Finishing and cementation. In Shillingburg HT Jr, Hobo S, Whitsett LD, et al (eds): *Fundamentals of Fixed Prosthodontics* (ed 3). Chicago, IL, Quintessence, 1997, p. 375.

6. Shillingburg HT Jr, Hobo S, Whitsett LD, et al: Investing and casting. In Shillingburg HT Jr, Hobo S, Whitsett LD, et al (eds): *Fundamentals of Fixed Prosthodontics* (ed 3). Chicago, IL, Quintessence, 1997, p. 401.

7. David AM, Laura M, Paul B: *Oxford Handbook of Clinical Dentistry* (ed 4). New York, NY, Oxford University Press, 2006, p. 290.

8. John GJ: *Self-Assessment Picture Tests in Dentistry—Operative Dentistry* (ed 1). St Louis, MO, Mosby, 1994, p. 102.

9. Trevor Burke FJ: Trends in indirect dentistry: 3. Luting materials. *Dental Update* 2005;32:251–260.

7

IMMEDIATE LOADING OF DENTAL IMPLANTS IN THE ESTHETIC REGION USING COMPUTER-GUIDED IMPLANT TREATMENT SOFTWARE AND STEREOLITHOGRAPHIC MODELS FOR A PATIENT WITH EATING DISORDERS

DANIEL F. GALINDO, DDS AND CAESAR C. BUTURA, DDS
Private Practice, ClearChoice Dental Implant Center, Phoenix, AZ

> The article is associated with the American College of Prosthodontists' journal-based continuing education program. It is accompanied by an online continuing education activity worth 1 credit. Please visit www.wileyhealthlearning. com/jopr to complete the activity and earn credit.

Keywords
Immediate loading; dental implants; implant-supported prosthesis; eating disorders; computer-guided implant treatment software; stereolithographic model.

Correspondence
Daniel Galindo, 20830 N. Tatum Blvd., Ste. 150, Phoenix, AZ 85050. E-mail: galindoprosthodontics@gmail.com

The authors deny any conflicts of interest.

Accepted March 28, 2013

Published in *Journal of Prosthodontics* February 2014; Vol. 23, Issue 2

doi: 10.1111/jopr.12077

ABSTRACT

This manuscript describes the reconstruction of a maxillary anterior segment using immediate implant placement and immediate implant loading techniques, aided by computer-guided implant treatment software and stereolithographic models and surgical templates, in a patient with a history of eating disorder. Her medical and dental histories did not make her a candidate for the use of conventional 2-stage implant surgery and restorative procedures along with an interim removable prosthesis.

Eating disorders are characterized by patterns of disturbances in eating behavior. Anorexia Nervosa (AN), Bulimia Nervosa (BN), and Eating Disorders Not Otherwise Specified (ED-NOS), which includes the provisional Binge-Eating Disorder (BED), are three formal diagnostic categories described by the American Psychiatric Association.[1] Eating disorders have been associated with increased suicide and mortality rates[2,3] and affect up to 24 million people of all ages and genders in the United States.[4] Several psychological and pharmacological treatment modalities have been described, such as family-based therapy, cognitive-behavior therapy, along with use of antidepressants, both in primary care settings and outpatient facilities.[5] Physical and psychosocial health consequences include, but are not limited to, limb and joint pain, headache, gastrointestinal problems, menstrual problems, shortness of breath, chest pain, anxiety, depression, and substance abuse.[6] Common oral and dental signs and symptoms include hypersensitivity, erythema, chemical erosion of the lingual surfaces of maxillary teeth, xerostomia, loss of enamel, gingival bleeding, caries, loss of occlusal vertical dimension, and angular cheilitis.[7–10] Few patients with eating disorders seek medical treatment,[11] and often the dentist is the first healthcare professional to detect the signs of eating disorders in an otherwise undiagnosed patient.[12] Several reports in the dental literature address the challenges of treating the consequences of this disease due to the complexity of the medical and dental clinical conditions. Most authors recommend that restorative therapy should begin once the patient's eating disorder is under control.[13,14] Treatment modalities vary depending on the extent of damage to the remaining dentition and supporting structures. Composite resin restorations have been recommended for the management of limited erosive lesions and caries along with the use of fluoride rinses and gels.[15] Lesions extending subgingivally or those where tooth foundation is compromised require the use of partial or full coverage restorations such as veneers, inlays, or crowns.[16]

Dental implants have been used successfully in the restoration of partially and fully edentulous patients for the past 30 years.[17–19] Methods and technologies have evolved to deliver highly functional and esthetic implant-supported restorations, especially in the maxillary anterior region[20] incorporating concepts such as immediate implant loading. Previously, dental implant treatment consisted of a two-stage surgical protocol where patients were asked to wear an interim removable prosthesis or remain partially edentulous during the healing phase.[21,22] At times, this was an inconvenience for the patient and forced clinicians to find a solution to this challenge. The concept of loading of implants immediately after surgical placement was introduced and defined as a restoration placed in occlusion with the opposing dentition within 48 hours of implant placement.[23] Multiple studies have reported successful outcomes when implants are immediately loaded through interim prostheses in edentulous arches[24,25] and later, in partially dentate arches.[26–28] The concept of immediate loading is based on three important principles: (1) micromotion of approximately 100 μm (with a range of 50 to 150 μm) may be the threshold value for implants to osseointegrate properly;[29] (2) implants need to be joined together through a rigid interim prosthesis to reduce micromotion and favor healing during immediate loading;[30,31] and (3)

micromotion between the implant and its osteotomy needs to be minimized through insertional torque values of at least 30 N cm at the time of implant placement.[32]

The original protocol for implant surgery required raising a flap to expose underlying bone, probably leading to a compromised esthetic result.[33] Several techniques were developed to minimize the impact of altering tissue attachment and position with modified flaps, mini flaps, and microflaps[34] as well as with enhanced suturing methods. Digital technologies have been developed to aid in the flapless surgical procedure, allowing for proper management of hard and soft tissues.[35,36] These technologies include computer-guided implant treatment software and stereolithographic models and surgical templates.

Computer-guided implant treatment software uses cone beam computed tomography (CBCT) files to create a 3D image of the patient's jaws. The software allows for the desired implants to be planned and positioned on the patient's image. Once the position has been finalized, stereolithographic models and surgical templates can be fabricated.[37] This allows for the fabrication of interim prostheses that will allow for adequate implant splinting with ideal esthetics and function.

Few reports describe the prognosis for dental implants and surrounding soft tissues in patients with eating disorders.[38] To our knowledge, no report in the literature addresses the use of immediately loaded dental implants in the management of a patient affected by eating disorders, incorporating the use of software for digital diagnostics and treatment planning along with virtual surgery and stereolithographic models.

CLINICAL REPORT

This clinical report presents a 29-year-old female patient with a 10+ year history of being diagnosed with an eating disorder. She received comprehensive medical and psychological treatment and was considered to be under remission. At the time of treatment, she continued to attend support meetings two times per week with her physicians and therapists. Prior to treatment, the patient underwent a thorough medical evaluation in conjunction with her attending physician. A full panel of laboratory values and a 12-lead electrocardiogram were obtained to determine her ability to undergo the surgical procedure. In light of the past longstanding eating disorder, her liver enzymes were elevated, thus precluding the use of general anesthesia. Her ECG was interpreted as normal. Based on this information, her physician cleared her for the procedure under local anesthesia. The treating physicians also deemed her fit for treatment, as she had not had any recurrences in the previous 18 months and had attended all scheduled support sessions.

The patient had been unsuccessfully restored several times in the anterior maxilla with full coverage restorations, which over time had to be replaced with more extensive restorations replacing extracted teeth. At the time of her

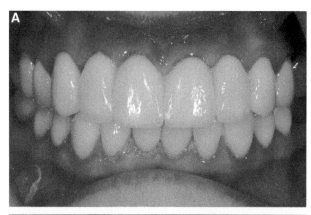

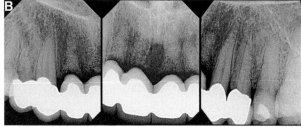

FIGURE 7.1 (A) Pretreatment dental condition and (B) preoperative periapical radiographs showing abutment teeth under fixed partial dental prosthesis.

examination, she presented with an eight-unit porcelain-fused-to-metal fixed partial denture (FPD) retained by maxillary canines and first premolars, which were failing due to recurrent decay (Fig 7.1). Her main concern had to do with

her inability to tolerate a removable prosthesis due to her sensitive gag reflex and the emotional and psychological effects of it on her overall condition. She was also unwilling to transition during the healing phase without teeth. After clinical and radiographic evaluation it was determined that the retaining teeth for her FPD had a questionable prognosis. The existing fixed restoration was removed to evaluate the condition of the canines and first premolars. The extent of decay compromised these teeth to the extent that endodontic treatment along with crown lengthening procedures, cast post and cores, and full coverage crowns were required. Past experiences with similar procedures on the now missing maxillary central and lateral incisors made her unwilling to proceed with such an alternative, and the option of dental implants was presented. To address the patient's chief complaint, the treatment plan included extraction of failing maxillary left and right canines and first premolars, immediate placement of dental implants on the sites of central incisors, canines, and first premolars, bilaterally, and two fixed four-unit implant-supported interim FPDs. After proper healing, the plan was to restore the patient with ceramic abutments and two four-unit ceramic FPDs.

CBCT was performed, and digital images reconstructed using computer-guided implant treatment software. Removal of teeth was done on the software, and buccolingual slides were evaluated for selected implant placement. The anterior and sagittal views ensured that the roots of adjacent teeth would not be compromised (Fig 7.2). Both a stereolithographic surgical guide and model were fabricated.

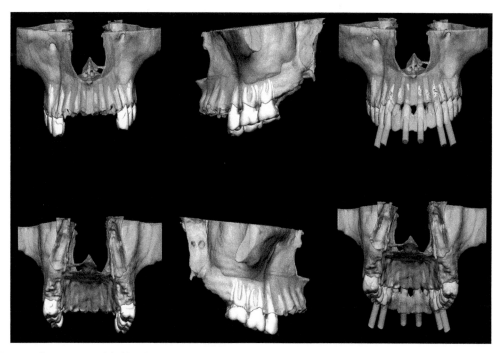

FIGURE 7.2 Images of computer-guided implant treatment software depicting selected implant position in relation to angulation and depth in residual bone and relation with remaining teeth. Design of definitive prosthesis imposed over planned implant position was used to evaluate abutment design and esthetics.

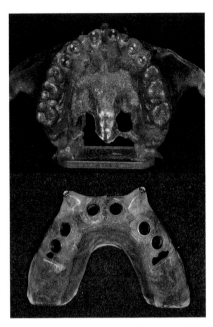

FIGURE 7.3 Stereolithographic model and surgical template were ordered. Implant analogs were set in model to allow for fabrication of abutments and interim prostheses.

Simulated surgery was completed on the model using NobelGuide instrumentation (Nobel Biocare, Yorba Linda, CA). The surgical guide was secured on the stereolithographic model, and implant placement was completed in the planned position (Fig 7.3). The stereolithographic model was duplicated using implant replicas, vinylpolysiloxane

(VPS) (Gingifast Rigid; Zhermack, Rovigo, Italy), and Type IV stone (GC Fujirock EP, GC Corporation, Tokyo, Japan). The cast with the implant replicas in the selected implant position was used for the design and fabrication of custom temporary abutments (Nobel Biocare) with the goal of providing proper guidance and support for the healing of the soft tissues. Four-unit cement- and screw-retained interim FPDs were fabricated using bis-acrylic temporization material (Protemp Plus, 3M ESPE, St. Paul, MN) to meet the esthetic and functional demands of the patient (Fig 7.4).

Actual surgery followed the same NobelGuide protocol. Failing teeth were removed, the surgical guide was seated, and site development was completed. Selected implants (Nobel Replace) were placed through the surgical template at a 35 N cm torque value. Temporary abutments were seated on the implants in the positions of central incisors and canines and torqued to 20 N cm. Screw access holes were sealed with Teflon tape and Fermit. Interim prostheses were modified as needed to develop the desired emergence profile and soft tissue contours. The four-unit interim FPDs were cemented over these abutments using RelyX luting cement (3M ESPE) while at the same time, screwed directly onto the implants in the first premolar position. The screw access holes were sealed in the previously described fashion. The occlusion on the interim FPD was adjusted to prevent loading during eccentric movements, while allowing maximum intercuspation loading in centric occlusion only on the first premolars. Radiographs were taken to verify implant, abutment, and prosthesis position. The patient was given postoperative instructions and recall appointments after

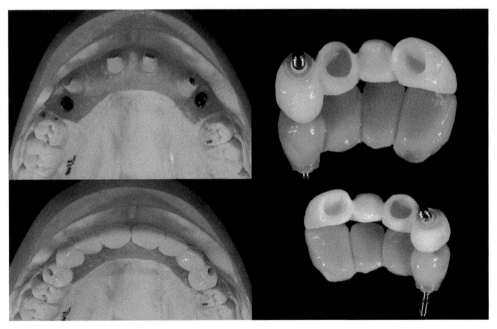

FIGURE 7.4 Temporary abutments were customized to develop proper emergence profile and esthetics. Two four-unit interim FPDs were fabricated; the restorations were cemented over the abutments in the central incisor and canine positions, while the first premolar was screw-retained directly on the implant. Ovate pontics were developed for the lateral incisors.

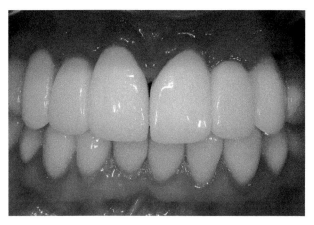

FIGURE 7.5 Intraoral labial view of interim prostheses after 1 week of healing.

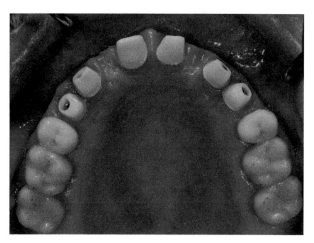

FIGURE 7.6 Zirconia abutments fabricated using CAD/CAM technology seated on implants.

1 week, 1 month, and 2 months. At each of these visits, implant and abutment stability, soft tissue health, and prosthesis appearance and function were evaluated (Fig 7.5). At 5 months, tissue health was considered optimal, and with no signs of prosthesis, abutment, or implant mobility, final restorative procedures were completed. The interim prostheses and abutments were removed, and impression copings connected to the implants. An open tray implant level impression was made using VPS impression material, making sure the healed soft tissue contour was adequately detailed. The soft tissue was reproduced in the impression using a VPS gingival mask (Gingifast Rigid), and the master cast was poured in Type IV stone (GC Fujirock EP). Abutment design and fabrication were completed with computer-aided design/computer aided manufacture (CAD/CAM) technology in zirconia (Procera, Nobel Biocare). Two four-unit zirconia frameworks were fabricated for the FPDs (Wieland ZENO, Pforzheim, Germany) (Figs 7.6 and 7.7). Both FPDs were cemented using temporary cement (Zone Temporary Cement, Dux Dental, Oxnard, CA). The fit of the abutments on the implants and of the FPDs on the

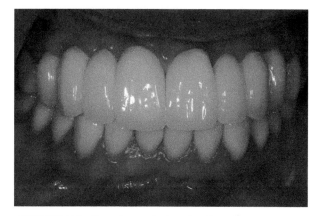

FIGURE 7.7 Two four-unit zirconia FPDs were cemented.

abutments was verified with periapical radiographs, and the marginal bone height was recorded. During the course of treatment and a follow-up period of 18 months, the patient has not presented with any complications (Fig 7.8).

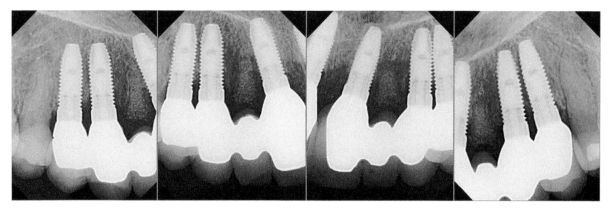

FIGURE 7.8 Periapical radiographs illustrating bone levels after 18 months in function in definitive prostheses.

SUMMARY

This clinical report describes rehabilitation using implant-supported FPDs on immediately placed and immediately loaded dental implants, aided by computer-guided implant treatment software, stereolithographic models, and surgical templates, of a partially dentate patient affected by eating disorders. The patient's anatomy was evaluated on CBCT scans to determine the ideal recipient sites for implant placement, as well as angulation and depth. Virtual surgery was done with the aid of computer-guided implant treatment software, and stereolithographic models, and surgical templates were obtained once the digital process was completed. Temporary abutments and interim prostheses were designed on the stereolithographic models to aid in soft tissue healing and enhance the final esthetic and functional result. Treatment for this patient with immediate implant placement and immediate implant loading kept her from having to use a removable prosthesis during the healing phase, thus avoiding the undesirable gag reflex.

ACKNOWLEDGMENTS

The authors thank Rick Durkee, CDT, and Sean Marchal, CDT, for their invaluable assistance in the laboratory procedures involved for the care of this patient, and Mariana Galindo for her assistance in preparation of the figures for this manuscript.

REFERENCES

1. American Psychiatric Association: *Diagnostic and Statistical Manual of Mental Disorders*. Washington, DC, American Psychiatric Association, 2000.

2. Crow SJ, Peterson CB, Swanson SA, et al: Increased mortality in bulimia nervosa and other eating disorders. *Am J Psychiatry* 2009;166:1342–1346.

3. Sullivan PF: Mortality in anorexia nervosa. *Am J Psychiatry* 1995;152:1073–1074.

4. The Renfrew Center Foundation for Eating Disorders: *Eating Disorders 101 Guide: A Summary of Issues, Statistics and Resources*. Philadelphia, Renfrew, 2003.

5. Allen S, Dalton WT: Treatment of eating disorders in primary care: a systematic review. *J Health Psychol* 2011;16: 1165–1176.

6. Johnson JG, Spitzer RL, Williams JB: Health problems, impairment and illnesses associated with bulimia nervosa and binge eating disorder among primary care and obstetric gynecology patients. *Psychol Med* 2001;31:1455–1466.

7. Montgomery MT, Ritvo J, Ritvo J, et al: Eating disorders: phenomenology, identification, and dental intervention. *Gen Dent* 1988;36:485–488.

8. Hazelton LR, Faine MP: Diagnosis and dental management of eating disorder patients. *Int J Prosthodont* 1996;9:65–73.

9. Abrahamsen TC: The worn dentition—pathognomonic patterns of abrasion and erosion. *Int Dent J* 2005;55(Suppl 1):268–276.

10. Schwarz S, Kreuter A, Rammelsberg P: Efficient prosthodontic treatment in a young patient with long-standing bulimia nervosas: a clinical report. *J Prosthet Dent* 2011;106:6–11.

11. Noordenbos G, Oldenhave A, Muschter J, et al: Characteristics and treatment of patients with chronic eating disorders. *Eat Disord* 2002;10:15–29.

12. Milosevic A: Eating disorders and the dentist. *Br Dent J* 1999;186:109–113.

13. Cowan RD, Sabates CR, Gross KB, et al: Integrating dental and medical care for the chronic bulimia nervosa patient: a case report. *Quintessence Int* 1991;22:553–557.

14. Bidwell HL, Dent CD, Sharp JG: Bulimia-induced dental erosion in a male patient. *Quintessence Int* 1999;30:135–138.

15. de Moor RJ: Eating disorder-induced dental complications: a case report. *J Oral Rehabil* 2004;31:725–732.

16. Schwarz S, Kreuter A, Rammelsberg P: Efficient prosthodontic treatment in a young patient with long-standing bulimia nervosa. *J Prosthet Dent* 2011;106:6–11.

17. Adell R, Lekholm U, Rockler B, et al: A 15-year study of osseointegrated implants in the treatment of the edentulous jaw. *Int J Oral Surg* 1981;10:387–416.

18. Albrektsson T, Zarb G, Worthington P, et al: The long-term efficacy of currently used dental implants: a review and proposed criteria of success. *Int J Oral Maxillofac Implants* 1986;1:11–25.

19. Lindquist LW, Carlsson GE, Jemt T: A prospective 15-year follow-up study of mandibular fixed prostheses supported by osseointegrated implants. Clinical results and marginal bone loss. *Clin Oral Implants Res* 1996;7:329–336.

20. Kamposiora P, Papavasiliou G, Madianos P: Presentation of two cases of immediate restoration of implants in the esthetic region, using Facilitate software and guides with stereolithographic model surgery prior to patient surgery. *J Prosthodont* 2012;21:130–137.

21. Brånemark PI, Adell R, Breine U, et al: Intraosseous anchorage of dental prostheses. I: experimental studies. *Scand J Plast Reconst Surg* 1969;3:81–100.

22. Brånemark PI, Hanson BO, Adell R, et al: Osseointegrated implants in treatment of the edentulous jaw. Experience from a 10-year period. *Scand J Plast Reconst Surg* 1977;16 (Suppl): 1–132.

23. Cochran DL, Morton D, Weber HP: Consensus statements and recommended clinical procedures regarding loading protocols for endosseous dental implants. *Int J Oral Maxillofac Implants* 2004;19(Suppl.):109–113.

24. Schnitman PA, Wohrle PS, Rubenstein JE, et al: Ten-year results for Branemark implants immediately loaded with fixed prosthesis at implant placement. *Int J Oral Maxillofac Implants* 1997;12:495–503.

25. Tarnow DP, Emtiaz S, Classi A: Immediate loading of threaded implants at stage 1 surgery in edentulous arches: ten consecutive

case reports with 1- to 5-year data. *Int J Oral Maxillofac Implants* 1997;12:319–324.

26. Ganeles J, Wismeijer D: Early and immediately restored and loaded dental implants for single-tooth and partial-arch applications. *Int J Oral Maxillofac Implants* 2004;19 (Suppl): 92–102.

27. Romanos GE, Nentwig GH: Immediate versus delayed functional loading of implants in the posterior mandible: a 2-year prospective clinical study of 12 consecutive cases. *Int J Periodont Rest Dent* 2006;26:459–469.

28. Zembic A, Glauser R, Khraisat A, et al: Immediate vs. early loading of dental implants: 3-year results of a randomized controlled clinical trial. *Clin Oral Implants Res* 2010;21: 481–489.

29. Brunski J: In vivo bone response to biomechanical loading at the bone/dental implant interface. *Adv Dent Res* 1999;13: 99–119.

30. Ericsson I, Randow K, Nilner K, et al: Early functional loading of Branemark dental implants. A 5 year follow up study. *Clin Implant Dent Relat Res* 2000;2:70–77.

31. Chow J, Hui E, Li D, et al: The Hong Kong Bridge Protocol. Immediate loading of mandibular Branemark fixtures using a fixed provisional prosthesis: preliminary results. *Clin Implant Dent Relat Research* 2001;3:166–174.

32. Drago C, Lazzara R: Immediate occlusal loading of Osseotite implant in mandibular edentulous patients: a prospective observational report with 18-month data. *J Prosthodont* 2006;15: 187–194.

33. Oh TJ, Shotwell JL, Billy EJ, et al: Effect of flapless implant surgery on soft tissue profile: a randomized controlled clinical trial. *J Periodontol* 2006;77:874–882.

34. Becker W, Goldstein M, Becker BE, et al: Minimally invasive flapless implant surgery: a prospective multi-center study. *Clin Implant Dent Relat Res* 2005;7(Suppl 1):S21–S27.

35. Marchack CB: CAD/CAM-guided implant surgery and fabrication of an immediately loaded prosthesis for a partially edentulous patient. *J Prosthet Dent* 2007;97:389–394.

36. Casap N, Tarazi E, Wexler A, et al: Intraoperative computerized navigation for flapless implant surgery and immediate loading in the edentulous mandible. *Int J Oral Maxillofac Surg* 2005;20:92–98.

37. Lal K, White GS, Morea DN, et al: Use of stereolithographic templates for surgical and prosthodontic implant planning and placement. Part I. The concept. *J Prosthodont* 2006;15:51–8.

38. Ambard A, Mueninghoff L: Rehabilitation of a bulimic patient using endosteal implants. *J Prosthodont* 2002;11:176–180.

8

A SCREWLESS AND CEMENTLESS TECHNIQUE FOR THE RESTORATION OF SINGLE-TOOTH IMPLANTS: A RETROSPECTIVE COHORT STUDY

Rainier A. Urdaneta, dmd,[1] Mauro Marincola, dds, msd,[2] Meghan Weed, rdh,[3] and Sung-Kiang Chuang, dmd, md, dmsc[4]

[1]Private Practice, Implant Dentistry Centre, Boston, MA
[2]University of Cartagena, Implant Dentistry Centre, Cartagena, Colombia and Private Practice, Rome, Italy
[3]Dental Hygienist, Implant Dentistry Centre, Boston, MA
[4]Assistant Professor in Oral & Maxillofacial Surgery, Harvard School of Dental Medicine and Massachusetts General Hospital, Boston, MA

Keywords
Locking taper implants; dental implants; dental crown; composite resins; Bicon implants.

Correspondence
Rainier A. Urdaneta, 25 Prairie Ave, Auburndale MA 02466.
E-mail: rainieru@yahoo.com

Paper presented at the 82nd General Exhibition of the International, American, and Canadian Association of Dental Research, Honolulu, HI, March 13, 2004; and the 19th Annual Meeting of the Academy of Osseointegration, San Francisco, CA, March 19, 2004.

This research is supported in part by the Oral and Maxillofacial Surgery Foundation (OMSF) Fellowship in Clinical Investigation Award (SKC).

Accepted July 30, 2007

Published in *Journal of Prosthodontics* October 2008; Vol. 17, Issue 7

doi: 10.1111/j.1532-849X.2008.00343.x

ABSTRACT

Purpose: The Integrated Abutment Crown™ (IAC) is a technique for the fabrication of single-tooth implant-supported crowns where the abutment and the crown are one unit. The abutment–crown complex is connected to the implant with a locking taper. This technique does not use cement to retain the crown or screws to retain the abutment. The purpose of this study was to evaluate the clinical outcome of screwless, cementless single implant-supported crowns (IACs) placed in a general dental practice.

Materials and Methods: A retrospective cohort study was conducted between July 2001 and August 2003. Patients were recalled between January and March 2004. The restorations were evaluated following the modified United States Public Health Service (USPHS) criteria. Several other variables, such as anatomic form, occlusion, soft tissue health, and reconstructive procedures, were also recorded. Descriptive statistics, univariate and multivariate marginal Cox Proportional Hazards Regression models, adjusted for multiple implants in the same patient, were used.

Results: During the chart review, 108 patients were identified. A cohort of 59 patients with a total of 151 IACs met the inclusion criteria. The Kaplan–Meier survival rate for IACs was 98.7%. Two IACs were removed, one due to implant failure; the other became loose several times and was replaced with a splinted restoration. Excellent marginal adaptation was observed with no clinically discernible interface between the veneer material and the abutment. Nine maxillary anterior IACs loosened on five patients; eight of them were reinserted and continued in function without further problems for the remainder of the study. An IAC located between a tooth and an implant was 2.65 times more likely to have postinsertion complications ($p = 0.05$). An IAC with incorrect anatomic form (overcontoured) was 3.26 times more likely to have postinsertion complications ($p = 0.01$). Maxillary anterior IACs adjacent to one tooth and one implant were 3.9 times more likely to come loose ($p = 0.05$).

Conclusions: The clinical outcome of this screwless and cementless system for single implant restorations compares favorably with the experience of screw- and cement-retained single implant restorations within the observation period.

Common techniques to achieve structural integrity of the crown/abutment and implant/abutment complexes in single-tooth implant restorations include screws and cement.[1–16]

When both the implant–abutment and crown–abutment complexes are retained with screws, long-term follow-up studies have reported several complications, including screw loosening, fracture, and other component failures.[17] Screw loosening appears to be a greater problem with single-tooth restorations replacing mandibular molars.[1,6,8,9] With regard to sulcular health, a screw-retained prosthesis does not seal the abutment-to-crown interface or margin, which harbors bacteria in the crevice. This may act as an endotoxin pump, encouraging the proliferation of micro-organisms in the sulcular region.[10–12]

When a crown is cemented onto an implant abutment, it is possible for excess cement to flow into the gingival sulcus.[13,14] Subgingival margins make it difficult to ensure the complete removal of excess cement,[14–16] and the possibility exists for residual cement to be forced into the sulcus as the restoration is being seated.[13,14,16] Incomplete cement removal from the gingival sulcus can lead to loss of peri-implant bone that may be visualized radiographically.[13,14] Furthermore, a gap between the crown and the implant or abutment has been associated with greater marginal bone loss during the first year of function.[5]

The Bicon Dental Implant™ system (Bicon, LLC, Boston, MA) is a screwless implant system. The implant and implant–abutment unit connect by means of a 3.0° locking taper. The high friction force created by the locking taper breaks down the titanium oxide layer, and the metals are fused together in a cold weld.[17] Therefore, there are no gaps between the implant and the abutment. The locking-taper connection provides a frictional seal shown to be hermetic to bacterial invasion[18] and clinically reliable.[19] A 10-year survival rate of 99.0% for Bicon implants restored with single-tooth restorations has been documented.[20]

The Integrated Abutment Crown™ (IAC) (Bicon, LLC) is an implant restoration where the implant abutment and the crown material are one unit[21] (Fig 8.1). A light-cured, highly filled composite resin material, such as Diamond Crown™ (DRM Research Laboratories, Branford, CT), is chemo-mechanically bonded in the laboratory to the coronal part of a titanium alloy abutment. This technique does not require cement or screws.

The purpose of this study was to examine the clinical outcome of single implant-supported IACs placed in a general practice and to create a basis for further long-term evaluation of this type of restoration. The hypothesis was that the screwless and cementless implant restoration presented in this study should have comparable performance to screw- and cement-retained single implant restorations.

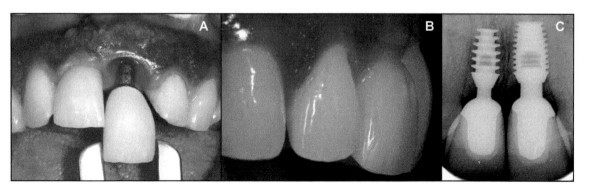

FIGURE 8.1 Insertion of an IAC. Both maxillary central incisors are IACs. A restoration is being inserted (A). Lateral view of the crowns after insertion (B). Periapical radiograph (C). (Picture courtesy Dr. Vincent Morgan, Implant Dentistry Centre, Boston, MA.)

MATERIALS AND METHODS

The present study was designed as a retrospective cohort study. The cohort was derived from the population of patients who had at least one IAC restored at the Implant Dentistry Centre, Faulkner Hospital (IDC-FH), Boston, MA between July 2001 and August 2003.

Patients of record treated at IDC-FH were selected if they satisfied the following inclusion criteria: (i) restored with at least one IAC and (ii) consented to participate after being fully informed of the conditions of the study. Exclusion criteria included inadequate or unavailable patient charts and/or patient unwilling or unable to attend the follow-up examination.

This study was approved by the Faulkner Hospital Institutional Review Board, Boston, MA.

This retrospective study involved the examination of patient records as well as clinical evaluations of the restorations during recall appointments between January and March 2004. Periapical and panoramic radiographs and clinical photographs were obtained.

Study Variables

Health Status Variables Demographic variables included age and gender. General health status was classified according to the American Society of Anesthesiology (ASA) system.[22] Patients were categorized as healthy (ASA 1), as having mild systemic disease (ASA 2), or as having moderate or severe systemic disease (ASA 3). Past history of smoking as well as current tobacco and alcohol use were documented.

Anatomic-Tooth Specific Variables These variables included implant position (maxilla, mandible, anterior, posterior), tooth type (incisor, canine, premolar, molar), bone quality (types 1–4), and proximity of the implant relative to other teeth or implants. The proximity of implants to other dento-alveolar structures were grouped into the following

categories: no teeth (edentulous), one natural tooth, two natural teeth, one implant, two implants, and one natural tooth-one implant.[23] The presence of endodontic treatment of the teeth immediately adjacent to the implant areas and the reasons for tooth loss were recorded.

Implant-Specific Variables These variables included size (width 3.5 to 6 mm, length 6 to 11 mm), coating [uncoated, titanium-plasma sprayed (TPS), hydroxyapatite (HA)], well size (2 or 3 mm), and surgical protocol (one vs. two stage). Immediate extraction and placement was recorded when a tooth was extracted on the same day as implant placement. When the implant restoration was placed in occlusion and splinted to adjacent structures on the same day of implant placement, it was recorded as immediate loading/stabilization (Fig 8.2).

Reconstructive Variables Bone graft augmentation procedures prior, at, or after implant placement were recorded.

Prosthetic-Soft Tissue Variables Stability of the implant and crown–abutment complex was determined by tapping back and forth between two instrument handles. Fractures and interproximal and occlusal contacts were documented. Fractures were defined as loss of core material, regardless of the amount and/or presence of cracks or fracture lines. Occlusal contacts were verified by the presence of marks and resistance to dislodgement of articulating paper (0.04 mm thick, Bausch Articulating Papers, Nashua, NH) when the patient's occlusion was in maximal intercuspation. A positive interproximal contact was recorded when resistance to dental floss and the presence of contact upon visual evaluation was observed.

Contact between opposing teeth on both right and left working sides during excursive jaw movements (lateral guidance) was documented as canine protected articulation or group function.[24] The contacts were verified twice by the presence of marks and resistance to dislodgement of articulating paper.

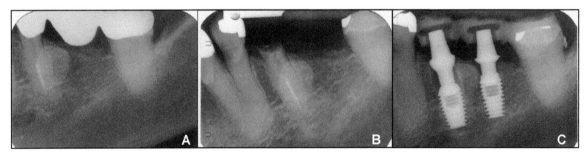

FIGURE 8.2 Periapical radiographs of a mandibular left bicuspid and first molar area, before treatment (A), after removal of the failing fixed partial denture (B), and after implant placement (C). The second mandibular left bicuspid was extracted, and an implant was placed on the same day. Implants on second premolar and first molar were splinted to adjacent teeth with composite resin and placed in occlusion on the day of implant placement (C).

Occlusion was classified on both right and left sides as class I, II, or III according to Angle's classification of occlusion.[24] If an IAC was located on the maxillary or mandibular right side, the type of occlusion and lateral guidance present on that side were recorded for that restoration. If an IAC had a positive working side contact, the restoration was recorded as guiding excursion. Furthermore, the structure of the opposing occlusal contact [tooth, implant, implant overdenture, removable partial denture (RPD), or complete denture (CD)] and the type of restorative material present on the opposing supporting cusp (tooth structure, porcelain, metal, acrylic, composite resin) were documented.

Using the modified United States Public Health Service (USPHS)[25] criteria, the crowns were evaluated for color match, surface texture, marginal adaptation, and anatomic form. Values of 0 (alpha) and 1 (bravo) were considered clinically acceptable. Values of 2 or higher required further treatment. For color match, an unrestored tooth in close proximity served as the comparison.

A restoration was considered an absolute failure when it could not remain in function as a consequence of implant loss or prosthetic malfunction.

Three soft tissue parameters were recorded for each implant site. The modified plaque index[26] and sulcular bleeding index[27] were recorded on the facial surfaces, and sulcular depth measurements were obtained on six surfaces (ml, l, dl, mf, f, df). A prosthodontist (first author) obtained the clinical measurements. To ensure consistency, several trial examinations were performed prior to the actual clinical measurements being recorded.

Complications Prosthodontic, surgical, or other complaints and all complications were noted.

Patient Questionnaire The patients' perceptions of esthetic results, satisfaction, and comfort were obtained using a standard questionnaire.[4] The survey was mailed to the patients after clinical evaluation had already been performed.

Data Management and Statistics

A database was created using Excel (Microsoft 2000, Seattle, WA) with appropriate checks to identify errors. Descriptive statistics were computed for all the study's variables. Univariate analyses were used to identify risk factors associated with complications after insertion of the IACs. Prosthetic risk factors with *p*-values ≤0.15 based on univariate analyses were entered into multivariate Cox proportional hazards regression models that adjusted for clustering failure-time observations within the same patient using the marginal approach.[28] Crown (IAC) survival rate was computed using the Kaplan–Meier Estimator.[29] Survival statistical computing methodologies used the SAS (Version 8.2, Cary, NC) programming environment in the PC-DOS operating system.

The procedure code "proc phreg" in SAS with the "cov-sandwich" or "covs" option was used.

RESULTS

A total of 108 patients were restored with 285 IACs between July 2001 and August 2003. All records of the 108 patients were reviewed. Among the 108 patients, 59 patients had subsequent follow-up visits and were included in the present study.

The cohort was composed of 151 Bicon implants restored with IACs on 59 patients with a mean age of 57.2 ± 14.3 years. Women made up 57.6% of the studied group.

The average time the IACs were in function was 16.7 months. The descriptive statistics for the study variables are summarized in Table 8.1.

The reason for tooth loss prior to implant placement was not available for 55 teeth. Of the remaining 96 teeth, 30 teeth (31.3%) were lost because of fractures or trauma, 42 teeth (43.8%) were extracted because of advanced dental caries, and 21 teeth (21.9%) were removed because of periodontal and/or endodontic reasons.

Two failures were documented. One IAC replacing a maxillary left second premolar was removed 1 month after insertion of the definitive restoration, due to the failure of the implant to become osseointegrated. The failed implant had been splinted to a previously integrated implant and placed in function with a temporary restoration immediately after placement. The implant was removed because of mobility and pain. An IAC replacing a maxillary lateral incisor was removed because it became loose several times. The new restoration was splinted to an adjacent implant to prevent further dislodgement. One hundred forty-nine IACs were in function at the last recall appointment and were classified as excellent for anatomic form (75.8%), marginal adaptation (98%), color match (64.1%), and surface texture (68.5%).

Fifty-one IACs had supragingival plaque recognizable with a periodontal probe (score 1, modified plaque index).[26]

The Kaplan–Meier[29] survival estimate for IACs was 98.7% with an associated 95% confidence interval between 96.8% and 100% (Table 8.2).

The patients' responses to their treatments were positive (Table 8.3). The majority of patients (95.7%) were extremely satisfied (score 0). Twelve patients did not return their questionnaire but were contacted by phone and reported having no problems.

In addition to the implant failure, the following complications were noted after insertion of the IACs, all of which occurred in the maxilla. A small fracture of the core material was documented on a maxillary left first premolar during the first year of function. After refinishing, the crown continued in function uneventfully for the remainder of the study. One patient complained of throbbing pain due to soft-tissue

TABLE 8.1 **Descriptive Statistics and Univariate Analysis for Risk Factors Associated with Complications After Insertion of the IACs (Total $n = 59$ Patients; Total $k = 151$ Implants)**

Variable	Number	Percent	HR (95% CI)	Robust p-Value
Age at implant placement ($n = 59$)	57.2 ± 14.3 (range 27.8–90.8)		0.98 (0.95, 1.01)	0.22
Gender ($n = 59$)				
Female	34	57.6	0.50 (0.19, 1.35)	0.17
Male	25	42.4	1.00 (Ref.)	
ASA status ($n = 59$)			1.09 (0.54, 2.22)[†]	0.80
ASA I	54	91.5		
ASA II	4	6.8		
ASA III	1	1.7		
Tobacco use ($n = 59$)				
Yes	7	11.9	0.73 (0.21, 2.52)	
No	52	88.1	1.00 (Ref.)	0.62
Jaw ($k = 151$)				
Mandible	57	37.8	‡	<0.0001*
Maxilla	94	62.3	1.00 (Ref.)	
Tooth type ($k = 151$)				
Incisor	34	22.5	7.46 (1.64, 33.92)	0.009
Canine	10	6.6	1.90 (0.18, 20.03)	0.59
Premolar	67	44.4	1.18 (0.22, 6.42)	0.85
Molar	40	26.5	1.00 (Ref.)	
Bone quality ($k = 109$)				
Type II	15	13.8	1.89 (0.73, 4.87)[†]	0.19
Type III	20	18.4		
Type IV	74	67.9		
Adjacent structures ($k = 151$)				
Adjacent to 1 tooth + 1 implant	63	41.7	2.25 (0.86, 5.92)	0.10
Not adjacent to 1 tooth + 1 implant	88	58.3	1.00 (Ref.)	
Diameter ($k = 151$)				
3.5 mm	16	10.6	0.88 (0.53, 1.47)[†]	0.63
4 mm	29	19.2		
4.5 mm	45	29.8		
5 mm	51	33.8		
6 mm	10	6.6		
Length ($k = 151$)				
6 mm	7	4.6	1.13 (0.85, 1.51)[†]	0.39
8 mm	85	56.3		
11 mm	59	39.1		
Coating ($k = 151$)				
Uncoated	5	3.3	2.00 (0.26, 15.35)	0.50
TPS	32	21.2	1.15 (0.36, 3.74)	0.81
HA	114	75.5	1.00 (Ref.)	
Surgical protocol ($k = 151$)				
2 stage	52	34.4	0.39 (0.11, 1.35)	0.14
1 stage	99	65.6	1.00 (Ref.)	
Immediate extraction ($k = 151$)				
Yes	47	31.1	1.69 (0.65, 4.38)	0.28
No	104	68.9	1.00 (Ref.)	
Immediate loading/stabilization ($k = 151$)				
Yes	55	36.4	2.94 (1.10, 7.89)	0.03
No	96	63.6	1.00 (Ref.)	

TABLE 8.1 *(Continued)*

Variable	Number	Percent	HR (95% CI)	Robust *p*-Value
Bone augmentation before implant (*k* = 151)				
Yes	7	4.6	‡	<0.0001*
No	144	95.4	1.00 (Ref.)	
Bone augmentation at implant (*k* = 151)				
Yes	47	31.1	0.66 (0.21, 2.05)	0.47
No	104	68.9	1.00 (Ref.)	
Interproximal contacts (*k* = 149)				
Yes	116	77.9	0.83 (0.27, 2.59)	0.75
No	33	22.1	1.00 (Ref.)	
Occlusal contacts (*k* = 149)				
Yes	116	77.9	1.00 (Ref.)	
No	33	22.1	3.02 (1.11, 8.17)	0.03
Type of occlusion (Angle) (*k* = 151)				
Class III	16	10.6	2.01 (0.41, 9.76)	0.39
Class II	48	31.8	1.51 (0.53, 4.31)	0.44
Class I	87	57.6	1.00 (Ref.)	
Lateral guidance (*k* = 151)				
No contact due to balancing interferences	2	1.3	‡	<0.0001
Group function	86	57.0	1.14 (0.43, 3.04)	0.79
Canine	63	41.7	1.00 (Ref.)	
IAC guiding excursion (*k* = 149)				
Yes	30	20.1	0.59 (0.14, 2.60)	0.49
No	119	80.0	1.00 (Ref.)	
Type of opposing structure (*k* = 151)				
None	3	2.0	‡	<0.0001
Tooth	107	70.9	1.00 (Ref.)	
Implant	37	24.5	0.15 (0.02, 1.17)	0.07
RPD/CD implant-supported	4	2.7	‡	<0.0001
Type of opposing material (*k* = 151)				
None	3	2.0	Not compared	
Tooth structure	66	43.7	1.000 (Ref.)	
Porcelain	44	29.1	0.45 (0.14, 1.39)	0.16
Metal	6	4.0	Not compared	
Acrylic/IPN	5	3.3	Not compared	
DC resin	27	17.9	‡	<0.0001
USPHS criteria (*k* = 149)				
Color match				
0-excellent match	91	64.1	2.32 (0.84, 6.45)†	0.11
1-minimal mismatch	51	35.9		
Surface texture				
0-smooth	102	68.5	0.50 (0.15, 1.69)†	0.27
1-dull	46	30.9		
2-rough, pitted	1	0.7		
Marginal adaptation				
0-no catch	146	98.0	1.000 (Ref.)	
1-catch	3	2.0	†,‡	<0.0001*
Anatomic form				
0-correct	113	75.8	2.94 (1.28, 6.75)†	<0.011
1-incorrect	35	23.5		
2-defective	1	0.7		

(continued)

TABLE 8.1   (Continued)

Variable	Number	Percent	HR (95% CI)	Robust *p*-Value
Mean modified plaque index	0.5 ± 0.6 (range 0–2)		0.45 (0.18, 1.15)	0.10
Mean sulcular bleeding index	0.2 ± 0.4 (range 0–2)		0.27 (0.04, 1.95)	0.19
Mean sulcular depth (mm)	3.0 ± 0.7 (range 1.5–5.0)		0.88 (0.44, 1.79)	0.72
Presence of complications (*k* = 151)				
No	134	88.7		
Yes	17	11.3		

*All complications occurred: in the maxilla, in patients with no augmentation procedures done before implant placement, and in restorations with good marginal adaptation.

†Modeled as a continuous variable with the HR for a linear trend.

‡HR was undetermined because there were no complications for this level of the covariate.

Note: Ref. means the "reference group" at each level of the covariate. The HR (hazard ratio) for the reference group is set at 1.00.

TABLE 8.2   Kaplan–Meier Survival for Integrated Abutment Crowns

Time After Insertion (Months)	*n* (At Risk)	%	95% CI	*K* (Failed)
0	151	100	100	0
6	113	98.7	96.8, 100.0	2
12	101	98.7	96.8, 100.0	0
18	61	98.7	96.8, 100.0	0
24	21	98.7	96.8, 100.0	0

TABLE 8.3   Descriptive Statistics for Patient Questionnaire (Score 0–5) (*n* = 47 Patients)

	Number	Percent
Satisfaction with implant crown		
0—extremely satisfied	45	95.7
1—somewhat satisfied	2	4.3
Satisfaction with appearance		
0—extremely satisfied	40	85.1
1—somewhat satisfied	3	6.4
2—no feeling either way	4	8.5
Would select same type of crown		
0—extremely satisfied	37	78.7
1—somewhat satisfied	8	17.0
2—no feeling	2	4.3
Would recommend procedure to a friend		
0—extremely satisfied	39	83.0
1—somewhat satisfied	7	15.0
2—no feeling	1	2.1
Appearance compared to teeth		
0—extremely satisfied	13	27.7
1—somewhat satisfied	16	34.0
2—no feeling	18	38.3

irritation around an IAC that had been in function for 1 year. Four occlusal contacts were adjusted due to biting sensitivity. An interproximal contact was added to an anterior IAC that had been in function for 5 months. Loosening of nine maxillary anterior IACs was documented.

The majority of the postinsertion complications occurred in restorations opposing natural teeth (16 out of 17, or 94%), immediately loaded implants (10 of 17, or 59%), and restorations adjacent to one tooth-one implant (10 of 17, or 59%).

Of the IACs that loosened, nine (100%) were opposing natural teeth, six (66%) were adjacent to one tooth-one implant, three (33%) were adjacent to two implants, and five (56%) implants had been immediately loaded. Of the eight IACs that loosened but remained in function, three (38%) had incorrect anatomic form and four (50%) lacked occlusal contacts.

Table 8.1 summarizes the univariate relationships between the study variables and complications after insertion of the IACs. During the univariate analysis, the following variables were identified as risk factors ($p \leq 0.15$) for complications after insertion of the IACs: adjacent structures, surgical protocol, immediate loading/stabilization, occlusal contacts, type of opposing structure, color match, anatomic form, and modified plaque index. Two clustered parsimonious multivariate regression models were developed (Table 8.4). Variables in the multivariate models were selected because they were statistically associated with complications in univariate analysis ($p \leq 0.15$) and were of prosthetic relevance. In the multivariate Cox models shown in Table 8.4, anatomic form, IAC adjacent to one tooth and one implant, and occlusal contacts remained statistically associated with complications after insertion of the IACs ($p \leq 0.05$). If an IAC had incorrect anatomic form, it was 3.26 times more likely to develop complications after insertion ($p = 0.01$; Table 8.4A). If an IAC was located between an implant and a tooth, it was 2.65 times more likely to have

TABLE 8.4 Multivariate Marginal Cox Regression Models for Risk Factors Associated with Complications After Insertion of IACs (Total $N = 59$ Patients; Total $k = 151$ Implants)

Variable	Hazard Ratio	95% CI	Robust p-Value
A. First multivariate model			
Adjacent to one tooth-one implant	2.65	(1.00, 7.15)	0.05*
Not adjacent to one tooth-one implant	1.00 (Ref.)		
USPHS, anatomic form	3.26	1.32, 8.07[†]	0.01*
B. Second multivariate model			
Immediate loading/stabilization			
Yes	2.53	0.90, 7.10	0.08
No	1.00 (Ref.)		
Occlusal contacts			
Yes	1.00 (Ref.)		
No	2.53	1.00, 6.42	0.05*
Type of opposing structure			
None	0.000	[‡]	<0.0001
Tooth	1.00 (Ref.)		
Implant	0.19	0.02, 1.52	0.12
RPD/CD implant-supported	0.000	[‡]	<0.0001

*Statistically significant at ($p \leq 0.05$).
[†]Modeled as a continuous variable with the HR for a linear trend.
[‡]HR was undetermined because there were no complications for this level of the covariate.
Note: Ref. means the reference group at each level of the covariate. The HR (hazard ratio) for the reference group is set at 1.00.

complications after insertion ($p = 0.05$; Table 8.4A). An IAC without contact in maximal intercuspation was 2.53 times more likely to have postinsertion complications ($p = 0.05$; Table 8.4B). Immediately stabilized implants were more likely to have postinsertion complications but not at a statistically significant level ($p = 0.08$; Table 8.4B).

To further evaluate the possible relationships of these risk factors with loosening of maxillary anterior IACs, a subgroup statistical analysis was performed. Maxillary anterior IACs adjacent to one tooth and one implant were 3.9 times more likely to come loose ($p = 0.05$).

DISCUSSION

The most common materials used for the restoration of both teeth and implants are ceramo-metal and all-ceramic crowns. According to Paul and Pietrobon[30] in their literature review, a single implant-retained metal–ceramic crown cemented on a metal abutment may be considered the standard selection.

The implant restorations evaluated in this study differ from cemented metal–ceramic crowns in that the metal abutments and the crown material were chemo-mechanically bonded in the laboratory; therefore, there was no need for cement. Also, the abutments were connected to the implants with a screwless locking taper, another significant difference. The concept of incorporating a screwless, locking taper

implant abutment with a crown material in a single integrated unit is new.

The IACs showed a 98.7% survival rate during a period of observation of up to 29 months with 71% of them restoring posterior areas.

These results compare favorably with the 12–18 month cumulative survival rate of 98.2% reported by Naert et al.[31] In a 5-year study with a lower cumulative success rate of 93.7% for implant-supported single crowns, two fractures of all-ceramic restorations were reported in the first 2 years where the majority of the crowns (79%) evaluated were placed in anterior areas.[32] Another study of implant-supported single-tooth replacements reported five fractured crowns during a period of up to 8 years where the majority of the restorations (31 of 49) were placed in anterior areas and the majority of the fractures (4 out of 5) occurred in posterior areas.[33]

Excellent marginal adaptation was observed with no clinically discernible interface between the veneer material and the implant abutment for 98% of the IACs. Even though the marginal adaptation showed no deterioration over time (Figs 8.3 and 8.4), the stability of the bond between the metal abutment and the resin veneering material will need to be demonstrated in long-term studies.

The surface texture rating was reduced in 47 IACs because of a slightly dull or granular surface appearance. Past research has shown that when polished, resin materials achieve higher roughness values than all-ceramic materials.[34]

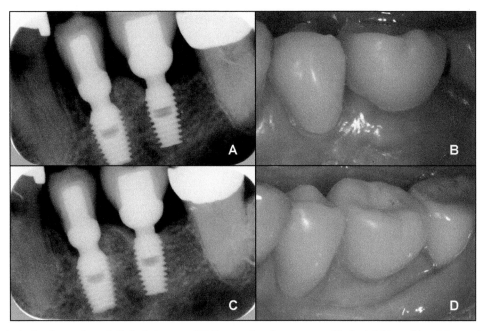

FIGURE 8.3   Periapical radiographs and clinical pictures of IACs restoring the same mandibular left bicuspid and first molar area presented in Figure 8.2. At crown insertion, June 2002 (A, B) and at a recall appointment, February 2004 (C, D).

The color remained stable during the period of observation. In a recent study,[35] Diamond Crown™ was shown to have significantly better color stability than Tetric Ceram™ (Ivoclar Vivadent AG, Liechtenstein).

The supragingival plaque accumulation observed around IACs was expected, because it has been consistently shown that resin-based materials accumulate plaque at a higher rate than tooth structure and all-ceramic restorations.[36–38]

The mean sulcular depth around IACs was 3.0 mm, whereas probing depths of 2.7 to 3.3 mm have been recorded for screw- and cement-retained single-tooth implant rehabilitations.[39]

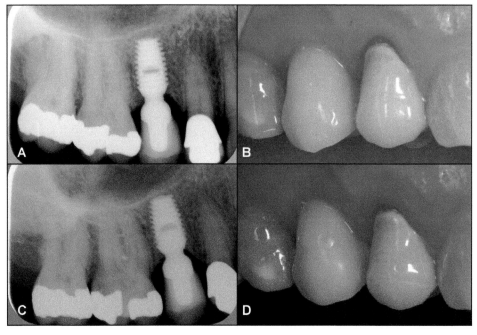

FIGURE 8.4   Clinical and radiographic view of an IAC on a maxillary right second premolar, at crown insertion (A, B), and at the recall appointment 27 months later (C, D).

The most common postinsertion complications were the need for the adjustment of occlusal contacts and loosening of maxillary anterior restorations. Nine maxillary anterior IACs loosened on five patients; eight of them were reinserted and continued in function without further problems for the remainder of the study. One IAC loosened several times. This IAC restoring a maxillary lateral incisor was replaced with a metal–ceramic restoration splinted to an adjacent implant. This patient's occlusion consisted of seven remaining mandibular teeth, six of which were mandibular anterior teeth and one of which was a mandibular molar with no opposing occlusion. Even though the anterior region of the mouth is characterized by reduced bite forces compared to the posterior region,[40] it is reasonable to conclude that the absence of posterior support caused most of this patient's functioning to occur in the maxillary anterior region and led to the loosening of this restoration. A poor occlusal scheme both increases the magnitude of loads and intensifies mechanical stresses. These factors increase the frequency of complications of implant restorations and/or bone support.[40]

To evaluate the potential risk factors associated with postinsertion complications, two multivariate Cox regression models were developed. The possible relationship between these risk factors and the most common complication, loosening of maxillary anterior IACs, was also investigated.

Based on the data shown in Table 8.4B, it can be concluded that IACs without contact in maximal intercuspation were 2.53 times more likely to have postinsertion complications ($p = 0.05$). Biting sensitivity was the second most common complication and required the adjustment of occlusal contacts in the weeks following the insertion of four IACs. These adjustments resulted in the fact that a majority of IACs with complications lacked occlusal contacts at the time of the recall examination. Therefore, the absence of occlusal contacts did not make the restorations more likely to have complications, but rather was a consequence of the treatment provided for biting sensitivity. No association was observed between presence of occlusal contacts and loosening of maxillary anterior IACs.

IACs with deficient anatomic form and IACs positioned between a tooth and an implant were more likely to have postinsertion complications (Table 8.4A); however, only positioning between a tooth and an implant was found to have a statistically significant effect on loosening of maxillary anterior IACs.

To explain the loosening of maxillary anterior IACs, two hypotheses are presented. The first theory is that the restorations loosened in response to masticatory forces. In class I occlusal relationships, mandibular anterior teeth occlude with the palatal surfaces of the maxillary anterior teeth, producing forces that are oblique to their long axis. For implants in the maxillary anterior area, these lateral loads make the crown height act as a lever and a force magnifier for any offset occlusal loads. This may lead to an increase in faciolingual microrotation[41] and could have caused the loosening of the maxillary anterior IACs.

Another possible explanation for the loosening of the IACs could have been the clinician's failure to properly engage the locking taper connection. This hypothesis appears to be supported by the fact that anatomic considerations in the maxillary anterior area limit a clinician's ability to effectively apply a seating force along the long axis of the implant during the insertion of the restoration.

The placement of a maxillary anterior implant rarely corresponds exactly to the crown-root position of the original tooth. After tooth loss, the thin labial bone remodels with the alveolar crest shifting palatally; therefore, necessitating the more palatal placement of the implant.[42] Hence, the long axis of a maxillary anterior implant crown frequently has a different trajectory than the long axis of its implant.

To effectively engage the locking taper connection, the seating forces must be directed in the long axis of the implant. Tapping on the incisal edges of most maxillary anterior IACs will not direct the forces along the long axis of the implant; whereas a similar force applied on the occlusal surface of a posterior IAC is more likely to be directed vertically in the same axis as the implant and, as a result, more effectively engage its taper connection.

The stability of the connection between locking-taper implants and the crown–abutment complexes for maxillary anterior IACs should be substantiated by a long-term evaluation of the study group.

CONCLUSIONS

The screwless and cementless implant restorations presented in this study showed a survival rate of 98.7%, excellent marginal adaptation with a cementless interface, color stability, and a reduced number of prosthetic components. Plaque accumulation was observed around the crown material. The surface texture had higher roughness. The duration of the follow-up did not allow for a long-term assessment of the IACs.

The results of this study demonstrate that IACs located between a tooth and an implant were 2.65 times more likely to have postinsertion complications ($p = 0.05$). IACs with incorrect anatomic form (overcontoured) were 3.26 times more likely to have postinsertion complications ($p = 0.01$).

The most common complication observed was loosening of nine maxillary anterior IACs. Of the IACs that loosened nine (100%) were opposing natural teeth, six (66%) were adjacent to one tooth-one implant, and five (56%) implants had been immediately loaded. Maxillary anterior IACs adjacent to one tooth and one implant were 3.9 times more likely to come loose ($p = 0.05$).

ACKNOWLEDGMENTS

The authors would like to recognize the clinicians and staff of the Implant Dentistry Centre at the Faulkner Hospital, Boston, MA for their cooperation in this study and their free and unfettered access to patient records.

REFERENCES

1. Becker W, Becker BE: Replacement of maxillary and mandibular molars with single endosseous implant restorations: a retrospective study. *J Prosthet Dent* 1995;74:51–55.

2. Enquist B, Nilson H, Astrand P: Single-tooth replacement by osseointegrated Branemark implants: a retrospective study of 82 implants. *Clin Oral Implants Res* 1995;6:238–245.

3. Henry PJ, Laney WR, Jemt T, et al: Osseointegrated implants for single-tooth replacement: a prospective 5-year multicenter study. *Int J Oral Maxillofac Implants* 1996;11:450–455.

4. Gibbard L, Zarb G: A 5-year prospective study of implant-supported single-tooth replacements. *J Can Dent Assoc* 2002;68:110–116.

5. Wannsfors K, Smedberg J-I: A prospective clinical evaluation of different single-tooth restoration designs on osseointegrated implants: a 3-year follow-up of Branemark implants. *Clin Oral Implants Res* 1999;10:453–458.

6. Bianco G, Di Raimondo R, Luongo G, et al: Osseointegrated implant for single tooth replacement: a retrospective multicenter study on routine use in private practice. *Clin Implant Dent Relat Res* 2000;2:152–158.

7. Mericske-Stern R, Grutter L, Rosch R, et al: Clinical evaluation and prosthetic complications of single tooth replacements by non-submerged implants. *Clin Oral Implants Res* 2001; 12:309–318.

8. Schwartz-Arad D, Samet N, Samet N: Single tooth replacement of missing molars: a retrospective study of 78 implants. *J Periodontol* 1999;70:449–454.

9. Eckert SE, Wollan PC: Retrospective review of 1170 endosseous implants in partially edentulous jaws. *J Prosthet Dent* 1998;79:415–421.

10. Misch CE: Principles of cement-retained fixed implant prosthodontics. In Misch CE (ed): *Contemporary Implant Dentistry* (ed 2). St. Louis, MO, Mosby, 1999, p. 554.

11. Quirynen M, Bollen CML, Eyssen H, et al: Microbial penetration along the implant components of the Branemark system, an in vitro study. *Clin Oral Implants Res* 1994;5:239–244.

12. Jansen VK, Conrads G, Richter EJ: Microbial leakage and marginal fit of the implant abutment interface. *Int J Oral Maxillofac Impl* 1997;12:527–540.

13. Pauletto N, Lahiffe BJ, Walton JN: Complications associated with excess cement around crowns on osseointegrated implants: a clinical report. *Int J Oral Maxillofac Implants* 1999;14:865–868.

14. Schwedhelm E, Lepe X, Aw T: A crown venting technique for the cementation of implant-supported crowns. *J Prosthet Dent* 2003;89:89–90.

15. Agar JR, Cameron SM, Hughbanks JC, et al: Cement removal from restorations luted to titanium abutments with simulated gingival margins. *J Prosthet Dent* 1997;78:43–47.

16. Dumbrigue HB, Abanomi AA, Cheng LL: Techniques to minimize excess luting agent in cement-retained implant restorations. *J Prosthet Dent* 2002;87:112–114.

17. Keating K: Connecting abutments to dental implants: "an engineer's perspective". *Irish Dentist* 2001; July 43–46.

18. Dibart S, Warbington M, Fan Su M, et al: In vitro evaluation of the implant-abutment bacterial seal: the locking taper system. *Int J Oral Maxillofac Implants* 2005;20:732–737.

19. Muftu A, Chapman RJ: Replacing posterior teeth with free-standing implant: four-year prosthodontic results of a prospective study. *J Am Dent Assoc* 1998;129:1097–1102.

20. Morgan K, Chapman RJ: Retrospective analysis of an implant system. *Compendium* 1999;20:601–625.

21. Urdaneta RA, Marincola M: The Integrated Abutment Crown™, a screwless and cementless restoration for single-tooth implants: a report on a new technique. *J Prosthodont* 2007;16:311–318.

22. American Academy of Anesthesiologists (ASA): Physical status classes. In *Clinical Anesthesia Procedures of the Massachusetts General Hospital*, Vol 5 (ed 3). Philadelphia, PA, Lippincott-Raven, 1998.

23. Truhlar RS, Orenstein IH, Morris HF, et al: Distribution of bone quality in patients receiving endosseous dental implants. *J Oral Maxillofac Surg* 1997;55(Suppl. 5):38–45.

24. The glossary of prosthodontic terms. *J Prosthet Dent* 1999; 81:39–110.

25. Ryge G, Cvar JF: Criteria for the clinical evaluation of dental restorative materials. US Public Health Service publication # 790–244. San Francisco, CA, Government Printing Office, 1971.

26. Silness J, Loe H: Periodontal disease in pregnancy II: correlation between oral hygiene and periodontal condition. *Acta Odontol Scand* 1964;22:121–135.

27. Muhlerman HR, Son S: Gingival sulcus bleeding: a leading symptom in initial gingivitis. *Helv Odontol Acta* 1971;15:107–113.

28. Chuang SK, Wei LJ, Douglas CW: Risk factors for dental implant failure: a strategy for the analysis of clustered failure-time observations. *J Dent Res* 2002;81:572–577.

29. Kaplan EL, Meier P: Nonparametric estimation from incomplete observations. *J Am Stat Assoc* 1958;53:467–481.

30. Paul SJ, Pietrobon N: Aesthetic evolution of anterior maxillary crowns. *Pract Periodontics Aesthet Dent* 1998;10:87–94.

31. Naert I, Koutsikakis G, Duyck J, et al: Biologic outcome of implant-supported restorations in the treatment of partial edentulism. Part I: a longitudinal clinical evaluation. *Clin Oral Implants Res* 2002;13:381–389.

32. Andersson B, Odman P, Lindvall AM, et al: Cemented single crowns on osseointegrated implants after 5 years: results from a prospective study on CeraOne. *Int J Prosthodont* 1998; 11:212–218.

33. Avivi-Arber L, Zarb GA: Clinical effectiveness of implant-supported single-tooth replacement: the Toronto Study. *Int J Oral Maxillofac Implants* 1996;11:311–321.

34. Jung M: Finishing and polishing of a hybrid composite and a heat-pressed glass ceramic. *Oper Dent* 2002;27:175–183.

35. De Lillo A, Lombardo S, Chiado Cutin D, et al: In vitro evaluation of chromatic stability in new-generation composites. *Minerva Stomatol* 2002;51:371–376.

36. Chan C, Weber H: Plaque retention on teeth restored with full ceramic crowns: a comparative study. *J Prosthet Dent* 1986;56:666–671.

37. Kostic L, Trifunovic D, Zelic O, et al: Microbiological investigation of supragingival dental plaque in patients treated with porcelain jacket and gold veneered resin crowns. *Stomatol Glas Srb* 1989;36:49–56.

38. Adamczyk E, Spiechowicz E: Plaque accumulation on crowns made of various materials. *Int J Prosthodont* 1990;3:285–291.

39. Puchades-Roman L, Palmer RM, Palmer PJ, et al: A clinical radiographic and microbiologic comparison of Astra Tech and Branemark single tooth implants. *Clin Implant Dent Relat Res* 2000;2:78–84.

40. Misch CE, Warren M: Occlusal considerations for implant supported prostheses: implant protective occlusion and occlusal materials. In Misch CE (ed): *Contemporary Implant Dentistry* (ed 2). St. Louis, MO, Mosby, 1999, pp. 610–622.

41. Bidez MW, Misch CE: Clinical biomechanics in implant dentistry. In Misch CE (ed): *Contemporary Implant Dentistry* (ed 2). St. Louis, MO, Mosby, 1999, pp. 310–314.

42. Misch CE: Prosthetic options in implant dentistry. In Misch CE (ed): *Contemporary Implant Dentistry* (ed 2). St. Louis, MO, Mosby, 1999, p. 68.

PART II

MANAGEMENT OF THE COMPLETELY EDENTULOUS PATIENT

9

EVIDENCE-BASED CRITERIA FOR DIFFERENTIAL TREATMENT PLANNING OF IMPLANT RESTORATIONS FOR THE MANDIBULAR EDENTULOUS PATIENT

STEVEN J. SADOWSKY, DDS, FACP, AND PETER W. HANSEN, DDS
Department of Integrated Reconstructive Dental Sciences, University of the Pacific Arthur A. Dugoni School of Dentistry, San Francisco, CA

Keywords
Implants; edentulous mandible; evidence-based dentistry.

Correspondence
Steven J. Sadowsky, University of the Pacific Arthur A. Dugoni School of Dentistry—Integrated Reconstructive Dental Sciences, 2155 Webster St. 400 M, San Francisco, CA 94115. E-mail: ssadowsky@pacific.edu

The authors deny any conflicts of interest.

Accepted March 28, 2013

Published in *Journal of Prosthodontics* February 2014; Vol. 23, Issue 2

doi: 10.1111/jopr.12085

ABSTRACT

Since the introduction of the ad modum Branemark prototype prosthesis for the mandibular edentulous patient more than 30 years ago, design permutations have met clinician and patient considerations. Dental student training and specialist continuing education often rely on anecdotal reports of success to determine the recommended design for patients. Decision-making algorithms for treatment are optimally predicated on the best available evidence. The purpose of this article is to elucidate the benefit/risk calculus of various implant modalities for the mandibular edentulous patient.

Since the advent of the implant fixed complete denture (IFCD) for the treatment of the mandibular edentulous patient more than 30 years ago, the ad modum Branemark prototype has prompted design innovations to address clinician- and patient-mediated concerns for the implant restoration of the edentate patient. Despite unsurpassed longitudinal implant and prosthetic survival of the IFCD,[1] outcome measures have emerged related to quality of life (QoL) concerns and have underscored the importance of developing new criteria for evidence-based differential implant treatment planning for the edentulous maxilla and mandible.[2,3] In accordance with the Commission on Dental Accreditation, which has mandated that dental graduates must be competent to assess, critically appraise, apply, and communicate scientific and lay literature as it relates to providing evidence-based patient care, the faculty at the University of the Pacific Arthur A. Dugoni School of Dentistry has reviewed these evidence-based guidelines for student clinical decision making. This article will discuss the indications for the implant-retained overdenture (IROD), the implant-supported overdenture (ISOD), IFCD, and implant-supported metal ceramic (MC) reconstructions.

The scientific rigor of the best available evidence varies and will be stratified in each section of this discussion based on a hierarchy designated by Sackett et al.[4] The hierarchy is outlined as follows:

Level 1A: Systematic review of randomized controlled trials (RCTs); 1B: RCTs with narrow confidence interval; 1C: All or none case series

Level 2A: Systematic review cohort studies; 2B: Cohort studies, low quality RCT; 2C: Outcomes research

Level 3A: Systematic review of case-controlled study; 3B: Case-controlled study

Level 4: Case series, poor cohort case-controlled study

Level 5: Expert opinion

A MEDLINE search was conducted along with a hand search for articles published within the last 20 years on implant restorative treatment for the edentulous patient.

GENERAL CONSIDERATIONS FOR IMPLANT TREATMENT

Three factors will govern the patient's suitability for implant therapy and the prosthetic design determinants: systemic conditions, local factors, and patient-mediated concerns. Multiple investigations have reviewed the systemic risks for implant therapy.[5–9] Details of these risk factors have been discussed in a previous article.[10] However, the level of evidence indicative of absolute and relative contraindications for implant therapy due to systemic diseases is low. Local factors dictating design considerations may include hard/soft tissue foundation, interarch space/relationship, applied forces, and antagonist dentition. Patient-mediated concerns may include cost, treatment time, morbidity, esthetics, retention security, phonetic concerns, and hygiene access. Studies on potential risk factors are restricted to retrospective cohort studies, clinical reports, and case series or level 3/4 evidence. More definitive studies, which will serve as a basis for consensus statements, will be predicated on future controlled studies.[11]

IMPLANT RESTORATION OF THE EDENTULOUS MANDIBLE

The rationale for placing implants in the edentulous mandible is to improve retention, stability, and chewing ability rendered by a complete denture and has been supported by the results of a prospective RCT evaluating patient satisfaction after 10 years of treatment.[11] Patients with a mandibular IROD, when compared to a conventional complete denture, revealed a higher mean satisfaction score. This was corroborated by a meta-analysis reporting mandibular IROD as more satisfactory at a clinically relevant level than complete dentures are.[12] Pan et al[13] demonstrated in an RCT of 214 patients that mandibular bone height had no effect on patient satisfaction with the function, chewing ability, and comfort of their prostheses. Regarding comparative patient satisfaction of edentulous patients when comparing a fixed complete denture to an implant overdenture (implant-supported or -retained) on the mandible, a number of studies failed to show a significant difference, and it has been postulated that subjective, patient-related factors are likely the main determinants of treatment outcomes.[14–16] However, selection of a fixed or removable prosthesis, number of implants, anchorage system, and loading protocol must be predicated on a review of the pertinent evidence, patient diagnostic data, and preferences. The evidence evaluating comparative patient satisfaction between conventional complete dentures and IROD treatment is level 1A. The evidence evaluating comparative patient satisfaction between the IFCD and ISOD modalities is level 1C.

IMPLANT OVERDENTURE

In the 1980s, a two-implant overdenture design was introduced. In a longitudinal study it was found to have cumulative implant and prosthetic survival rates of 96.4% and 100%, respectively, over 15 years.[17] Similar results were found using a nonsplinted or splinted anchorage system.[18] In 2002, The McGill Consensus Statement purported that as a minimum treatment objective, mandibular two-implant overdentures should be the first-choice standard of care for edentulous patients.[19] However, in a systematic review of the literature, Fitzpatrick[20] underscored the importance of clinician- and patient-mediated determinants for selecting a successful treatment modality as well as informing the patient of the risk/ benefit calculus of the prosthodontic options.[21] In fact, evidence suggests that 75% of all patients treated with implants receive insufficient information regarding treatment limitations, complications, costs, and alternatives.[22]

Overdenture prostheses are either implant-supported or combined implant-retained and tissue-supported. The mucosal support can best be achieved if there is some hinging movement of the superstructure by using two solitary anchors or a splinted design with a round/ovoid bar and single clip. With more than two implants or more than one bar segment, no rotational axis is present, and the overdenture is mainly implant-supported.[23] Despite findings that there are no significant differences in peri-implant health,[24–26] masticatory forces,[27–29] or patient satisfaction[30–32] with either a splinted or nonsplinted anchorage system or between two or four implants, there are indications for a bar design and/or more than two implants. In patients with sensitive mucosa over the mental foramina region, a bar design allows for a protective cantilever extension. Distal extensions also provide a high level of stability against lateral forces and improve retention.[33] The cantilever bar should not, however, extend beyond the position of the first premolar and cannot compensate for a short central segment.[33] In scenarios with a dentate maxilla, high muscle attachments, sharp mylohyoid ridges, and narrow tapered arches, more than two implants are recommended to enhance prosthetic stability.[34–36] Patient-mediated factors, such as cost of treatment, maintenance, and ease of cleaning, may impact the selection of anchorage system and number of implants. The solitary anchor attachment system initially is a more economical treatment modality than the bar construction.[36] However, as a result of the need for significantly more aftercare appointments for the 2-IROD retained with a ball attachment, an overdenture with a bar may be more cost effective.[37–39] Over a 3-year follow-up, with 2-IROD using the Locator attachment system, approximately 40% required denture adjustments, 34% needed improvement in retention, and 12% presented with loose implant abutments.[40] Mackie et al[41] found slightly less than 20% of the Locator overdentures on two implants required a reline after 3 years, and also noted food impaction in the occlusal rim of the abutment prevented complete seating for nearly half of the patients after 7 years. The need for relines for IROD as well as ISOD, regardless of design, has been reported to vary from 8% to 30%.[42] When the ball design was used, a greater ease of cleaning was reported for solitary anchors compared to bar attachments.[43] For patients restored with a two-implant bar overdenture with up to a 4-year follow-up, the most frequently observed complication was hyperplasia (38.3%), bar unscrewing (6.4%), and loss of retention (2.8%).[44] It is noteworthy that the burden of prosthodontic maintenance of overdentures with two, three, or four implants using a round bar was found to be statistically similar.[45] However, when four interforaminal implants are used to anchor the overdenture, a rigid milled bar substructure capitalizing on retention security of swivel latches[46] with a metal reinforced denture framework required less prosthodontic aftercare than a resilient bar (e.g., Dolder bar) over 5 years.[47] In summary, the decision to place more than two implants for an overdenture or a splinted/nonsplinted design will be predicated on the patient's jaw morphology and anatomy, antagonist arch, retention needs, hygiene, and cost considerations.[25] When

opting for multiple implants, a rigid anchorage system, although requiring a larger initial investment, is more cost effective than the resilient bar.[48,49] The interarch space (from soft tissue to antagonist occlusal contact) needed for solitary abutments (Locator), Hader bar, or milled bar design with secondary framework require 8 to 9 mm, 12 mm, and 10 mm, respectively.[50,51]

The evidence evaluating IROD and ISOD designs ranges from level 2 to 4. Controlled clinical trials evaluating patient satisfaction and QoL with the IROD and ISOD designs given specific risk factors of jaw morphology, anatomic limitations, and dentate antagonist would enhance the rigor of the available literature.

Immediate Loading Protocols

Indications for immediate load on the edentulous mandible include morphological, functional and psychologic factors,[52] but the patient's systemic status, loading forces, anatomic/surgical presentation, and level of oral hygiene will dictate the patient's candidacy.[53–55] Patients with wound healing delays such as hyperparathyroidism, diabetes, heavy smoking habits (>20 cigarettes/day), current chemotherapeutic therapy, or history of radiation to head or neck are poor candidates for this regimen.[56,57] Heavy bruxers or clenchers are also best excluded from immediate load protocols.[58] Primary stability (35 N cm), at least 10 mm implant length, and surgical skill appear to be important for success.[56,59–61]

A systematic review reported that immediate loading of implant overdentures in the edentulous mandible (1 to 2 days) is scientifically and clinically validated with implant survival rates ranging from 96 to 100% (1 to 13 years) and prosthodontic survival rates ranging from 88.3 to 100%.[62] The number of implants (2 to 4), splinted, or single had no effect on implant survival.[63–68] Prosthetic maintenance with a small patient sample (8) immediately loaded with unsplinted implants supporting a Locator mandibular overdenture with a 3-year follow-up revealed similar complications to those seen with delayed-loading patients. Most frequent incidences of aftercare burden were replacement of attachment inserts, abutment loosening, and reline.[69] QoL (phonetics, comfort, masticatory performance, nutritional condition) and patient satisfaction (lack of movement of the prosthesis when talking or laughing) have been demonstrated with immediate load of the bar 2-IROD.[70] Using an early loading protocol (2 weeks), Ma et al used strong methodological rigor to investigate the mandibular 2-IROD using the unsplinted design and noted no marginal bone loss differences compared to delayed loading protocols over 10 years.[71] However, it should be noted that more RCTs comparing outcomes between delayed and immediate load and splinted and unsplinted designs, with long-term treatment outcomes and larger sample sizes are necessary to further validate immediate loading protocols for mandibular overdentures.[72] The level of evidence has been represented by 2B/3B.

IMPLANT FIXED COMPLETE DENTURE

A 20-year follow-up investigation on the mandibular IFCD design has yielded an implant survival rate of 99.2% (using machined surfaces and 2-stage surgical protocol).[73] Although implant survival with this design is exceptional, prosthetic maintenance was not uncommon when evaluated with an 8-year follow-up period.[74] The most prevalent complications were chipping or fracturing of the veneering material, prosthetic tooth fracture, tooth wear, maxillary hard relines, and screw complications. Patients were 52.5 times more likely to need posterior tooth replacement at 5 years than at 2 years.[74] However, significantly more aftercare treatment was required by implant overdenture patients in comparison with fixed complete denture patients.[75,76] The decision to provide a fixed complete denture vs. an overdenture design is predicated on a number of clinician- and patient-mediated factors. Patients with combination syndrome,[77] TMD,[78] tapered mandibular arch form,[79] or marked residual ridge resorption[80–82] would benefit from an IFCD. On the other hand, patients with off-ridge relations,[83] facial or dental esthetic concerns,[84] hygiene access considerations,[85] or economic concerns[86] may be optimally treated with an ISOD. However, long-term costs of overdentures due to maintenance may surpass the initial savings in upfront fees compared to an IFCD.[75,87]

Guidelines for treatment planning an IFCD include a minimum of 10 mm alveolar dimension, a minimum of 10 mm interocclusal dimension measured from soft-tissue ridge crest to occlusal plane, and an anterior-posterior (A-P) distribution of at least 10 mm.[88] This span would allow a 15 mm cantilever using a formula by English.[79] When a square arch would preclude a centimeter A-P span of straight implants placed in the interforaminal region, the use of tilted terminal implants will allow for a longer occlusal table with reduced cantilever and improved distribution of implants.[89,90] In a meta-analysis, Monje et al demonstrated no significant differences in marginal bone loss when comparing splinted tilted and straight implants with up to a 5-year follow-up.[91] While there has been controversy regarding the importance of at least 2 mm of peri-implant keratinized mucosa,[92–94] Schrott et al[95] conducted a 5-year evaluation of keratinized mucosa on peri-implant health and concluded that an increased soft tissue recession over time has to be expected circumferential to implants with insufficient keratinized mucosa.

Few comparative prospective controlled studies have investigated patient satisfaction with a fixed versus a removable prosthetic design on the edentulous mandible.[96] Quirynen et al[97] assessed clinical and patient satisfaction outcomes with mandibular 2-IROD and IFCD after 10 years of function and reported that both prostheses provided favorable long-term outcomes. The IFCD group scored only slightly higher for chewing comfort and general satisfaction. Feine et al[98] used a 2-month crossover design to compare a long bar ISOD on four implants with an IFCD in experienced denture users. The results of this study revealed no treatment modality superiority in general satisfaction, ability to chew and to speak, satisfaction with esthetics and self-confidence, and masticatory function. Patient preference appeared to be dependent on many factors. The removable design group rated ease of cleaning and esthetics high in their choice, and the fixed group rated stability the most important factor. The level of evidence on IFCD is level 1B/2B. Randomized clinical long-term data would enhance evaluation of patient-mediated responses to treatment.

Immediate Load Protocols

Immediate loading of the completely edentulous mandible with an IFCD has been widely documented.[99–101] An immediate load IFCD design on three straight implants for the edentulous mandible was reported with a 98% implant survival rate with up to 3-year follow-up using the Branemark Novum concept and later with a longer follow-up of up to 5 years at 91% implant survival.[102,103] However, this design used prefabricated surgical and prosthetic components and did not have universal application. Capelli et al[104] found no implant failure in immediate rehabilitation of the edentulous mandible with upright or tilted implants with up to 40 months of follow-up. Recently, the All-on-4 concept has been shown to be effective using tilted implants with a prosthesis survival rate of 99.2% over 10 years.[105] Maximum insertion torque values of failed implants were significantly lower than those in successful cases of immediately loaded edentulous mandibles.[106] Mechanical complications such as resin veneer fracture and tooth fracture were more prevalent during the initial 6-month loading period using the recommended protocol of fixed provisional prostheses.[107] Implant placement immediately postextraction has been shown to be a predictable procedure.[108,109] Artzi et al[110] compared the efficacy of full-arch, immediately restored implant-supported reconstructions in extraction and healed sites over a 3-year period. Cross-arch immediate loading of implants placed in extraction sites or in healed sites were comparable in respect to crestal bone levels; however, when cervical augmented sites were compared to nonaugmented sites there was significantly greater crestal bone loss at augmented sites. In a recent systematic review, immediate loading in the edentulous mandible shows encouraging results, but appropriate patient selection, primary implant stability, at least 10 mm long implants, splinting of implants, and the expertise of surgeons all seem to be important for predictable prognosis.[61] Indications for an immediately loaded IFCD are similar to the immediately loaded implant overdenture prosthesis.[53,55] Few studies report QoL and patient satisfaction data for this treatment modality.[111,112] Babbush[113] performed a post-treatment evaluation of patient experiences with immediately loaded full-arch prostheses. He reported on responses from 250 patients who filled out a self-administered 20-question edentulous patient impact questionnaire. Ninety five percent described themselves as extremely satisfied (74%) or satisfied (21%) with their prostheses.

The highest level of evidence is presently level 2A. Larger prospective RCTs or systematic reviews of RCTs are needed comparing immediate and delayed loading outcomes. RCTs of low methodological quality can alter interpretation of the benefit of intervention when incorporated in a systematic review.[114]

METAL CERAMIC FIXED DENTAL PROSTHETIC DESIGN

Restoration of the edentulous mandible with an MC is optimally indicated for patients with limited alveolar resorption. As opposed to the ISOD/IROD or IFCD design, which require a composite defect, either by resorptive process or alveoplasty, the FDP is a replacement for a tooth-only defect (without requiring pink porcelain).[115] There is a dearth of articles detailing the implant survival and prosthetic success rates of MC restorations on a large cohort with 5- to 10-year follow-up.[116] Ferrigno et al evaluated 40 patients, each supporting an MC restoration on six implants in the mandible, and reported a 96.2% implant survival rate and 100% prosthetic success.[117] A 5-year follow-up investigation of MC prostheses in 22 mandibles confirmed a high implant survival rate (98.5%) when the mean number of implants was 7.2, mean length of implants was 14.7 mm, and mean diameter of implants 3.8 mm.[118] Implants of at least 10 mm with textured microtopography have been shown to be comparable to longer machined implants and confirmed by a meta-analysis.[119,120] Furthermore, the appropriate number and length of implants is patient-dependent and is determined by the quality/quantity of bone, and anticipated force to be placed on the restoration and the arch form. At least six implants are recommended.[121] In narrow tapered arches, the addition of an implant in the central incisor position will improve the mechanical retention of cement-retained anterior FDPs and the implant distribution, and counter the anterior cantilever.[122] Regardless of the morphological diversity of patients' jaws, there is a premium on experienced surgeons placing the implants congruent with the restorative crown with the least latitude for error for the MC design.[123]

A systematic review addressed the paucity of reports on complications with observations of at least 5 years of rehabilitation of the mandibular edentate population with MC restorations.[124] Pjetursson et al[125] noted that implant-supported FDPs in partially edentulous patients have a 38.7% complication rate after only 5 years. Fracture of the ceramic veneer material, abutment or screw loosening, and loss of retention were the most frequently encountered technical complications. Given this high aftercare burden incidence in the partially edentulous scenario, design of the full-arch restoration into shorter segments will reduce casting errors and facilitate repair. The number of prostheses per edentulous arch has not been shown to be significant in prosthetic survival rate.[126] Short-span FDPs (two three-unit FDPs and one six-unit dental prosthesis) facilitate a passive fit, ceramic veneering, and re-intervention if needed.[121] Additionally, screw-retained designs are preferable for retrievability unless cementation of MC restorations can be done with provisional cements, assuming sufficient mechanical retention in the abutment design.[127] The level of evidence ranges from 1B to 3B, but there are only a handful of clinical trials, marred by their heterogeneity, and although the implant and prosthodontics survival rate has been reported as high, meager data on specific design, complications, and patient satisfaction are available.

Immediate Load Protocols

A compilation of current literature on the MC restoration of the edentulous mandible with immediate loading of implants points to implant survival rates comparable to delayed loading, but suffers from limited sample size and observation periods.[128–131] Furthermore, no prosthetic failures were reported in these four studies in follow-up from 1 to 3 years.[62] However, data on specific prosthetic complications are lacking. A systemic review on immediate loading of immediately placed implants on the edentulous mandible, while promising, reported that the conclusions of these articles are based on a low level of evidence, poor data on complications, and no more than 5-year follow-up.[61,132] Similar criteria have been outlined for immediate load of MC and IFCD restorations, including the absence of wound healing delays, an implant of sufficient micro- and macro-structure to meet primary stability requirements in a given bone density, and a minimum number of implants.[53] For the edentulous mandible, the minimum recommendation is six implants.[126] Rigid splinting provided by metal-reinforced provisional fixed prostheses or by acrylic resin is still controversial.[133,134]

The evidence on immediate loading of MC restorations is characterized at best by level 2B. Longer follow-ups and larger sample sizes with more granularity on the design considerations, prosthetic aftercare burden, and patient satisfaction outcomes are recommended.

SUMMARY

When assessing the strength of the evidence on the implant restoration of the edentulous mandible, there is a notable lack of RCT studies. Randomization to intervention and the presence of a control group are considered important determinants of quality of the methodology, because biased results are reduced compared to prospective studies. Since the selection of treatment is dependent on both clinician- and patient-related factors, true randomization may be complicated by ethical issues; however, more longitudinal comparative studies with prosthetic success data and QoL outcomes would be instrumental in a comprehensive informed consent for patients. Based on the present evidence, investigations with improved scientific rigor are most needed in the area of MC restorations because of the heterogeneity in number of implants, arch form, and length of implants, as well as loading protocols.

REFERENCES

1. Astrand P, Ahlqvist J, Gunne J, et al: Implant treatment of patients with edentulous jaws: a 20-year follow-up. *Clin Implant Dent Rel Res* 2008;10:207–217.

2. Emami E, Heydecke G, Rompre PH, et al: Impact of implant support of mandibular denture on satisfaction, oral and general health-related quality of life: a meta-analysis of randomized controlled trials. *Clin Oral Implants Res* 2009;20:533–544.

3. Assuncao WG, Zardo GG, Delben JA, et al: Comparing efficacy of mandibular implant-retained overdentures among elderly edentulous patients: satisfaction and quality of life. *Gerontology* 2007;24:235–238.

4. Sackett DL, Rosenberg WM, Gray JA, et al: Evidence-based medicine: what it is and what it isn't. *Br Med J* 1996;312:71–72.

5. Bornstein MM, Cionca N, Mombelli A: Systemic conditions and treatments as risks for implant therapy. *Int J Oral Maxillofac Implants* 2009;24 (Suppl): 12–27.

6. Moy PK, Medina D, Shetty V, Aghaloo TL: Dental implant failure rates and associated risk factors. *Int J Oral Maxillofac Implants* 2005;20:569–577.

7. Ekfeldt A, Christansson U, Eriksson T, et al: A retrospective analysis of factors in the maxillae. *Clin Oral Implants Res* 2001;12:462–467.

8. Hellstein JW, Adler RA, Edwards B, et al: Managing the care of patients receiving antiresorptive therapy for prevention and treatment of osteoporosis. *J Am Dent Assoc* 2011;142:1243–1251.

9. Grant BT, Amenedo C, Freeman K, et al: Outcomes of placing dental implants in patients taking oral bisphosphonates: a review of 115 cases. *J Oral Maxillofac Surg* 2008;66:223–230.

10. Sadowsky SJ, Bedrossian E: Evidence-based criteria for differential treatment planning of implant restorations for the partially edentulous patient. *J Prosthodont* 2013;22:319–329.

11. Cochran DL, Schou S, Heitz-Mayfield LJ, et al: Consensus statements and recommended clinical procedures regarding risk factors in implant therapy. *Int J Oral Maxillofac Implants* 2009;24 (Suppl): 86–89.

12. Meijer HJA, Raghobar GM, Van't Hof MA: Comparison of implant-retained mandibular overdentures and complete dentures: a 10-year prospective study of clinical aspects and patient satisfaction. *Int J Oral Maxillofac Implants* 2003;18:879–885.

13. Pan S, Dagenais M, Thomasen JM, et al: Does mandibular edentulous bone height affect prosthetic treatment success? *J Dent* 2010;38:899–907.

14. Emami E, Heydecke G, Rompre PH, et al: Impact of implant support for mandibular dentures on satisfaction, oral and general health-related quality of life: a meta-analysis of randomized-controlled trials. *Clin Oral Implants Res* 2009;20:533–544.

15. de Gradmont P, Feine JS, Tache R, et al: Within-subject comparisons of implant-supported mandibular prostheses: psychometric evaluation. *J Dent Res* 1994;73:1096–1104.

16. De Kok IJ, Chang KH, Lu TS, et al: Comparisons of three-implant-supported fixed dentures and two-implant-retained overdentures in the edentulous mandible: a pilot study of treatment efficacy and patient satisfaction. *Int J Oral Maxillofac Implants* 2011;26:415–428.

17. Attard NJ, Zarb GA: Long-term treatment outcomes in edentulous patients with implant overdentures: the Toronto Study. *Int J Prosthodont* 2004;17:425–433.

18. Gotfredsen K, Holm B: Implant supported mandibular overdentures retained with ball or bar attachments: a randomized prospective 5-year study. *Int J Prosthodont* 2000;13: 125–130.

19. Feine JS, Carlsson GS, Awad MA, et al: The McGill consensus statement on overdentures. *Int J Prosthodont* 2002;15:413–414.

20. Fitzpatrick B: Standard of care for edentulous mandible: a systematic review. *J Prosthet Dent* 2006;96:71–78.

21. Zarb GA, Albrektsson T: Consensus report: towards optimized treatment outcomes for dental implants. *J Prosthet Dent* 1998;80:641.

22. Strietzel FP: Patient's informed consent prior to implant-prosthodontic treatment: a retrospective analysis of expert opinions. *Int J Oral Maxillofac Implants* 2003;18: 433–439.

23. Zitzmann NU, Marinello CP: A review of clinical and technical considerations for fixed and removable implant prostheses in the edentulous mandible. *Int J Prosthodont* 2002;15: 65–72.

24. Batenburg RH, Raghobar GM, Van Oort RP, et al: Mandibular overdentures supported by two or four endosteal implants. A prospective, comparative study. *Int J Oral Maxillofac Surg* 1998;27:435–439.

25. Sadowsky SJ: Mandibular implant-retained overdentures: a literature review. *J Prosthet Dent* 2001;86:468–473.

26. Ueda T, Kremer U, Katsoulis J, et al: Long-term results of mandibular implants supporting an overdenture: implant survival, failures, and crestal bone level changes. *Int J Oral Maxillofac Implants* 2011;26:365–372.

27. Geertman ME, Slagter AP, van't Hof MA, et al: Masticatory performance and chewing experience with implant-retained mandibular overdentures. *J Oral Rehabil* 1999;26:7–13.

28. Fontijn-Tekamp FA, Slagter AP, van't Hof MA, et al: Bite forces with mandibular implant-retained overdentures. *J Dent Res* 1998;77:1832–1839.

29. Bilhan H, Geckili O, Mumcu E, et al: The influence of implant number and attachment type on maximum bite force of mandibular overdentures: a retrospective study. *Gerodontology* 2012;29:116–120.

30. Wismeijer D, van Waas MA, Vermeeren JI, et al: Patient satisfaction with implant-supported mandibular overdentures. A comparison of three treatment strategies with ITI-dental implants. *Int J Oral Maxillofac Surg* 1997;26:263–267.

31. Mumcu E, Bilhan H, Geckili O: The effect of attachment type and implant number on satisfaction and quality of life of mandibular implant-retained overdenture wearers. *Gerodontology* 2012;29:618–623.

32. Cune M, Burgers M, van Kampen F, et al: Mandibular overdentures retained by two implants: 10-year results from a crossover clinical trial comparing ball-socket and bar-clip attachments. *Int J Prosthodont* 2010;23:310–317.

33. Mericske-Stern R: Prosthodontic management of maxillary and mandibular overdentures. In Feine JS, Carlsson GE (eds.): *Implant Overdentures. The Standard of Care for Edentulous Patients.* Hanover Park, IL, Quintessence, 2003, p. 33.

34. Batenburg RH, Meijer HJ, Raghobar GM, et al: Treatment concept for mandibular overdentures supported by endosseous implants: a literature review. *Int J Oral Maxillofac Implants* 1998;13:539–545.

35. Mericske-Stern R, Taylor TD, Belser U: Management of the edentulous patient. *Clin Oral Implants Res* 2000;11:108–125.

36. Kuoppala R, Napankangas R, Raustia A: Outcome of implant-supported overdenture treatment-a survey of 58 patients. *Gerodontology* 2012;29:577–584.

37. Stoker GT, Wismeijer D, van Waas MAJ: An eight-year follow-up to a randomized clinical trial of aftercare and cost analysis with three different types of mandibular implant-retained overdentures. *J Dent Res* 2007;86:276–280.

38. Klemetti E: Is there a certain number of implants needed to retain an overdenture? *J Oral Rehabil* 2008;35:80–84.

39. Dudic A, Mericske-Stern R: Retention mechanisms and prosthetic complications of implant-supported mandibular overdentures: long-term results. *Clin Implant Dent Relat Res* 2002;4:212–219.

40. Vere J, Patel R, Wragg P: Prosthodontic maintenance requirements of implant-retained overdentures using the Locator attachment system. *Int J Prosthodont* 2012;25:392–394.

41. Mackie A, Lyons K, Thomson WM, et al: Mandibular two-implant overdentures: three-year prosthodontics maintenance using the Locator attachment system. *Int J Prosthodont* 2011;24:328–331.

42. Payne AG, Solomons YF: The prosthodontics maintenance requirements of mandibular mucosa- and implant-supported overdentures: a review of the literature. *Int J Prosthodont* 2000;13:238–245.

43. Cune MS, de Putter C, Hoogstraten J: Treatment outcome with implant-retained overdentures: part II—patient satisfaction and predictability of subjective treatment outcome. *J Prosthet Dent* 1994;72:152–158.

44. Bressan E, Tomasi C, Stellini E, et al: Implant-supported mandibular overdentures: a cross-sectional study. *Clin Oral Implants Res* 2012; 814–819.

45. Payne AG, Solomons YF: Mandibular implant-supported overdentures: a prospective evaluation of the burden of prosthodontics maintenance with 23 different attachment systems. *Int J Prosthodont* 2000;13:246–253.

46. Toljanic JA, Antoniou D, Clark RS, et al: A longitudinal clinical assessment of spark erosion technology in implant-retained overdenture prostheses: a preliminary report. *J Prosthet Dent* 1997;78:490–495.

47. Krennmair G, Krainhofner M, Piehslinger E: The influence of bar design (round versus milled bar) on prosthodontics maintenance of mandibular overdentures supported by 4 implants: a 5-year prospective study. *Int J Prosthodont* 2008;21:514–520.

48. Weinlander M, Piehslinger E, Krennmair G: Removable implant-prosthodontic rehabilitation of the edentulous mandible: five-year results of different prosthetic anchorage concepts. *Int J Oral Maxillofac Implants* 2010;25:589–597.

49. Dudic A, Mericske-Stern R: Retentive mechanisms and prosthetic complications of implant supported overdentures: long-term results. *Clin Implant Dent Rel Res* 2002;4:212–219.

50. Phillips K, Wong KM: Space requirements for implant-retained bar-and-clip overdentures. *Compend Contin Educ Dent* 2001;22:516–518.

51. Schmitt SM: Spark erosion for precise fitting of implant retained restorations. *J Dent Technol* 1998;15:15–19.

52. Misch CE, Wang H-L, Misch CM, et al: Rationale for the application of immediate load in implant dentistry: part I. *Implant Dent* 2004;13:207–217.

53. Gapski R, Wang HL, Mascarenhas P, et al: Critical review of immediate loading. *Clin Oral Implants Res* 2003;14:515–527.

54. Attard NJ, David LA, Zarb GA: Immediate loading of implants with mandibular overdentures; one year clinical results of a prospective study. *Int J Prosthodont* 2005;18:463–470.

55. Sadowsky SJ: Immediate load on the edentulous mandible: treatment planning considerations. *J Prosthodont* 2010;19:647–653.

56. Esposito M, Grusovin MG, Willings M, et al: The effectiveness of immediate, early, and conventional loading of dental implants: a Cochrane systematic review of randomized controlled trials. *Int J Oral Maxillofac Implants* 2007;22:893–904.

57. Chiapasco M, Abati S, Romeo E, et al: Implant-retained mandibular overdentures with Branemark system MKII implants: a prospective comparative study between delayed and immediate loading. *Int J Oral Maxillofac Implants* 2001;16:537–546.

58. Jaffin RA, Kumar A, Berman CL: Immediate loading of implants in partially and fully edentulous jaws: a series of 27 case reports. *J Periodontol* 2000;71:310–319.

59. Horiuchi K, Uchida H, Yamamoto K, et al: Immediate loading of Branemark system implants following placement in edentulous patients: a clinical report. *Int J Oral Maxillofac Implants* 2000;15:824–830.

60. Esposito M, Grusovin MG, Willings M, et al: Interventions for replacing missing teeth: different times for loading dental implants. *Cochrane Database Syst Rev* 2009;4:CD003607.

61. Strub JR, Jurdzik BA, Tuna T: Prognosis of immediately loaded implants and their restorations: a systematic review. *J Oral Rehabil* 2012;39:704–717.

62. Gallucci GO, Morton D, Weber H-P: Loading protocols for dental implants in edentulous patients. *Int J Oral Maxillofac Implants* 2009; (Suppl): 132–146.

63. Chiapasco M, Gatti C, Rossi E, et al: Implant-retained mandibular overdentures with immediate loading. A retrospective multicenter study on 226 consecutive cases. *Clin Oral Implants Res* 1997;8:48–57.

64. Marzola R, Scotti R, Fazi G, et al: Immediate loading of two implants supporting a ball attachment-retained mandibular overdenture. A prospective clinical study. *Clin Implant Dent Relat Res* 2007;9:136–143.

65. Stephan G, Vidot F, Noharet R, et al: Implant-retained mandibular overdentures. A comparative pilot study of immediate loading versus delayed loading after two years. *J Prosthet Dent* 2007;97(Suppl 6): S138–S145.

66. Grandi T, Guazzi P, Samarani R, et al: Immediate loading of two unsplinted implants retaining the existing complete denture in elderly edentulous patients: 1-year results from a multicenter prospective cohort study. *Eur J Oral Implantol* 2012;5:61–68.

67. Striker A, Gutwald R, Schmelzeisen R, et al: Immediate loading of 2 interforaminal dental implants supporting an overdenture. Clinical and radiographic results after 24 months. *Int J Oral Maxillofac Implants* 2004;19:868–872.

68. Liddelow GJ, Henry PJ: A prospective study of immediately loaded single implant-retained mandibular overdentures: preliminary one-year results. *J Prosthet Dent* 2007;97(Suppl 6): S126–S137.

69. Roe P, Kan JY, Rungcharassaeng K, et al: Immediate loading of unsplinted implants in anterior mandible for overdentures: 3-year results. *Int J Oral Maxillofac Implants* 2011;26:1296–1302.

70. Borges Tde F, Mendes FA, de Oliveira TR, et al: Mandibular overdentures with immediate loading: satisfaction and quality of life. *Int J Prosthodont* 2011;24:534–539.

71. Ma S, Tawse-Smith A, Thomson WM, et al: Marginal bone loss with mandibular two-implant overdentures using different loading protocols and attachment systems: 10-year outcomes. *Int J Prosthodont* 2010;23:321–332.

72. Alsabeeha N, Atieh M, Payne AGT: Loading protocols for mandibular implant overdentures: a systematic review with meta-analysis. *Clin Implant Dent Rel Res* 2010;12(Suppl 1): 28–38.

73. Astrand P, Ahlqvist J, Gunne J, et al: Implant treatment of patients with edentulous jaws: a 20-year follow-up. *Clin Implant Dent Relat Res* 2008;10:207–217.

74. Purcell BA, McGlumphy EA, Holloway JA, et al: Prosthetic complications in mandibular metal-resin implant-fixed complete dental prosthesis: a 5- to 9-year analysis. *Int J Oral Maxillofac Implants* 2008;23:847–857.

75. Watson RM, Davis DM: Follow up and maintenance of implant supported prostheses: a comparison of 20 complete mandibular overdentures and 20 complete mandibular fixed cantilever prostheses. *Br Dent J* 1996;181:321–327.

76. Goodacre CJ, Bernal G, Rungcharassaeng K, et al: Clinical complications with implants and implant prostheses. *J Prosthet Dent* 2003;90:121–132.

77. Henry PJ, Bower RC, Wall CD: Rehabilitation of the edentulous mandible with osseointegrated dental implants: a 10-year follow-up. *Aust Dent J* 1995;40:1–9.

78. Bergendal T, Magnusson T: Changes in signs and symptoms of temporomandibular disorders following treatment with implant-supported fixed prosthesis: a prospective 3-year follow-up. *Int J Prosthodont* 2000;13:392–398.

79. English CE: Critical A–P spread. *Implant Soc* 1990;1:2–3.

80. Davis WH, Lam PS, Marshall MW, et al: Using restorations borne totally by anterior implants to preserve the edentulous mandible. *J Am Dent Assoc* 1999;130:1183–1189.

81. Jacobs R, Schotte A, van Steenberghe D, et al: Posterior jaw bone resorption in osseointegrated implant-supported overdentures. *Clin Oral Implants Res* 1992;3:63–70.

82. Wright PS, Glantz PO, Randow K, et al: The effects of fixed and removable implant-stabilized prostheses on posterior mandibular residual ridge resorption. *Clin Oral Implants Res* 2002;13:169–174.

83. Naert I, van Steenberghe D, Worthington P (eds): *Osseointegration in Oral Rehabilitation*. London, Quintessence, 1993, pp. 105–107.

84. Tang I, Lund JP, Tache R, et al: A within-subject comparison of mandibular long-bar and hybrid implant-supported prostheses: psychometric evaluation and patient preference. *J Dent Res* 1997;76:1675–1683.

85. Feine JS, de Grandmont P, Boudrias P, et al: Within-subject comparisons of implant-supported mandibular prostheses: choice of prosthesis. *J Dent Res* 1994;73:1105–1111.

86. Attard NJ, Zarb GA, Laporte A: Long-term treatment costs associated with implant supported mandibular prostheses in edentulous patients. *Int J Prosthodont* 2005;18:117–123.

87. Walton JN, MacEntee MI: A retrospective study on maintenance and repair of implant-supported prostheses. *Int J Prosthodont* 1993;6:451–455.

88. Cooper LF, Limmer BM, Gates WD: "Rules of 10"—guidelines for successful planning and treatment of mandibular edentulism using dental implants. *Compend Contin Educ Dent* 2012;33:328–334.

89. Kim KS, Kim YL, Bae JM, et al: Biomechanical comparison of axial and tilted implants for mandibular full-arch fixed prostheses. *Int J Oral Maxillofac Implants* 2011;26:976–984.

90. Krekmanov L, Kahn M, Rangert B, et al: Tilting of posterior mandibular and maxillary implants for improved prosthesis support. *Int J Oral Maxillofac Implants* 2000;15:405–415.

91. Monje A, Chan HL, Suarez F, et al: Marginal bone loss around tilted implants in comparison to straight implants: a meta-analysis. *Int J Oral Maxillofac Implants* 2012;27:1576–1583.

92. Wennstrom JL, Bengazi F, Lekholm U: The influence of the masticatory mucosa on peri-implant soft tissue condition. *Clin Oral Implants Res* 1994;5:1–8.

93. Bengazi F, Wennstrom JL, Lekholm U: Recession of the soft tissue margin at oral implants. A 2-year longitudinal prospective study. *Clin Oral Implants Res* 1996;7:303–310.

94. Myshin HL, Wiens JP: Factors affecting soft tissue around dental implants: a review of the literature. *J Prosthet Dent* 2005;94:440–444.

95. Schrott AR, Jimenez M, Hwang J-W, et al: Five-year evaluation of the influence of keratinized mucosa on peri-implant soft-tissue health and stability around implants supporting full-arch mandibular fixed prostheses. *Clin Oral Implants Res* 2009;20:1170–1177.

96. Raghobar GM, Meijer HJA, Stellingsma K, et al: Addressing the atrophied mandible: a proposal for a treatment approach involving endosseous implants. *Int J Oral Maxillofac Implants* 2011;26:607–617.

97. Quirynen M, Alsaadi G, Pauweis M, et al: Microbiological and clinical outcomes and patient satisfaction for two treatment options in the edentulous lower jaw after 10 years of function. *Clin Oral Implants Res* 2005;16:277–287.

98. Feine JS, de Grandmont P, Boudrias P, et al: Within-subject comparisons of implant-supported mandibular prostheses: choice of prosthesis. *J Dent Res* 1994;73:1105–1111.

99. Schnitman PA, Wohrle PS, Rubenstein JE, et al: Ten-year results for Branemark implants loaded with fixed prostheses at implant placement. *Int J Oral Maxillofac Implants* 1997;12:495–503.

100. Testori T, Melter A, Del Fabbro M, et al: Immediate occlusal loading of Osseotite implants in the lower edentulous jaw. A multicenter prospective study. *Clin Oral Implants Res* 2004;15:278–284.

101. Randow K, Ericsson J, Nilner K, et al: Immediate functional loading of Branemark dental implants. An 18-month study. *Clin Oral Implants Res* 1999;10:8–15.

102. Branemark PI, Engstrand P, Ohrnell LO, et al: Branemark Novum: a new treatment concept for rehabilitation of edentulous mandible. Preliminary results from a prospective clinical follow-up study. *Clin Implant Dent Rel Res* 1999;1:2–16.

103. Gualini F, Gualini G, Cominelli R, et al: Outcome of Branemark Novum implant treatment in edentulous mandibles: a retrospective 5-year follow-up study. *Clin Implant Dent Relat Res* 2009;11:330–337.

104. Capelli M, Zuffretti F, Del F, et al: Immediate rehabilitation of completely edentulous jaw with fixed prostheses supported by either upright or tilted implants: a multicenter clinical study. *Int J Oral Maxillofac Implants* 2007;22:639–644.

105. Malo P, de Araujo Nobre M, Lopes A, et al: A longitudinal study of the survival of All-on-4 implants in the mandible with up to 10 years of follow-up. *J Am Dent Assoc* 2011;142:310–320.

106. Li W, Chow J, Hui E, et al: Retrospective study on immediate functional loading of edentulous maxillas and mandibles with 690 implants, up to 71 months of follow-up. *J Oral Maxillofac Surg* 2009;67:2653–2662.

107. Hinze M, Thalmair T, Bolz W, et al: Immediate loading of fixed provisional prostheses using four implants for the rehabilitation of the edentulous arch: a prospective clinical study. *Int J Oral Maxillofac Implants* 2010;25:1011–1018.

108. Esposito MA, Koukoulopoulou A, Coulthard P, et al: Interventions for replacing missing teeth: dental implants in fresh extraction sites (immediate, immediate-delayed and delayed implants). *Cochrane Database Syst Rev* 2006;18:CD005968.

109. Quirynen M, Van Assche N, Botticelli D, et al: How does the timing of implant placement to extraction affect outcome. *Int J Oral Maxillofac Implants* 2007;22 (Suppl): 203–223.

110. Artzi Z, Kohen J, Carmeli G, et al: The efficacy of full-arch immediately restored implant-supported reconstructions in extraction and healed sites: a 36-month retrospective evaluation. *Int J Oral Maxillofac Implants* 2010;25:329–335.

111. Cochran DL, Morton D, Weber HP: Consensus statements and recommended clinical procedures regarding loading protocols for endosseous dental implants. *Int J Oral Maxillofac Implants* 2004;19 (Suppl): 109–113.

112. Weber HP, Morton D, Gallucci GO, et al: Consensus statements and recommended clinical procedures regarding loading protocols. *Int J Oral Maxillofac Implants* 2009;24 (Suppl): 180–183.

113. Babbush CA: Posttreatment quantification of patient experiences with full-arch implant treatment using a modification of the OHIP-14 questionnaire. *J Oral Implantol* 2012;38:251–260.

114. Ioannidou E, Doufexi A: Does loading time affect implant survival? A meta-analysis of 1266 implants. *J Periodontol* 2005;76:1252–1258.

115. Bedrossian E, Sullivan RM, Fortin Y, et al: Fixed-prosthetic implant restoration of the edentulous maxilla: a systematic pretreatment evaluation method. *J Oral Maxillofac Surg* 2008;66:112–122.

116. Rasmusson L, Roos J, Bystedt H: A ten-year follow-up study of titanium dioxide-blasted implants. *Clin Implant Dent Relat Res* 2005;7:36–42.

117. Ferrigno N, Laureti M, Fanali S, et al: A long-term follow-up study of non-submerged ITI implants in the treatment of totally edentulous jaws. Part 1: ten-year life table analysis of a prospective multicenter study with 1286 implants. *Clin Oral Implants Res* 2002;13:260–273.

118. Schwartz-Arad D, Chaushu G: Full-arch restoration of the jaw with fixed ceramometal prosthesis. *Int J Oral Maxillofac Implants* 1998;13:819–825.

119. Renouard F, Nisand D: Impact of implant length and diameter on survival rates. *Clin Oral Implants Res* 2006;17(Suppl 2): 35–51.

120. Kotsovillis S, Fourmousis I, Karoussis IK, et al: A systematic review and meta-analysis on effect of implant length on

survival of rough-surface dental implants. *J Periodontol* 2009;80:1700–1718.

121. Gallucci GO, Bernard J-P, Belser UC: Treatment of completely edentulous patients with fixed implant-supported restorations: three consecutive cases of simultaneous immediate loading in both maxilla and mandible. *Int J Periodontics Restorative Dent* 2005;25:27–37.

122. Ogawa T, Dhaliwal S, Naert I, et al: Impact of implant number, distribution and prosthesis material on loading on implants supporting fixed prostheses. *J Oral Rehabil* 2010;37:525–531.

123. Lambert PM, Morris HF, Ochi S: Positive effect of surgical experience with implants on second-stage implant survival. *J Oral Maxillofac Surg* 1997;55(12 Suppl 5): 12–18.

124. Papaspyridakos P, Chen Chun-Jung, Chuang S-K, et al: A systematic review of biologic and technical complications with fixed implant rehabilitations for edentulous patients. *Int J Oral Maxillofac Implants* 2012;27:102–110.

125. Pjetursson BE, Bragger U, Lang NP, et al: Comparison of survival and complication rates of tooth-supported fixed dental prostheses (FDP) and implant-supported FDPs and single crown (SCs). *Clin Oral Implants Res* 2007;18(Suppl 3): 97–113.

126. Lambert FE, Weber HP, Susaria SM, et al: Descriptive analysis of implant and prosthodontics survival rates with fixed implant-supported rehabilitations in the edentulous maxilla. *J Periodontol* 2009;80:1220–1230.

127. Bernal G, Okamura M, Munoz CA: The effects of abutment taper, length, and cement type on resistance to dislodgement of cement-retained, implant-supported restorations. *J Prosthodont* 2003;12:111–115.

128. Ganeles J, Rosenberg MM, Holt RL, et al: Immediate loading of implants with fixed reconstructions in the completely edentulous mandible. Report of 27 patients from a private practice. *Int J Oral Maxillofac Implants* 2011;16:418–426.

129. Testori T, Meltzer A, Del Fabbro M, et al: Immediate occlusal loading of Osseotite implants in the lower edentulous jaw. A multicenter prospective study. *Clin Oral Implants Res* 2004;15:278–284.

130. Degidi M, Perrotti V, Piattelli A: Immediately loaded titanium implants with a porous anodized surface with at least 36 months of follow-up. *Clin Implant Dent Relat Res* 2006;8:169–177.

131. DeBruyn H, Van de Velde T, Collaert B: Immediate functional loading of TiOblast dental implants with at least 36 months of follow-up. *Clin Oral Implants Res* 2008;19:717–723.

132. Schwartz-Arad D, Gulayev N, Chaushu: Immediate versus non-immediate implantation for full-arch fixed reconstruction following extraction of all residual teeth. *J Periodontol* 2000;71:923–928.

133. Strietzel FP, Karmon B, Lorean A, et al: Implant-prosthetic rehabilitation of the edentulous maxilla and mandible with immediately loaded implants: preliminary data from a retrospective study, considering time of implantation. *Int J Oral Maxillofac Implants* 2011;26:139–147.

134. Gallucci GO, Bernard JP, Bertosa M, et al: Immediate loading with fixed screw-retained provisional restorations in edentulous jaws. The pick-up technique. *Int J Oral Maxillofac Implants* 2004;19:524–533.

10

MANDIBULAR IMPLANT OVERDENTURE TREATMENT: CONSENSUS AND CONTROVERSY

DAVID R. BURNS, DMD
Associate Professor, Department of Prosthodontics, Virginia Commonwealth University, School of Dentistry, Richmond, VA

Keywords
Dental implant; denture; edentulism; combination syndrome; peri-implant; patient satisfaction; treatment complications.

Correspondence
Dr. David R. Burns, Virginia Commonwealth University, MCV Campus, School of Dentistry, Department of Prosthodontics, P.O. Box 980566, Richmond, VA 23298-0566.
E-mail: Dburns@den1.den.vcu.edu

Supported in part by National Institutes of Health grant 1R01DE12204-01A1.

Presented in part at the American College of Prosthodontists Annual Session, October 22, 1999, New York, NY.

Accepted February 16, 2000

Published in *Journal of Prosthodontics* March 2000; Vol. 9, Issue 1

doi: 10.1053/jd.2000.6782

ABSTRACT

A literature review of implant overdenture treatment for the edentulous mandible is presented. The report focuses on the knowledge base for this treatment modality, in an effort to distinguish between areas that are well characterized and enjoy a higher level of consensus among practitioners as compared with those that are more controversial and not clearly understood.

Researchers and clinicians must address many diverse aspects of knowledge in understanding and providing mandibular implant overdenture treatment. The areas supported by research generally embrace a higher level of consensus among practitioners. Research data, however, is not available to support all of the considerations necessary to predict successful clinical treatment outcome. There are voids in our knowledge base in which objective information does not exist.

Some areas are either unable to be tested or have not been considered using a strict research protocol. Additionally, it is not uncommon to find contradictory results and conclusions from related research efforts, even when strict research protocols are followed. In the absence of unequivocal evidence-based knowledge, these questions are often addressed using nonscientific data, clinical experience, and the opinions, assumptions, and inferences of clinicians. These contributions can be useful and clinically relevant, but should be considered controversial and subject to interpretation. To properly critique the understanding of mandibular implant overdenture treatment, clinicians must distinguish areas of consensus from areas of controversy.

The purpose of this report is to review the literature, addressing some of the current issues influencing our understanding of mandibular implant overdenture treatment, and to distinguish between areas of consensus of opinion and controversy. This awareness becomes increasingly important with a growing acceptance of this treatment modality and a possible paradigm shift in therapeutic philosophy, in which implant overdenture treatment could become the future standard of care for mandibular edentulism.

EDENTULISM

In considering this treatment modality and to understand the extent of the clinical problem, it is necessary to first explore the treatment diagnosis: edentulism. According to National Institute of Dental and Craniofacial Research epidemiological data, approximately 10% of the US adult population is completely edentulous.[1] The estimated number of edentulous individuals ages 18 to 74 using complete denture prostheses in this country is nearly 14 million.[2] With people living longer, the demographics of the United States are shifting to a progressively larger older adult subgroup. As a result, it is estimated that within the population over the next 30 years, the number of edentulous individuals over age 65 will remain constant at around 9 million, despite a decrease in the percentage who are edentulous.[3]

CONVENTIONAL DENTURE TREATMENT

Numerous factors are involved in the successful delivery of conventional complete denture treatment.[4,5] Patients perceive improved treatment success in terms of increased prosthesis retention and stability.[6] Redford et al[2] showed that over 50% of mandibular complete dentures have problems with stability and retention. Across-arch comparisons indicated that mandibular denture treatment produced significantly more problems than did maxillary denture treatment. A "lack of retention" was found to be the driving force behind this differential.[2] Perhaps the most significant biological condition associated with mandibular complete denture retention is physiological alveolar ridge resorption, resulting in diminishing oral tissue volume for denture

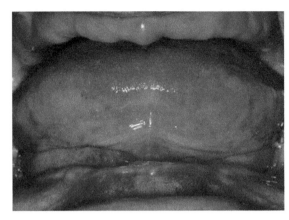

FIGURE 10.1 Diminished supporting tissue volume can have a negative influence on mandibular complete denture stability and retention. Alternatives to conventional denture treatment may be necessary when this occurs.

support (Fig 10.1). In some cases, it is not possible to achieve optimal results using conventional complete denture treatment alone, and alternatives must be considered. When satisfactory denture support is present, denture adhesives can improve treatment outcome, but they are also subject to misuse or abuse.[7] When problems arise from inadequate supporting tissue volume for mandibular denture treatment, denture adhesives can sometimes prove inadequate. In the past, treatment solutions have generally focused on providing increased supporting tissue volume. Alveolar ridge augmentation using a variety of natural and synthetic materials has been used for this purpose. Similarly, alveoloplasty and tissue extension procedures have been used to expose additional intraoral tissues and reposition muscle attachments for denture support. These treatments have provided mixed long-term success and have occasionally introduced significant complications and morbidity.[8,9]

DENTAL IMPLANT UTILIZATION

Within the dental profession over the past 15 years, the consideration of dental implants has shifted from a peripheral position to one of central importance. When the Brånemark dental implant philosophy was first formally introduced in the United States in 1982, research focused on the bone-implant interface and biological considerations. These areas had been previously identified as the weak link for the predictability and success of dental implant treatment. Research in implant prosthodontics for the edentulous patient initially received little interest. It was shown, however, that the use of dental implants could provide predictable prosthodontic results.[10,11] During this initial time period, the most common implant prosthodontic treatment of choice for an edentulous mandible involved the placement of 5 or 6 implants and fabrication of a fixed-detachable, all-implant supported prosthesis (Fig 10.2).[12]

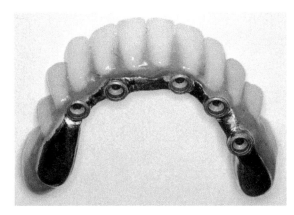

FIGURE 10.2 The totally implant-supported prosthesis in the anterior mandible was the treatment of choice when the Brånemark dental implant philosophy was first formally introduced in the United States in 1982.

Today, important improvements have been made in understanding the prosthodontic aspects of implant-related treatment.[13] Research efforts have focused on materials, treatment design, and methodology. As a result, treatment methods have changed as dental implant systems have been improved.

IMPLANT OVERDENTURE TREATMENT

With time, mandibular implant overdenture treatment has gained considerable acceptance. It is an especially attractive treatment option because of its relative simplicity, minimal invasiveness, and affordability.[14–19] The prosthesis is supported by both implant and mucosa and generally requires fewer implants when compared with the totally implant-supported prosthesis design. Fewer implants and a removable prosthesis offer a less complex and less expensive option for an edentulous patient.[19]

Van der Wijk et al[20] compared the financial costs of different treatment strategies for an edentulous mandible. They compared first-year treatment costs associated with conventional denture treatment, mandibular implant overdenture treatment using either endosseous or transmandibular implant systems, and conventional denture treatment in combination with preprosthetic surgery. Results indicated that the costs for overdenture treatment supported by a transmandibular implant were 7 times those of conventional denture therapy. Both endosseous implant overdenture treatment and conventional denture treatment after preprosthetic surgery resulted in patient costs that were 3 times those of conventional dentures.

Investigations have concluded that mandibular implant overdenture treatment can show significantly improved retention and stability characteristics as compared with conventional mandibular complete dentures. Additionally, a direct relationship has been shown between prosthesis retention and stability and patient satisfaction.[6,16,21] In fact, even

with otherwise successful conventional complete denture treatment in the mandible, it has been shown that it is possible to achieve a higher clinical standard for success with the implant overdenture.[21]

NATURAL TEETH VERSUS DENTAL IMPLANTS

Treatment decisions regarding the restoration of compromised mandibular teeth can be difficult. When teeth require significant prosthodontic or periodontal treatment or when occlusal relationship problems exist, information and guidelines on tooth maintenance versus dental implant use are sparse and controversial (Fig 10.3). In one of the few published reports comparing overdenture treatment using natural tooth roots and implants, Mericske-Stern[22] concluded that the data indicate a higher probability of success in the mandible when overdentures are supported by implants rather than tooth roots. The author could not recommend significant endodontic, periodontic, and/or prosthodontic treatment to save a few remaining teeth when dental implant treatment was possible. She concluded that the cost effectiveness of dental implants in combination with the mandibular implant overdenture would generally provide a more favorable treatment outcome.

PRESERVATION OF BONE

Longitudinal studies have shown that a mean yearly alveolar ridge height reduction of around 0.4 mm can be expected in the edentulous anterior mandible, resulting from physiological changes.[23,24] Additionally, the rate of resorption is 4 times greater in the mandible, compared with the maxilla.

In comparison, Quirynen et al[25] studied the degree of bone loss associated with dental implant treatment. Clinically examining patients with a total of 509 implants, they found the mean annual marginal bone loss (scored on standardized radiographs) to be 0.9 mm during the first year after implant placement and

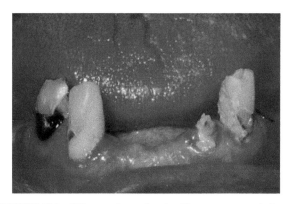

FIGURE 10.3 When teeth require significant treatment, information and guidelines for tooth maintenance versus dental implant use are sparse and controversial.

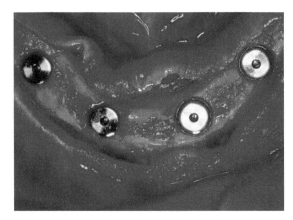

FIGURE 10.4 Four dental implants located within the anterior mandibular alveolar bone. Dental implant use can have a significant positive influence in maintaining residual alveolar bone in the edentulous mandible (Nobel Biocare, Inc., Yorba Linda, CA).

0.1 mm in following years. Other studies have documented similar results.[26,27] The data are significant when considering the ability of implants to preserve alveolar bone (Fig 10.4).

This data comparison supports the conclusion that after the first year, implants have a significant positive influence in maintaining alveolar bone. Evidence indicates that physiological residual ridge resorption occurs in the anterior edentulous mandible at a rate 4 times greater than bone resorption occurring in the same location when dental implants have been used.

NUMBER OF IMPLANTS REQUIRED: INTERCONNECTED VERSUS INDEPENDENT IMPLANTS

If a practitioner concludes that a patient would be best treated with an implant overdenture, how many implants should be placed? The answer is controversial because adequate data to address this concern are lacking. Some practitioners believe that using more implants for overdenture treatment results in a better treatment outcome, but supporting evidence is limited. Similarly, from a prosthodontic treatment perspective, practitioners must decide between a rigid bar fixation connecting 2 or more implants and an independent implant attachment system. Guidelines to assist with this treatment decision are also limited and controversial.

Two dental implants are usually considered the minimum number necessary for mandibular implant overdenture treatment.[18,21] The mucosa and implants provide support, retention, and stability for implant overdentures. As more implants are used, responsibility for these functions shifts from the mucosa to the implants. The improvements to the overall performance of the prosthodontic treatment provided by using additional implants are not clearly understood.

Published reports describe 2 general technical methods for using implants as the foundation beneath an

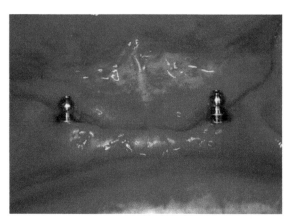

FIGURE 10.5 Two independent dental implants with O-ring attachments in the anterior mandible (Nobel Biocare, Inc.).

overdenture.[15,17,28–30] The first method uses implants as independent units, connected individually to an overdenture with components such as ball or ERA (Sterngold-Implamed, Inc., Attleboro, MA) attachments. While the denture base properly contacts the mucosa, the simultaneous interlocking of attachment components provides the retentive quality for these systems. This technique is more commonly selected when 2 implants are used. This may be because of the desire to simplify treatment. Additionally, abutment parallelism can be more critical with independent implant systems, and this necessity can be increasingly more difficult to achieve as greater numbers of implants are involved (Fig 10.5). The evolution of some attachment systems such as the ERA has provided angled abutments, which allow additional latitude in this regard.

The second method employs a rigid interconnection between implants using a cast metal bar attachment. The overdenture is fabricated to passively fit and attach to the bar while simultaneously resting on adjacent mucosa for support. The connection between the bar and denture base provides the attachment's retentive quality. This method is suitable for 2 or more implants, but is the method of choice when more than 2 implants are used (Figs 10.6 and 10.7).

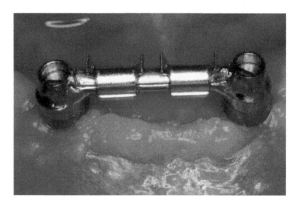

FIGURE 10.6 Two dental implants with bar attachment in the anterior mandible (Nobel Biocare, Inc.).

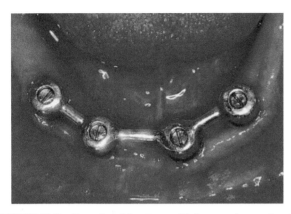

FIGURE 10.7 Four dental implants with bar attachment fixation in the anterior mandible (Nobel Biocare, Inc.).

From a biomechanical perspective, Misch[13] discussed the rationale and theory for rotational movement of a prosthesis around a bar attachment. He indicated that by allowing an attachment clip, located in the denture base, to freely rotate around a bar, prosthesis movement can compensate for the resilience of the supporting mucosa and reduce the transference of torsional forces to the implants. The 2-implant, single bar attachment works best when this is desired. The bar is fabricated with reasonable alignment perpendicular to the posterior edentulous arches, and parallel to the plane of occlusion. When more than 2 implants and multiple bars between implants are used, the attachment clips located on each bar are frequently not parallel to one another or perpendicular to the posterior ridges. According to Misch,[13] when this occurs, the clips can bind in function, limiting prosthesis movement. This can produce a reduced range of motion between the prosthesis and bar attachment, increased prosthesis support from the implants, and increased applied torsional forces to the implants. In clinical situations involving poor posterior ridge form, reducing posterior mucosal support in this manner may be advantageous. The importance, however, of a specific prosthesis range of motion requirement is controversial and needs additional study to provide better understanding of its clinical implications.

Treatment involving 2 independent implants without rigid interconnection is an important consideration with mandibular overdenture treatment. Data support the use of independent implants for a mandibular overdenture.[17,29,30] When existing conventional dentures are directly altered to accommodate implant overdenture attachments, the treatment is usually easier and more predictable with independent implants that require less alteration of the denture base.[15,21]

There is clear evidence indicating a significant negative correlation between socioeconomic status and edentulism.[31–33] For those edentulous individuals who can benefit from implant-retained/supported prostheses, treatment costs are considerably higher when additional implants and/or bar fixation between implants are used. An impelling, but

controversial, consideration suggests that if these variable treatment modalities have equivalent treatment outcomes, the 2-independent-implant treatment is the method of choice because patients can receive the same or similar treatment benefit for less patient expense, treatment involvement, and complexity.

Kenny and Richards[34] evaluated the photoelastic stress patterns produced by implant-retained overdentures. They found that independent O-ring attachments transferred less stress to implants than the bar-clip attachments when their model was subjected to posterior vertical load. Menicucci et al,[35] in an in vivo study, used strain gauges placed within abutments to measure force distribution differences between the independent ball and the connected bar attachment treatment modalities. They concluded that the ball attachments seemed to provide greater stability with the load more evenly distributed onto the distal mucosa on both sides of the dental arch. Axial load on the working-side abutment increased when the bar-anchored attachment was used.

This controversial concept was also addressed by Batenburg et al.[36] They studied 60 mandibular implant overdenture patients who were divided into 2 groups, 1 treated with 2 endosteal implants and the other with 4. They found no significant differences with regard to the peri-implant health. The authors suggested that additional study is necessary, but based on their finding, concluded that there seemed to be no need to insert more than 2 endosteal implants to support an overdenture.

Wismeijer et al[37] studied 110 patients who had received mandibular implant overdenture treatment. Subjects received either 2 implants with ball attachments, 2 implants with an interconnecting bar, or 4 interconnected implants. Subjects completed questionnaires designed to elicit opinion regarding individual treatment outcome. Sixteen months after treatment, almost all subjects were generally satisfied. No significant difference was found between the 3 treatment strategies. The study concluded that implant treatment using the 2-implant ball attachment is sufficient, but the authors emphasized the need for additional clinical studies.

In a retrospective study, Mericske-Stern[17] examined 67 patients divided into 3 groups: 27 with 2 implants using a ball attachment, 29 with 2 implants connected with a bar, and 11 as the control group with 3 or 4 implants, all splinted with a bar. Evaluation included assessments of occlusion, the need for denture remounting, and the need for relining and replacement of attachment retainers. The author concluded that the retention, stability, and occlusal equilibration of dentures improved slightly with increasing numbers of implants. Using three-dimensional finite-element analysis, Meijer et al[38] studied the stress distribution in the anterior mandibular bone around implants under conditions in which either 2 or 4 implants were used. They concluded that there was no reduction of the principal stresses in bone when the occlusal load was distributed over an increasing number of implants.

Fontijn-Tekamp et al,[39] in an in vivo study, analyzed the difference in masticatory forces using conventional maxillary denture treatment, and in the mandible, either conventional denture treatment or implant-supported denture treatment using either a transmandibular implant or 2 anteriorly placed endosseous implants. They found that both implant treatments produced significantly higher masticatory forces compared with conventional denture treatment, but that forces did not differ between the mainly implant-borne and the mucosa-implant borne implant treatments. Chao et al[40] conducted a literature review to analyze survival rates of loaded implants, occlusal forces, and stress distributions of implant overdenture prostheses in the edentulous mandible. This report concluded that the number of implants supporting a prosthesis seems to have less influence on stress distribution than does prosthesis design and the related direction of forces.

Zarb and Schmitt[18] indicated from their study that the major determinant of success in complete denture prosthodontics is patient-perceived denture stability, which can be achieved irrespective of the number of implants successfully integrated. This theory supports the concept that fewer implants can be equally effective for the overdenture prosthesis. The placement of additional implants beyond that necessary for the proposed prosthodontic treatment provides a means for contingency planning against the loss of implants, if tissue integration fails. Zarb and Schmitt[41] reported a clinical success rate in excess of 96% for implants supporting overdentures. Other authors have reported similar results.[19,42–45] These findings support the view that the high degree of predictability of implant integration in the anterior mandible may preclude the contingency placement of additional implants in anticipation of potential loss.

COMBINATION SYNDROME ASSOCIATED WITH DENTAL IMPLANTS

Several authors have reported the response of supporting soft tissues for implant overdentures and opposing prostheses.[6,15,16,46–52] In situations in which mandibular implant overdentures oppose maxillary complete dentures, some authors contend that conditions may be produced at the prosthesis-tissue interface that are similar to those observed with combination syndrome. This condition usually is associated with mandibular distal extension removable partial denture and maxillary complete denture treatments in situations in which mandibular posterior prosthesis support is lost.[46,48,51,52] This situation can lead to the transference of significant occlusal forces into the anterior maxilla with subsequent maxillary alveolar bone resorption and soft tissue inflammation.

Jacobs et al[50] and Burns et al,[6] on the other hand, documented improved tissue health and reduced annual residual ridge resorption in supporting tissues of prostheses

that oppose a mandibular implant overdenture. They concluded that a more stable occlusion provides a better distribution of occlusal forces and protects the maxillary anterior edentulous ridge. Jacobs pointed out the need for regular recall and routine prosthesis reline to maintain proper occlusal relationships.

It is possible that in association with mandibular implant overdenture treatment, reduced posterior prosthesis support caused by alveolar bone resorption could set the stage for pathological complications similar to combination syndrome. Under conditions of adequately maintained posterior prosthesis support, however, the stabilizing influence of implants may promote tissue health. Additionally, Johns et al[19] found a significant decrease in soreness, stomatitis, and ulceration in the anterior mandibular tissues with the use of implant overdenture treatment, when compared with conventional dentures.

PERI-IMPLANT RESPONSE

The peri-implant osseous and gingival tissue response to mandibular implant overdenture treatment has been documented in the literature.[17,19,41–45,47,53,54] Gene rally, favorable results have been reported concerning peri-implant tissue response. Geertman et al[42] evaluated several peri-implant parameters including the plaque index, bleeding index, gingival index, probing depth, quantitative assessment of the keratinized mucosa, and radiographic evaluation of bone level. The authors recorded favorable results for these assessments among 3 implant systems. Mericske-Stern[17] concluded that implants supporting overdentures may be maintained in a healthy and stable condition, independent of the retentive device used for overdenture anchorage.

Johns et al[19] reported on a controversial issue by stating that a healthy soft tissue response is possible, regardless of whether the implants were placed in areas of alveolar mucosa or attached gingiva. Both Zarb and Schmitt[41] and Jemt et al[43] indicated that bone level maintenance around isolated overdenture implant abutments seemed to parallel that reported for natural tooth abutments in the general fixed prosthodontic literature. Wright et al[53] studied the influence of attachment bar design on implant overdenture treatment and documented hyperplasia of the mucosal tissue around implants and the bar in 35% of the patients they observed. Improving oral hygiene and adjusting the dentures in conjunction with the surgical removal of hyperplastic tissue resolved these problems.

TREATMENT COMPLICATIONS

Treatment complications associated with implant overdentures have been discussed in numerous studies.[15,16,19,28,42,43,55–59] Geertman et al[42] evaluated complications using a clinical implant performance scale. This method identified a range of complications using a criterion-defined 5-point scale. Most complications were not serious. Loosening of coping screws and the need for replacement of attachment clips were the most common. Gingival hyperplasia, maxillary denture reline requirements, and occlusal adjustment were also noted, but infrequent.

Walton and MacEntee[58] retrospectively evaluated treatment maintenance requirements for 156 patients who received overdenture treatment over a 6-year period. They found problems with loose, lost, or broken retentive clips that accounted for the most common overdenture repairs. More importantly, they found that the vast majority of repairs were needed within the first year of prosthesis service. Hemmings et al[55] compared the complications and maintenance requirements for fixed implant prostheses and implant overdentures in edentulous mandibles over a 5-year period. They found that overdentures required more adjustment than the fixed prostheses, but that the adjustments were usually performed within the first year post-insertion. The main complications associated with mandibular implant overdenture treatment involved the peri-implant mucosa, abutment and gold screws, acrylic resin components, and retentive clips (Fig 10.8).

Jemt et al[43] studied implant overdenture treatment in a 5-year prospective, multicenter study. They found that the success rates for implants and overdenture prostheses in the mandible were 94.5% and 100%, respectively. Most (79%) of the failed implants in the mandible were identified before or during the first year of function. Similarly, Kucey[56] retrospectively studied implant placement and prosthodontic treatment over a 5-year period. He found that implant overdenture treatment showed no implant loss and 100% restoration retention during this period. Muftu and Karabetou[60] warned that complications associated with implant overdenture treatment cannot be dismissed and managing these complications may require extra clinical time and expense, a fact that should be taken into account when identifying the patient's total financial commitment for this type of treatment.

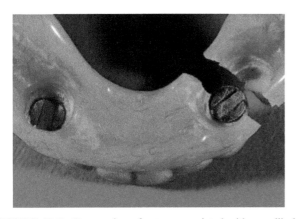

FIGURE 10.8 Denture base fracture associated with mandibular implant overdenture treatment.

PATIENT SATISFACTION

An understanding of patient satisfaction associated with mandibular implant overdenture treatment has received considerable acknowledgement in the literature.[6,15,37,43,61–73] Burns et al[6] and Boerrigter et al[65,69] showed a significant increase in patient satisfaction with this treatment when compared with conventional dentures. Burns concluded that mandibular implant overdenture treatment provided patients with a more predictable treatment outcome and a potentially higher standard of success than is possible with most treatments using conventional complete dentures. Feine et al[61] compared patient satisfaction between implant-supported fixed prosthodontic treatment and implant overdenture treatment in the mandible. After subjects experienced each treatment type, an equal number preferred the removable to the fixed treatment. For the categories of prosthesis stability and the ability to chew, the fixed treatment received a higher rating. The removable treatment was rated superior for ease of cleaning and esthetics. In terms of reducing patient complaints, Cune et al[64] suggested that treatment with dental implants in combination with an overdenture is very effective. In particular, for the mandibular implant prosthesis, patient comfort was significantly improved. Geertman et al[68] compared the 2 endosseous implant and transmandibular implant overdenture treatments in the mandible in terms of patient satisfaction, complaints, and subjective chewing ability, and found no statistical difference. They suggested that their results were unexpected, because the transmandibular treatment provides a greater degree of implant support for the prosthesis compared with the 2 endosseous implant treatments.

Grogono et al[73] studied the differential of importance between function and esthetics, reporting data collected from 61 questionnaires completed by patients with existing implant prosthodontic treatment. The most common reason for choosing a dental implant prosthesis was to improve eating ability. Eighty-two percent of respondents reported improved eating ability after implant utilization. Function and confidence were more important than esthetics. This information is of particular interest because the esthetic outcome of treatment with a mandibular implant overdenture is similar to that of a conventional denture.

CONCLUSIONS

The information presented in this report represents a portion of the knowledge base available for mandibular implant overdenture treatment. Some information is well documented and supported by evidence, and some is not. Conclusions for this material, based on the consideration of consensus of opinion versus controversy, are as follows.

Areas of General Consensus

- Edentulism is a significant health problem in the United States and will continue to be of concern in the future.
- Patients experience greater difficulties with mandibular conventional dentures than with maxillary dentures.
- Retention and stability problems have significant negative influence on treatment outcomes for conventional mandibular dentures.
- The success of dental implants in the anterior mandible is generally excellent.
- Dental implants, when used with mandibular overdenture treatment, have demonstrated many benefits compared with conventional denture treatment.
- Implants in the anterior mandible can slow the process of physiological bone resorption.
- Peri-implant and osseous response to mandibular implant overdenture treatment has proven favorable.
- Treatment complications are a concern, especially during the first year of treatment service.
- The potential for complications points to the need for routine recall and follow-up evaluation and treatment.
- Data indicate significant increases in patient satisfaction with mandibular implant overdenture treatment when compared with conventional denture treatment.

Areas of Controversy

- When complex treatment is required to restore a few remaining natural teeth in the anterior mandible, extraction of the teeth and replacement using implant overdenture treatment may be the best option, but decision guidelines are needed.
- The number of implants required to provide adequate mandibular implant overdenture treatment outcome remains open to debate.
- The necessity for rigid interconnection between implants in the anterior mandible has not been definitively determined.
- Negative influence of mandibular implant overdenture treatment on the anterior maxilla (combination syndrome) requires additional understanding.
- The necessity for placement of dental implants in attached keratinized gingiva rather than alveolar mucosa is unresolved.
- Dentistry may be experiencing a paradigm shift in which the mandibular implant overdenture treatment could become the future standard of care for the edentulous mandible.

REFERENCES

1. Marcus SE, Drury TF, Brown LV, et al: Tooth retention and tooth loss in the permanent dentition of adults: United States 1988–1991. *J Dent Res* 1996;75(Spec Iss):684–695.
2. Redford M, Drury TF, Kingman A, et al: Denture use and the technical quality of dental prostheses among persons 18–74 years of age: United States, 1988–1991. *J Dent Res* 1996;75 (Spec Iss):714–725.
3. Douglas CW: Review of the literature (from Prosthodontics 21 Symposium). *J Prosthet Dent* 1990;64:275–283.
4. Brill N: Full denture retention: factors in the mechanism of full denture retention—a discussion of selected papers. *Dent Pract Dent Rec* 1967;18:9–19.
5. Mack AO: *Full Dentures*. Bristol, England, John Wright and Sons, 1971, p. 94.
6. Burns DR, Unger JW, Elswick RK, et al: Prospective clinical evaluation of mandibular implant overdentures. Part II: patient satisfaction and preference. *J Prosthet Dent* 1995; 73:364–369.
7. Slaughter A, Katz RV, Grasso JE: Professional attitudes toward denture adhesives: a Delphi technique survey of academic prosthodontists. *J Prosthet Dent* 1999;82:80–89.
8. Jennings DE: Treatment of the mandibular compromised ridge: a literature review. *J Prosthet Dent* 1989;61:575–579.
9. Matras H: A review of surgical procedures designed to increase the functional height of the resorbed alveolar ridge. *Int Dent J* 1983;33:332–338.
10. Laney WR, Tolman DE, Keller EE, et al: Dental implants: tissue-integrated prosthesis utilizing the osseointegration concept. *Mayo Clin Proc* 1986;61:91–97.
11. Albrektsson T, Zarb G, Worthington P, et al: The long term efficacy of currently used dental implants: a review and proposed criteria of success. *Int J Oral Maxillofac Implants* 1986;1:11–24.
12. Brånemark P, Zarb GA, Albrektsson T (eds): *Tissue Integrated Prosthesis* (ed 1). Chicago, IL, Quintessence, 1985, pp. 211–232.
13. Misch CE: *Contemporary Implant Dentistry* (ed 2). St. Louis, MO, Mosby, 1999.
14. Parel SM: Implants and overdentures: the osseointegrated approach with conventional and compromised applications. *Int J Oral Maxillofac Implants* 1986;1:93–99.
15. Engquist B, Bergendal T, Kallus T, et al: A retrospective multicenter evaluation of osseointegrated implants supporting overdentures. *Int J Oral Maxillofac Implants* 1988;3:129–134.
16. Naert I, Quirynen M, Theuniers G, et al: Prosthetic aspects of osseointegrated fixtures supporting overdentures. A 4-year report. *J Prosthet Dent* 1991;65:671–680.
17. Mericske-Stern R: Clinical evaluation of overdenture restorations supported by osseointegrated titanium implants: a retrospective study. *Int J Oral Maxillofac Implants* 1990;5: 375–383.
18. Zarb GA, Schmitt A: The longitudinal clinical effectiveness of osseointegrated dental implants: the Toronto study. Part II: the prosthetic results. *J Prosthet Dent* 1990;64:53–61.

19. Johns RB, Jemt T, Heath MR, et al: A multicenter study of overdentures supported by Brånemark implants. *Int J Oral Maxillofac Implants* 1992;7:513–522.

20. Van der Wijk P, Bouma J, van Waas MA, et al: The cost of dental implants as compared to that of conventional strategies. *Int J Oral Maxillofac Implants* 1998;13:546–553.

21. Burns DR, Unger JW, Elswick RK, et al: Prospective clinical evaluation of mandibular implant overdentures. Part I: retention, stability and tissue response. *J Prosthet Dent* 1995;73:354–363.

22. Mericske-Stern R: Overdentures with roots or implants for elderly patients: a comparison. *J Prosthet Dent* 1994;72:543–550.

23. Atwood DA, Coy WA: Clinical, cephalometric, and densitometric study of reduction of residual ridges. *J Prosthet Dent* 1971;26:280–295.

24. Tallgren A: The continuing reduction of the residual alveolar ridges in complete denture wearers: a mixed-longitudinal study covering 25 years. *J Prosthet Dent* 1972;27:120–131.

25. Quirynen M, Naert I, van Steenberghe D, et al: Periodontal aspects of osseointegrated fixtures supporting a partial bridge. An up to 6-years retrospective study. *J Clin Periodontol* 1992;19:118–126.

26. Adell R, Lekholm U, Rockler B, et al: A 15-year study of osseointegrated implants in the treatment of the edentulous jaw. *Int J Oral Surg* 1981;10:387–416.

27. Naert I, Quirynen M, Theuniers G, et al: Prosthetic aspects of osseointegrated fixtures supporting overdentures. A 4-year report. *J Prosthet Dent* 1991;65:671–680.

28. Naert I, Quirynen M, Hooghe M, et al: A comparative prospective study of splinted and unsplinted Brånemark implants in mandibular overdenture therapy: a preliminary report. *J Prosthet Dent* 1994;71:486–492.

29. Jennings KJ: ITI hollow-cylinder and hollow-screw implants: prosthetic management of edentulous patients using overdentures. *Int J Oral Maxillofac Implants* 1991;6:202–206.

30. Donatsky O: Osseointegrated dental implants with ball attachments supporting overdentures in patients with mandibular alveolar ridge atrophy. *Int J Oral Maxillofac Implants* 1993;8:162–166.

31. Marcus SE, Kaste LM, Brown LJ: Prevalence and demographic correlates of tooth loss among the elderly in the United States. *Special Care Dent* 1994;14:123–127.

32. Caplan DJ, Weintraub JA: The oral health burden on the United States: a summary of recent epidemiologic evidence. *J Dent Educ* 1993;57:853–862.

33. Jack SS, Bloom B: National Center for Health Statistics. Use of Dental Services and Dental Health: United States, 1986. Vital Health Stat 10(165). DHHS Pub. No. (PHS) 88-1593. Washington, DC, US Government Printing Office, 1988, pp. 1–84.

34. Kenny R, Richards MW: Photoelastic stress patterns produced by implant-retained overdentures. *J Prosthet Dent* 1998;80:559–564.

35. Menicucci G, Lorenzetti M, Pera P, et al: Mandibular implant-retained overdenture: a clinical trial of two anchorage systems. *Int J Oral Maxillofac Implants* 1998;13:851–856.

36. Batenburg RHK, Raghoebar GM, Van Oort RP, et al: Mandibular overdentures supported by two or four endosteal implants. *Int J Oral Maxillofac Surg* 1998;27:435–439.

37. Wismeijer D, Van Waas MA, Vermeeren JI, et al: Patient satisfaction with implant-supported mandibular overdentures. A comparison of three treatment strategies with ITI-dental implants. *Int J Oral Maxillofac Surg* 1997;26:263–267.

38. Meijer HJ, Starmans FJ, Steen WH, et al: A three-dimensional finite element study on two versus four implants in an edentulous mandible. *Int J Prosthodont* 1994;7:271–279.

39. Fontijn-Tekamp FA, Slagter AP, van't Hof MA, et al: Bite forces with mandibular implant-retained overdentures. *J Dent Res* 1998;77:1832–1839.

40. Chao YL, Meijer HJ, Van Oort RP, et al: The incomprehensible success of the implant stabilized overdenture in the edentulous mandible: a literature review on transfer of chewing forces to bone surrounding implants. *Eur J Prosthodont Restor Dent* 1995;3:255–261.

41. Zarb GA, Schmitt A: The edentulous predicament II: the longitudinal effectiveness of implant-supported overdentures. *J Am Dent Assoc* 1996;127:66–72.

42. Geertman ME, Boerrigter EM, Van Waas MA, et al: Clinical aspects of a multicenter clinical trial of implant-retained mandibular overdentures in patients with severely resorbed mandibles. *J Prosthet Dent* 1996;75:194–204.

43. Jemt T, Chai J, Harnett J, et al: A 5-year prospective multicenter follow up report on overdentures supported by osseointegrated implants. *Int J Oral Maxillofac Implants* 1996;11:291–298.

44. Donatsky O: Osseointegrated dental implants with ball attachments supporting overdentures in patients with mandibular alveolar ridge atrophy. *Int J Oral Maxillofac Implants* 1993;8:162–166.

45. Cune MS, de Putter C, Hoogstraten J: Treatment outcome with implant-retained overdentures: part I—clinical findings and predictability of clinical treatment outcome. *J Prosthet Dent* 1994;72:144–151.

46. Lechner SK, Mammen A: Combination syndrome in relation to osseointegrated implant-supported overdentures: a survey. *Int J Prosthodont* 1996;9:58–64.

47. Batenburg RH, van Oort RP, Reintsema H, et al: Overdentures supported by two IMZ implants in the lower jaw. A retrospective study of peri-implant tissues. *Clin Oral Implants Res* 1994;5:207–212.

48. Thiel CP, Evans DB, Burnett RR: Combination syndrome associated with a mandibular implant-supported overdenture: a clinical report. *J Prosthet Dent* 1996;75:107–113.

49. Denissen HW, Kalk W, van Waas MA, et al: Occlusion for maxillary dentures opposing osseointegrated mandibular prostheses. *Int J Prosthodont* 1993;6:446–450.

50. Jacobs R, van Steenberghe D, Nys M, et al: Maxillary bone resorption in patients with mandibular implant-supported overdentures or fixed prostheses. *J Prosthet Dent* 1993;70:135–140.

51. Maxson BB, Powers MP, Scott RF: Prosthodontic considerations for the transmandibular implant. *J Prosthet Dent* 1990;63:554–558.

52. Barber HD, Scott RF, Maxson BB, et al: Evaluation of anterior maxillary alveolar ridge resorption when opposed by the trans-mandibular implant. *J Oral Maxillofac Surg* 1990;48:1283–1287.

53. Wright PS, Watson RM, Heath MR: The effects of prefabricated bar design on the success of overdentures stabilized by implants. *Int J Oral Maxillofac Implants* 1995;10:79–87.

54. Spiekermann H, Jansen VK, Richter EJ: A 10-year follow-up study of IMZ and TPS implants in the edentulous mandible using bar-retained overdentures. *Int J Oral Maxillofac Implants* 1995;10:231–243.

55. Hemmings KW, Schmitt A, Zarb GA: Complications and maintenance requirements for fixed prostheses and overdentures in the edentulous mandible: a 5-year report. *Int J Oral Maxillofac Implants* 1994;9:191–196.

56. Kucey BK: Implant placement in prosthodontics practice: a five-year retrospective study. *J Prosthet Dent* 1997;77:171–176.

57. Carlson B, Carlsson GE: Prosthodontic complications in osseointegrated dental implant treatment. *Int J Oral Maxillofac Implants* 1994;9:90–94.

58. Walton JN, MacEntee MI: Problems with prostheses on implants: a retrospective study. *J Prosthet Dent* 1994;71:283–288.

59. Hutton JE, Heath MR, Chai JY, et al: Factors related to success and failure rates at 3-year follow-up in a multicenter study of overdentures supported by Brånemark implants. *Int J Oral Maxillofac Implants* 1995;10:33–42.

60. Muftu A, Karabetou S: Complications in implant-supported overdentures. *Compendium* 1997;18:493–504.

61. Feine JS, de Grandmont P, Boudrias P, et al: Within-subject comparisons of implant-supported mandibular prostheses: choice of prosthesis. *J Dent Res* 1994;73:1105–1111.

62. Jonkman RE, van Waas MA, Kalk W: Satisfaction with complete immediate dentures and complete immediate overdentures. A 1 year survey. *J Oral Rehabil* 1995;22:791–796.

63. de Grandmont P, Feine JS, Tache R, et al: Within-subject comparisons of implant-supported mandibular prostheses: a psychometric evaluation. *J Dent Res* 1994;73:1096–1104.

64. Cune MS, de Putter C, Hoogstraten J: Treatment outcome with implant-retained overdentures: part II—patient satisfaction and predictability of subjective treatment outcome. *J Prosthet Dent* 1994;72:152–158.

65. Boerrigter EM, Geertman ME, Van Oort RP, et al: Patient satisfaction with implant-retained mandibular overdentures. A comparison with new complete dentures not retained by implants—a multicentre randomized clinical trial. *Br J Oral Maxillofac Surg* 1995;33:282–288.

66. Harle TJ, Anderson JD: Patient satisfaction with implant-supported prostheses. *Int J Prosthodont* 1993;6:153–162.

67. Humphris GM, Healey T, Howell RA, et al: The psychological impact of implant-retained mandibular prostheses: a cross-sectional study. *Int J Oral Maxillofac Implants* 1995;10:437–444.

68. Geertman ME, van Waas MA, van't Hof MA, et al: Denture satisfaction in a comparative study of implant-retained mandibular overdentures: a randomized clinical trial. *Int J Oral Maxillofac Implants* 1996;11:194–200.

69. Boerrigter EM, Stegenga B, Raghoebar GM, et al: Patient satisfaction and chewing ability with implant-retained mandibular overdentures. *J Oral Maxillofac Surg* 1995;53:1167–1173.

70. Geertman ME, Boerrigtor EM, Van't Hof MA: Two-center clinical trial of implant-retained mandibular overdentures versus complete dentures—chewing ability. *Community Dent Oral Epidemiol* 1996;24:79–84.

71. Wismeijer D, Vermeeren IJH, van Waas MAJ: Patient satisfaction with overdentures supported by one-stage TPS implants. *Int J Oral Maxillofac Implants* 1992;7:51–55.

72. Wismeyer D, van Waas MA, Vermeeren JI: Overdentures supported by ITI implants: a 6.5-year evaluation of patient satisfaction and prosthetic aftercare. *Int J Oral Maxillofac Implants* 1995;10:744–749.

73. Grogono AL, Lancaster DM, Finger IM: Dental implants: a survey of patient's attitudes. *J Prosthet Dent* 1989;62:573–576.

11

EVIDENCE-BASED CRITERIA FOR DIFFERENTIAL TREATMENT PLANNING OF IMPLANT RESTORATIONS FOR THE MAXILLARY EDENTULOUS PATIENT

STEVEN J. SADOWSKY, DDS, FACP,[1] BRIAN FITZPATRICK, BDSC, MDSC, FRACDS,[2] AND DONALD A. CURTIS, DMD, FACP[3]

[1]Department of Integrated Reconstructive Dental Sciences, University of the Pacific, Arthur A. Dugoni School of Dentistry, San Francisco, CA
[2]Prosthodontist in Private Practice, Brisbane, Australia
[3]Department of Preventive & Restorative Dental Sciences, UCSF School of Dentistry, San Francisco, CA

Keywords
Implants; edentulous maxilla; evidence-based dentistry.

Correspondence
Steven J. Sadowsky, University of the Pacific, Arthur A. Dugoni School of Dentistry Integrated Reconstructive Dental Sciences, 2155 Webster 400 M, San Francisco, CA 94115. E-mail: ssadowsky@pacific.edu

The authors deny any conflicts of interest.

Accepted May 25, 2014

Published in *Journal of Prosthodontics* online October 13, 2014

doi: 10.1111/jopr.12226

ABSTRACT

Since the introduction of the endosseous concept to North America in 1982, there have been new permutations of the original ad modum Branemark design to meet the unique demands of treating the edentulous maxilla with an implant restoration. While there is a growing body of clinical evidence to assist the student, faculty, and private practitioner in the algorithms for design selection, confusion persists because of difficulty in assessing the external and internal validity of the relevant studies. The purpose of this article is to review clinician- and patient-mediated factors for implant restoration of the edentulous maxilla in light of the hierarchical level of available evidence, with the aim of elucidating the benefit/risk calculus of various treatment modalities.

Restoration of the maxillary edentulous patient with implants is often more challenging than the mandibular arch due to anatomic, biomechanical, and esthetic considerations. Maxillary bone density is predominantly quality 3, as opposed to the mandible, characterized more commonly as quality 2, using the Lekholm-Zarb classification, which has been correlated to primary implant stability.[1,2] Microcomputed tomography has recently shown the mandible to have 1.8 times the bone mineral density of the maxilla.[3] The resorptive pattern of the edentulous maxilla is superiorly and medially directed, resulting in limitations in both height and width of the bony foundation for implants. In contrast, the progressive atrophy of the mandible often leaves a significant depth and width of basal bone anteriorly to accommodate implants.[4] Biomechanically, the antagonist jaw of a maxillary implant prosthesis is more frequently opposed by anterior teeth or implants than mandibular implant restorations are, leading to higher loading forces.[5] In addition, the rigid maxilla does not have the shock-absorbing effect seen in the cantilevered mandible and may not tolerate applied forces equally.[6] Esthetically, a maxillary implant reconstruction is more demanding due to the impact on appearance of maxillary lip support, lip line, and the gingival and tooth display.[7] The resorptive pattern of the maxilla, when extensive, may also lead to dissatisfaction with certain prosthetic designs, since almost 90% have a smile extended to second premolars,[8] which impacts buccal corridor esthetics.[9] Given these risk factors, it is not surprising that the survival rate and patient satisfaction of maxillary implant prostheses is lower than similar data reported on the mandible.[10–13] Because of these challenges, there continues to be controversy on the appropriate implant treatment for the edentulous maxilla.

Our purpose is to review the indications and prosthetic design recommendations when considering the overdenture (IOD), fixed complete denture (IFCD), and metal ceramic (MC) options.[14] The faculty at the University of the Pacific Arthur A. Dugoni School of Dentistry (San Francisco, CA) has reviewed these guidelines for evidence-based student clinical decision-making in accordance with the Commission on Dental Accreditation (CODA) mandates. The level of evidence varies in each section of the discussion and will be quantified based on Sackett et al's[15] hierarchy (Table 11.1). A MEDLINE search was conducted along with a hand search for articles published over the last 25 years on implant restorative treatment for the maxillary edentulous patient and reviewed by each author.

GENERAL CONSIDERATIONS FOR IMPLANT THERAPY

Complete denture principles are the foundation for determining the anatomic, functional, and esthetic blueprint for an

TABLE 11.1 Sackett's Hierarchy of Evidence[15]

Level of Evidence	Description
1A	Systematic review of randomized controlled trials (RCTs)
1B	RCTs with narrow confidence interval
1C	All or none case series
2A	Systematic review cohort studies
2B	Cohort study/low quality RCT
3A	Systematic review of case-controlled studies
3B	Case-controlled study
4	Case series, poor cohort case controlled study
5	Expert opinion

implant rehabilitation of an edentulous patient. Systemic, local, and patient-mediated concerns are the triad of factors that will influence the suitability and design preference for an implant restoration of the edentulous maxilla, given the available evidence. Systemic risks for implant therapy have been elucidated in a number of publications,[16–23] although the level of evidence indicative of absolute and relative contraindications is low, due to heterogeneity of studies and lack of standardization of populations.[20,24] Emerging evidence, although weak, suggests a correlation between genetic traits and disruption of osseointegration.[25] Local factors influencing implant treatment include bone quality,[26] degree of bone resorption,[27] previous implant failure,[28,29] jaw classification,[30] lip and facial support needs,[31] intermaxillary space,[32] exposure on smile of the transition line between prosthesis and mucosa,[33] and discrepancy of the arches.[34] Patient-mediated factors impacting prosthetic design options may include financial estimates,[35] total risk analysis including adjunctive procedures,[36,37] treatment time,[38] aftercare burden,[39,40] hygiene access,[14] morbidity,[41] phonetics,[27,32] and esthetics.[6,42] The evidence that documents systemic risks is predominantly from level 2B and 3A. The evidence supporting the influence of local factors ranges from level 2B to 5. Patient-mediated factors affecting design options are documented mainly with level 2A to 3B evidence.

INDICATIONS FOR IMPLANT RESTORATION OF THE EDENTULOUS MAXILLA

Quality of life (QoL) outcomes were evaluated in a systematic review, including 18 randomized controlled trials, comparing complete dentures and IODs for the edentulous maxilla.[43] Although high satisfaction ratings were reported for maxillary implant prostheses, the overall ratings were not significantly greater than for a complete denture. In a crossover study by de Albuquerque et al,[44] 13 patients were restored first with a new maxillary and mandibular denture and then with a maxillary IOD (with or without palatal coverage) opposing an IFCD; however, ratings with the implant prostheses were not significantly higher than for new conventional maxillary prostheses. While there have been conflicting reports comparing patient satisfaction of IOD and CD,[45,46] indications for an implant prosthesis include anatomic morphological limitations precluding adequate stability and retention for a CD, patient intolerance for palatal coverage, and treatment of the refractory gagger.[47] Evidence supporting the indications for an implant prosthesis on the edentulous maxilla range from level 2A to 3B.

SELECTION OF FIXED OR REMOVABLE IMPLANT PROSTHETIC DESIGN

While there has been ambiguity in the literature regarding patient preferences for a fixed or removable implant prosthesis,[14,48] each has advantages. Removable designs allow for facial scaffolding and dental esthetics for certain jaw and lip morphologies,[14,30,49] improved hygiene access (except with the MC design),[48,50] latitude in positioning of implants,[32,49] ease in reconciling arch discrepancies,[32] and initial cost savings.[14,27] Fixed prostheses offer retention security,[34] enhanced chewing of hard foods (compared to implant- and tissue-borne overdentures),[48] and reduced maintenance.[40] When MC restorations were compared to IFCD prostheses, the QoL ratings were higher for the former design due to esthetic and functional assessments.[51] Given the relative benefits of these designs, a comprehensive examination and diagnosis is of utmost importance to guide the patient in making appropriate treatment decisions. Selection of fixed or removable designs is documented by level 2B to 3B evidence.

Three assessments are critical to a proper selection of prosthetic design: esthetic factors, occlusal vertical dimension (OVD), and radiographic data.[11,12,14,30,48,52,53] The preference of a removable design will be influenced by the need for lip and cheek support, which often can be predicted by the thickness of a buccal flange of an existing complete denture.[54] Duplicating the complete denture and removing the anterior flange can be diagnostic in determining if the maxillary anterior teeth are sufficient to provide lip and facial support (Fig 11.1). If the anterior/posterior resorption exceeds 10 mm, a removable design is indicated.[55] Secondly, maximum upper lip elevation on smiling will divulge if the prosthetic-tissue junction will be hidden (Fig 11.2A), or if there may be potential esthetic problems with this fixed design.[56] Without the denture in place, if the alveolar ridge is displayed during smiling, the use of a buccal flange in a removable prosthesis may be advisable (Fig 11.2B).[30] However, an IFCD may be selected if an ostectomy has been well planned and executed before implant placement to assure that

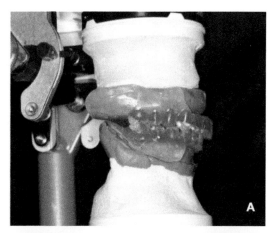

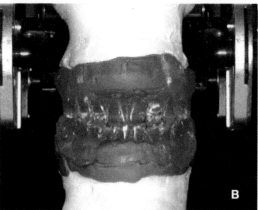

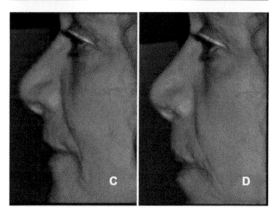

FIGURE 11.1 (A) Sagittal view of horizontal defect of pre-maxilla region using an anterior flangeless duplicated denture. If the teeth are appropriately placed for lip support, a metal ceramic (MC) restoration is not advised. (B) Frontal view of vertical extent of residual ridge resorption. (C) Facial profile with no prosthesis in place. (D) Facial profile with flangeless denture in place demonstrating excessive lip support. With appropriate anterior set-up, an MC restoration is feasible.

the bony platform is superior to the most apical position of the lip on exaggerated smile.[57] Bidra[7] also reported that class II division 2 patients with a terminal maxillary dentition would benefit from orthodontic intrusion of the anterior sextant before extraction, availing them of an IFCD option

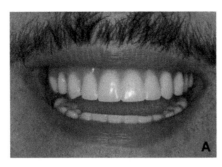 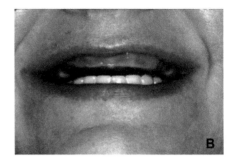

FIGURE 11.2 (A) Exaggerated smile of patient with maxillary fixed complete denture (IFCD) hiding the prosthetic-tissue junction. (B) Display of residual alveolar ridge without any prosthesis in place.

after extraction. A high smile line may also be challenging in an MC restoration because of the difficulty of achieving natural-appearing papillae and symmetrical gingival scalloping.[58,59] This feature is more commonly found in females who demonstrate a higher lip line (1.5 mm on average[60]) than males. Esthetic factors critical to prosthetic design selection are supported by level 3B to 5.

The OVD will often have functional and esthetic ramifications when treatment planning the patient with a maxillary edentulous arch.[61] While no single method has been established to determine OVD, the use of physiologic rest position (VDR), swallowing, phonetic, esthetic, and facial measurements all may contribute to the analysis.[62,63] The appropriate interocclusal distance (facial vertical space between VDR and OVD) is about 3 mm for a skeletal class I, but may be less for a class III and more for a class II.[64] If the existing maxillary denture has been constructed at the appropriate OVD, and the anterior and posterior planes of occlusion are suitable, based on esthetic,[65] phonetic,[66] and biometric references,[67] a duplicate denture/radiographic and surgical template can be fabricated.[68] If the existing denture is not acceptable, an idealized wax-up is required before duplication. AbuJamra et al[69] described a laboratory technique to visualize the interarch space available for implant prosthetic restoration of an edentulous patient. Silicone putty impression material was used to form a resilient cast and an external mold from an approved denture. The denture and resilient cast were mounted on an articulator at the prescribed OVD, and spatial relationships visualized in 3 dimensions when removing the denture from the resilient cast (Fig 11.3). For a Locator-retained IOD (Zest Anchors, Inc., Escondido, CA; Fig 11.4), 8 to 9 mm of intermaxillary space (from crest of soft tissue to antagonist occlusal plane) is recommended; for a resilient bar IOD (Dolder bar; Sterngold, Attleboro, MA; Fig 11.5), 12 mm; for a milled bar IOD (Spark-eroded milled bar; Dental Arts Laboratory, Peoria, IL; Fig 11.6), 11 mm; for an IFCD (Fig 11.7), 11 to 12 mm, and for the MC design (Fig 11.8), 7 mm.[70,71] If insufficient space is available to house the prosthetic components for a desired design, an alveoplasty using a surgical template will be required, based on these measurements.[72] When there is insufficient space, Fajardo

et al,[73] using an in vitro study, demonstrated the effective use of glass fibers to strengthen thin acrylic areas, but planning for appropriate acrylic thickness is recommended. The impact of OVD on pretreatment protocols, anchorage selection, and maintenance is supported mainly by level 4 and 5 evidence.

Treatment planning the patient with an edentulous maxillary arch benefits from the use of a radiographic template in conjunction with an orthopantomogram and/or a CBCT scan, using appropriate selection criteria.[74,75] This allows a prosthetically driven treatment plan and assessment of the available bony height, width, and possibly density.[76,77] The Hounsfield scale has been used to evaluate bone density (with the aid of software programs) along with resonance frequency analysis and insertion torque measurements to make a more objective assessment of the bone quality.[78] When the volume of bone is compromised, sinus augmentation has been commonly used to increase the alveolar bone height prior to implant placement in the posterior maxilla.[79–81] However, the intermaxillary relationship should always be kept in mind, as sinus grafting may represent only part of the reconstructive procedure to rectify limited bone volume.[37] Wallace and Froum,[82] in a systematic review on sinus grafting, reported a mean implant survival rate of 91.8%; more favorable outcomes with roughened implants; particulate versus block grafts; use of a membrane over the lateral window; but not with the use of platelet-rich plasma. In a retrospective multicenter review on sinus grafting, smoking habits of >15 cigarettes/day and residual ridge height <4 mm were significantly associated with reduced implant survival.[83] Given the paucity of evidence evaluating short implants[84] in the restoration of maxillary edentulous patients, as opposed to the partially edentate or mandibular edentulous patients,[84–86] it is still unclear when sinus lift procedures are needed. A Cochrane systematic review noted that, while conclusions are based on small trials with short follow-up, if the residual native bone height is 3 to 6 mm, a crestal approach to lift the sinus lining and place 8 mm implants may lead to fewer complications than a lateral window approach to place longer implants.[87] No significant relationship between crown-to-implant ratio and marginal bone loss has been established, at least when the C:I is

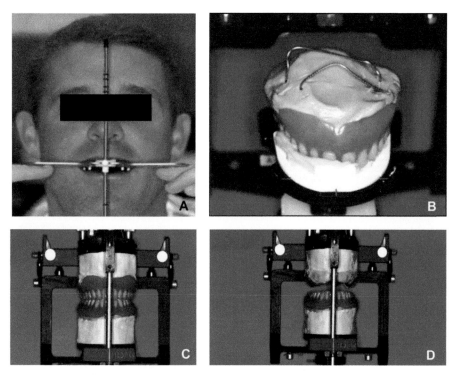

FIGURE 11.3   (A) Facebow registration using Kois Facial Analyzer (Panadent Corp, Grand Terrace, CA). (B) Mounting of the maxillary denture with laboratory putty in the intaglio surface with paper clips to retain mounting stone. This will allow a resilient cast. (C) Maxillary and mandibular dentures on resilient casts, mounted on the articulator at the appropriate occlusal vertical dimension (OVD). (D) Measurement of space allowance before prosthetic design is selected. If insufficient space, the amount of required alveoloplasty can be visualized.

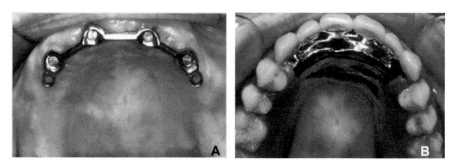

FIGURE 11.4   (A) Locator abutments evenly distributed for maxillary overdenture. (B) Suprastructure overdenture in place over locator abutments. Metal reinforcement adds fracture resistance.

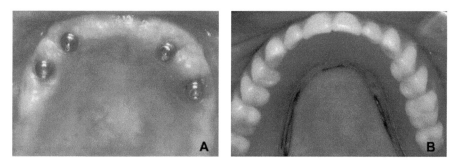

FIGURE 11.5   (A) Dolder bar anchorage system. (B) Suprastructure in place over Dolder bar.

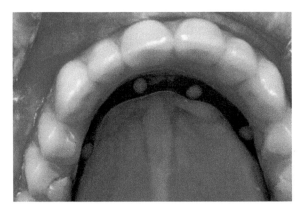

FIGURE 11.6 Implant fixed complete denture.

<3:1.[88] However, esthetic consequences of altering normal anatomic relations may be problematic.[89] Assessment of radiographic data and its influence on treatment planning of implants in the edentulous maxilla is documented predominantly by level 2A to 3B.

Consensus statements on surgical techniques to augment the deficient maxillary edentulous ridge for implants noted that most studies are retrospective in nature.[90] Autogenous onlay bone grafting procedures supporting implants have survival rates slightly lower than those placed in native bone.[37,90] Implants placed in augmented sites opposing unilateral occlusal support showed the highest implant failure rate.[90] Split-ridge and expansion techniques are effective for correction of moderately resorbed edentulous ridges in selective cases, and survival rate of implants following this technique are similar to success in native bone.[90] The use of a graftless approach with pterygomaxillary implants,[91,92] zygomatic implants,[93–96] and/ or tilted implants,[97–99] has been used with high reported success when there is inadequate vertical bone for orthodox implant placement; however, in a 2009 review, Att et al[96] reported that more than half of the 42 studies culled failed to detail the prosthetic outcomes. It is also important to keep in mind that successful implant/prosthodontic outcomes are linked to the level of operator experience.[100,101] Most importantly, when there is a need for additional surgical or interdisciplinary intervention to optimize the site for implants for a particular prosthetic design, a risk, benefit, cost, alternative

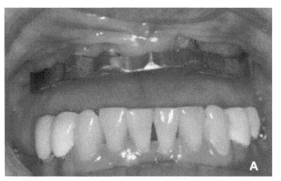

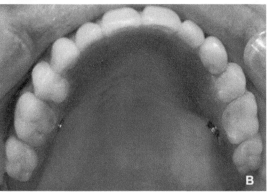

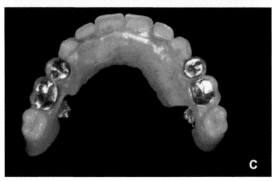

FIGURE 11.7 (A) Milled bar mesostructure for overdenture. (B) Suprastructure milled bar overdenture with swivel latches engaged on palatal shelf in first molar region. (C) Gold occlusal design on posterior teeth to thwart attrition.

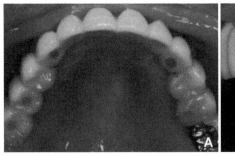

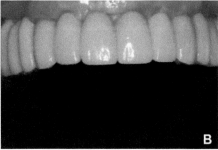

FIGURE 11.8 (A) Screw-retained metal ceramic (MC) design. (B) Gingival-cervical crown junction of the MC design.

analysis is recommended as part of the patient's informed consent. Surgical procedures to augment the deficient edentulous maxilla are documented with level 2A to 3A.

THE IMPLANT OVERDENTURE

In a systematic review, the survival of maxillary implant overdentures was reported to be 93% after at least a 5-year follow-up.[9] The level of evidence is low because of the heterogeneity of the prosthetic methodologies in the included studies, which have varying implant type and number, anchorage systems, and suprastructure designs. Implant overdentures can be classified as either implant-mucosa or implant-supported prostheses. Implant-supported overdentures do not have a mucosal rest and do not allow movement.[49] The advantage of an implant-supported prosthesis is a decrease in prosthetic maintenance, which may compensate over time for initial higher costs.[85,102,103] Decisions regarding the optimal number of implants, anchorage system, suprastructure design, expected maintenance, and immediate loading protocols remain controversial.

Number of Implants

In a recent systematic review, Roccuzzo et al[104] found no studies on the optimal number of implants for maxillary implant-supported overdentures. In a recent consensus report, Gotfredsen et al[105] noted that there were no RCTs available to demonstrate that a particular number of implants for maxillary IODs offered better biological, technical, or patient-mediated outcomes. However, Balaguer et al[11] in a longitudinal prospective study (36- to 159-month follow-up) of 107 maxillary overdentures reported a significantly higher implant survival with six implants compared to four. In a meta-analysis on maxillary IODs, Slot et al[106] also reported a statistical difference in four- and six-implant designs. Varying conclusions may be due to heterogeneity in inclusion criteria and overdenture design as well as the low quality of evidence in maxillary IOD studies.[9] Notwithstanding these data, there appears to be a consensus that a minimum of four implants is recommended for a maxillary IOD, evenly distributed over the arch, for a palateless design.[4,32,107] The distribution and number of implants may have a significant impact on applied load, as was demonstrated by an in vitro study.[108] When the patient presents with a heavy smoking habit, previous failure with implants, or bruxism, more than 4 implants are advised.[10,29] The evidence supporting the number of implants appropriate for an implant overdenture ranges mainly from 1A to 2C, with consensus statements from level 5.

Anchorage Design/Maintenance

In a systematic review, an assessment was made on the influence of maxillary IOD splinted and unsplinted anchorage systems on peri-implant indices and patient satisfaction.[109] There were no significant differences between these designs, except the bar group had reduced maintenance. These data were replicated by an earlier systematic review, a recent Cochrane review, and a 5- to 8-year retrospective clinical study.[49,53,110] Despite these conclusions, there is a lack of standardization of the anchorage design and superstructure, limiting the strength of the evidence.[111] For example, ball and Locator (Zest anchors) attachments have been shown to have different rates of prosthodontic complications, but without reference to number or distribution of implants, palatal coverage, or status of opposing arch.[112] Rigid overdenture designs, with a milled bar and a frictional overcasting that prevents prosthesis rotation, have reduced maintenance in comparison to resilient anchorage designs.[47,102,113] Furthermore, with this system, a number of attachments allow for a biomechanical behavior similar to a fixed prosthetic implant restoration including a spark-eroded swivel latch (Fig 11.7B).[114,115] One overarching problem has been quantification of what constitutes maintenance. Some have classified it in terms of number of appointments,[107] others on the basis of severity: major non-retrievable, major retrievable, and minor retrievable.[116] In summary, for patients requiring facial scaffolding, hygiene access, and retention security, a rigid overdenture design with locking attachments has demonstrated high patient satisfaction as long as the patient has adequate dexterity.[102] In vitro studies have demonstrated reduced center point deviation with milled titanium versus heavier cast frameworks,[117,118] but there seems to be no significant impact on long-term function of restorations.[119] Solitary anchorage designs, on the other hand, may be helpful in patients with limited financial resources, poor oral hygiene, and limited keratinized tissue.[120] Overall, a bar has been recommended when restoring divergent implants of more than 10°.[121] With the resilient designs, a 17% to 22% loosening or fracture rate has been reported in the first year.[4,107,122] Regardless of the anchorage design, the IOD is prone to denture tooth attrition, and a number of materials have been recommended to resist wear (Fig 11.7C).[123,124] Finally, it is apparent that controlled trials on a larger number of participants comparing types of attachments, superstructure designs (including cast metal-[125,126] or fiber-reinforced[127,128] denture bases for resilient superstructures), status of opposing arch, palatal contour, and cost and time analyses are lacking for the maxilla.[13,115] The evidence supporting anchorage design decision making is mainly level 1A to 3A.

Immediate Load Protocols

While there are numerous advantages in immediately loading a maxillary overdenture, including shortening the provisional prosthetic period and overall treatment time, few patient-mediated benefits are documented.[129] The shortcomings in fitting the superstructure to soft tissues that will change weeks later, need for multiple relines, and contamination of the surgical site with impression material or methyl methacrylate all need to be considered in the clinical decision making. Early loading (between 7 days and 8 weeks) has been more frequently used with the selection of roughened implant surfaces and may avoid many of the drawbacks of immediate loading.[129] Systematic reviews have noted that early and conventional loading protocols are better documented than immediate loading and seem to result in fewer failures compared to immediate loading.[129–131] Loading protocols are documented mainly with level 2A to 3B evidence.

THE IMPLANT FIXED COMPLETE DENTURE

Two groups comprising 76 and 109 patients were treated with 450 and 670 implants, respectively, for an IFCD, 15 years apart, and followed for 5 years.[132,133] The two cohorts reflected changes in the implant and prosthetic protocol from 1987 to 2001. Approximately half of the implants in the second cohort received a roughened implant, and all other patients received machined implants. For the late group, the prosthesis was designed more for esthetics by using shorter abutment cylinders and placing the prosthesis closer to the tissue. The 5-year cumulative implant/prosthetic survival rate was 93.4%/97.1% and 97.3%/100.0% for the early and late group, respectively. Patients in the late group had fewer complications with diction and veneer fracture. This underscores the questionable validity of combining results from different time periods.[134] These data were based on patients receiving an average of 6 implants. Assessments regarding the optimal number of implants, framework design, expected maintenance, and immediate loading protocols will facilitate decisions regarding the IFCD, given the best available evidence. The data on IFCDs is supported by level 2A to 2B.

Number of Implants

No comparative trials, let alone RCTs, were available to assess the optimal number and position of implants for a maxillary IFCD. Most of the included studies in a systematic review reported on complication rates for IFCDs supported by 4 to 6 implants without addressing how many reconstructions had 4, 5, or 6 implants.[135] A descriptive study reviewing long-term evidence on implant and prosthodontic survival rates of fixed rehabilitations and reported prosthetic protocols with ≥6 implants showed a higher survival rate than those with <6 implants.[136] The failure of one of the implants with <6 implants could jeopardize the prosthodontic survival and may explain why selected articles showed a lower survival rate with this number.[136] Risk factors such as compromised quality/quantity of bone and high applied forces should also be considered when determining the number of implants.[4] The number of implants for an IFCD is documented by level 2A evidence.

Framework Design

Framework fracture continues to be reported during follow-up periods with IFCDs.[137–139] The most common reasons for these findings were insufficient cross-sectional dimension distal to the terminal implant, poor alloy choice, excessive cantilever length for the anterior/posterior span, and inadequately designed frameworks.[140] Stewart and Staab[141] showed that the "I" and the "L" shaped configurations had the most fracture resistance for cantilevered frameworks. The recommendations that cantilevers may extend at most to 1.5× the anterior/posterior span was empirically established and should be modified by the estimated applied forces (e.g., parafunction, skeletal form, opposing dentition) and number of implants.[140,142] Given that the population of IFCD patients may generate as much as 240 N,[143] current materials are able to accommodate these loads without deformation, as long as the height of the bar is adequate.[143] Optimal thickness will depend on type of metal, number of implants, supporting bone, and loading forces. A broad range of recommendations has been published for the dimensional protocol of cast bars (3–7 mm) and milled bars (2.5 mm).[140] However, a minimum of 4 × 4 mm appears to be a safe dimension for both. Cast noble alloys (gold, silver, palladium, and platinum) and titanium alloys have been used widely and have similar yield strength (825–900 MPa) with similar long-term outcomes.[119,144] Retentive elements (nailhead features, loops, and undercut areas) for denture base materials should be incorporated in the framework design, including posts for anterior teeth, and primed with a silicoater. A framework can only be fabricated after an idealized wax-up dictates its appropriate three-dimensional location by the use of a matrix. Different designs have been investigated. A retrospective study on all-ceramic crowns cemented onto a CAD/CAM titanium framework, with pink ceramic, has reported a 92.4% prosthetic survival rate with a 10-year follow-up, albeit on only 28 maxillary prostheses.[145] Clinical long-term data are lacking for the use of extensive implant-borne zirconia frameworks.[146–148] Framework design principles for the IFCD are documented with predominantly level 2B to 3A evidence.

Maintenance

A systematic review of the biologic and technical complications with IFCDs reported a prosthesis success rate (free of complication) of 8.6% after 10 years.[149] The most common prosthesis-related complication was chipping or fracture of the veneering material (33.3% at 5 years and 66.6% at 10 years).[149] This has been attributed to material failure, framework misfit, inadequate prosthetic space, excessive cantilevers, and laboratory errors. The most common implant-related complication was peri-implant bone loss (>2 mm) at a rate of 40.3% after 10 years. The most frequent prosthesis-related biologic complication was hypertrophy of the tissue around the IFCD (13.0% and 26.0% after 5 and 10 years, respectively).[149] Ten-year results from two separate studies quantified framework fracture at 9.8%.[119,150] A prospective RCT 10-year study on cast titanium-resin prostheses on 24 patients reported a total of 4.7 resin-related complications per prosthesis, which lingual gold onlays reduced.[151] Purcell et al,[152] in a retrospective chart review with an average recall time of almost 8 years, found that patients were 50 times more likely to replace posterior teeth at the 5-year mark than at the 2-year mark. The use of urethane dimethacrylate teeth has been suggested to reduce wear (SR Phonares NHC anterior, SR Phonares NHC posterior; Ivoclar Inc., Amherst, NY).[153] Moffitt et al[154] also speculated that tooth debonding or fracture will continue to be a formidable challenge with this design. Both antagonist occlusal plane evaluation and occlusal equilibration, especially in excursions (including lateral protrusive pathways), are critical to reduce mechanical complications. Maintenance data ranges mainly between level 1A and 2B.

Immediate Loading Protocol

With assiduous patient selection, use of roughened implant surfaces, immediate loading (given a 30 N cm insertion torque) with an IFCD has been shown in a recent meta-analysis to have the same effect on implant survival (90.4% to 100% from 1 to 10 years of follow-up) and complications as with early or conventional loading.[155] Nevertheless, most follow-up times are short, and the investigations demonstrate heterogeneity, including number of implants, which point to the need for comparative studies on different loading protocols reporting complications over a period of greater longevity.

The effective use of tilted implants for terminal abutments for an All-on-4 IFCD has enabled this design to be more universally applied. A meta-analysis demonstrated that there are no more biomechanical or biologic complications with tilted implants as compared to vertically placed implants.[97] Long tilted implants parallel to the anterior wall of the sinus allow for high levels of primary stability, a longer occlusal table, and a shorter cantilever when posterior native bone is unavailable for vertical implants.[156] Patzelt et al[157] completed a systematic review, including 1201 All-on-4 immediately loaded prostheses (within 48 hours), and reported a 99% implant and prosthesis survival rate for 36 months for the maxilla or mandible. Seventy-four percent of the implant failures were documented in the first year. The major prosthetic complication was fracture of the all-acrylic transitional prosthesis, similar to Hinze et al's findings.[158] The conclusions of the systematic review, however, were that the evidence was limited by the quality of the available studies and the lack of long-term outcomes. For example, Browaeys et al[159] reported 30% of the implants in an All-on-4 concept

had almost 2 mm of marginal bone loss after 3 years, but the study was marred by a small sample size, and a multivariate analysis on host factors could not be assessed.

A retrospective analysis of the associated risk factors when restoring 285 maxillae with an All-on-4 approach revealed a number of associated risk factors.[160] Opposing natural dentition (unstable occlusal plane), reduced bone density, male gender, and parafunction were linked to implant failure. The author recommended patient profiling for treatment planning additional implants and/or delayed loading. The evidence supporting the All-on-4 concept is Level 2A-2B.

The Metal Ceramic Design

For patients with sufficient resources and limited alveolar resorption, an MC design can offer a highly esthetic, biocompatible, functional, and hygienic restoration with reduced bulk and maintenance as compared to the IOD and IFCD designs.[34,161] However, both surgical and prosthodontic acumen is required, since the implants must be congruent with the crowns, and the creation of a natural morphology of the tooth/tissue junction is rigorous. Complete fixed, segmented rehabilitations supported by 6 to 8 rough surface implants have been documented in a review with a 96.4% prosthodontic survival rate at the 10-year endpoint.[137] No statistical differences have been reported between segmented and one-piece full-arch maxillary reconstructions and in the interest of protocol simplification, passive fit, laboratory steps, and repair; 1 or 2 anterior and 2 posterior splinted segments are practical.[136,162] In an ovoid dental arch, implants in the canine positions and at least one additional implant in the central incisor position will resist forces created by an anterior lever arm, reducing stress on the abutment screws.[161] Early approaches with machined implants achieved a 5-year cumulative implant survival rate of 98.5% with immediate implantation, without immediate loading.[163] Immediate loading of immediately placed implants suffers from a lack of scientific validation by clinical data.[130] Following a maximum observation period of 10 years (median 29 months) on 25 patients, immediate loading of rough-surfaced, screw-type implants in the healed edentulous maxilla for a MC restoration demonstrated a 98.2% success rate for implants and 88% for patients.[164] The time of implantation did not influence survival or success rates. The authors did express caution when using more than 10 implants or lengths of 10 mm or less.[164] The evidence documenting the MC restoration is level 2A to 3B.

Maintenance

There is a dearth of studies on complications with the MC design with observation periods of at least 5 years on

TABLE 11.2   Algorithm for Decision Making in Treatment Planning the Implant Restoration of the Edentulous Maxilla

	Limited Alveolar Resorption	Moderate-to-Advanced Alveolar Resorption	
Prosthetic design	Metal ceramic design	Fixed complete denture	Overdenture
Intermaxillary space allowance	Ideally 7 mm	≥11–12 mm	Locator (≥8–9 mm), bar and clip (≥12 mm), milled bar with overcasting (≥11 mm)
Local factors	Sufficient bone for implants congruent with crowns positioned for segmented prostheses, esthetic approval of smile design	No display of the prosthetic/tissue junction, facial esthetic approval without flange	Requires anterior flange, discrepant arches easier to reconcile, severe resorption may need adjunctive surgical augmentation or tilted/ zygomatic implants
Patient-related factors	Financial acceptance	Preference for fixed, accepting of limited hygiene access	Accepting of a removable design although possibility of a latching device, hygiene access priority
Number of implants	6–8 implants	Five to six implants depending on bone quality/quantity, bruxism, heavy smoking, opposing natural dentition, previous failure with implants	Five to six implants depending on bone quality/quantity, bruxism, heavy smoking, opposing natural dentition, previous failure with implants
Anchorage design	Preferably screw-retained	4 × 4 mm framework with retentive features and tribochemical preparation	Solitary anchors may be indicated if imitations in financial resources, home care facility, or keratinized tissue. A rigid bar system is recommended if divergence of implants and/or high retention needs

Ultimately, clinical judgment and emerging evidence of sound scientific rigor will govern decision making.

conventionally, early, or immediately loaded implants in the completely edentulous patient.[149] Two studies investigating mainly partially edentulous patients have reported a dominant and costly complication. Bragger et al[165] calculated a threefold increase in ceramic veneer fracture on implant MC FDPs compared to tooth-supported restorations, after 4 to 5 years of service. Kinsel and Lin[166] found a sevenfold increase in ceramic fracture when the opposing dentition was implant-supported or when the patient was a bruxer. Patients who did not wear an orthotic had twice the odds of porcelain fracture.[166] The impact of occlusal scheme has not been established. Other technical problems, such as prosthetic/abutment screw loosening, of retention of cemented prostheses have been less prevalent than veneer fracture.[167] Biological complications are mostly patient-based and can be related to heredity, susceptibility to peri-implantitis, and poor oral hygiene; when operator error is not an overriding factor.[168] Despite substantial improvements in implant dentistry over time, technical, biological, and esthetic complications are still frequent.[169] This places a premium on retrievability, and if cement-retained units are designed, radiopaque provisional cements are recommended. Longitudinal studies reporting on adverse clinical outcomes are necessary to provide practitioners with evidence-based treatment planning and patients with informed consent.[170] Level 2A to 5 evidence supports the discussion on maintenance of the MC restoration.

SUMMARY

An algorithm has been generated to provide an overview of the decision-making criteria when considering restoring the edentulous maxilla with an IOD, IFCD, or MC prosthesis (Table 11.2). The implant restoration of the edentulous maxilla continues to be demanding in light of the density and volume of bone, anatomic limitations, antagonist arch presentation, esthetic considerations, and the frequency of biologic and technical complications. Design considerations have been described to assist in treatment planning decision making to improve cost-effectiveness and patient satisfaction. The hierarchical level of evidence supporting the discussion in each section has been graded, and gives credence to the need for more randomized controlled trials and longitudinal comparative studies on larger cohorts.

REFERENCES

1. Truhlar RS, Orenstein IH, Morris HF, et al: Distribution of bone quality in patients receiving endosseous dental implants. *J Oral Maxillofac Surg* 1997;55(12 Suppl 5):38–45.
2. Farre-Pages N, Auge-Castro ML, Alaejos-Algarra F, et al: Relation between bone density and primary implant stability. *Med Oral Patol Oral Cir Bucal* 2011;16:e62–e67.

3. Kim YJ, Henkin J: Micro-computed tomography assessment of human alveolar bone: bone density and three-dimensional micro-architecture. *Clin Implant Dent Rel Res* 2013; doi: 10.1111/cid.12109.

4. Reich KM, Huber CD, Lippnig WR, et al: Atrophy of the residual alveolar ridge following tooth loss in an historical population. *Oral Dis* 2011;17:33–44.

5. Sadowsky SJ: Treatment considerations for maxillary implant overdentures: a systematic review. *J Prosthet Dent* 2007;97: 340–348.

6. Rodriguez AM, Orenstein IH, Morris HF, et al: Survival of various implant-supported prosthesis designs following 36 months of clinical function. *Ann Periodontol* 2000;5:101–108.

7. Bidra AS: Three-dimensional esthetic analysis in treatment planning for implant-supported fixed prosthesis in the edentulous maxilla: review of the esthetics literature. *J Esthet Restor Dent* 2011;23:219–236.

8. Dong JK, Jin TH, Cho HW, et al: The esthetics of the smile: a review of some recent studies. *Int J Prosthodont* 1999; 12:9–19.

9. Malhotra S, Sidhu MS, Prabhakar M, et al: Characterization of a posed smile and evaluation of facial attractiveness by panel perception and its correlation with hard and soft tissue. *Orthodontics (Chic.)* 2012;13:34–45.

10. Rohlin M, Nilner K, Davidson T, et al: Treatment of adult patients with edentulous arches: a systematic review. *Int J Prosthodont* 2012;25:553–567.

11. Balaguer J, Ata-Ali J, Penarrocha-Oltra D, et al: Long-term survival rates of implants supporting overdentures. *J Oral Implantol* 2013 Jun 10 [Epub ahead of print].

12. Brennan M, Houston F, O'Sullivan M, et al: Patient satisfaction and oral health-related quality of life outcomes of implant overdentures and fixed complete dentures. *Int J Maxillofac Implants* 2010;25:791–800.

13. Andreiotelli M, Att W, Strub JR: Prosthodontic complications with implant overdentures: a systematic literature review. *Int J Prosthodont* 2010;23:195–203.

14. Zitzmann NU, Marinello CP: Treatment outcomes of fixed or removable implant-supported prostheses in the edentulous maxilla. Part I: patients' assessments. *J Prosthet Dent* 2000;83:424–433.

15. Sackett DL, Rosenberg WM, Gray JA, et al: Evidence-based medicine: what it is and what it isn't. *Br Med J* 1996;312: 71–72.

16. Esser E, Wagner W: Dental implants following radical oral cancer surgery and adjuvant radiotherapy. *Int J Oral Maxillofac Implants* 1997;12:552–557.

17. Wagner W, Esser E, Ostkamp K: Osseointegration of dental implants in patients with and without radiotherapy. *Acta Oncol* 1998;37:693–696.

18. Koka S, Babu NM, Norell A: Survival of dental implants in post-menopausal bisphosphonate users. *J Prosthodont Res* 2010;54:108–111.

19. Hellstein JW, Adler RA, Edwards B, et al: Managing the care of patients receiving antiresorptive therapy for prevention and treatment of osteoporosis: executive summary of recommendations from the American Dental Association Council on Scientific Affairs. *J Am Dent Assoc* 2011;142:1243–1251.

20. Cochran DL, Schou S, Heitz-Mayfield LJ, et al: Consensus statements and recommended clinical procedures regarding risk factors in implant therapy. *Int J Oral Maxillofac Implants* 2009;24 Suppl:86–89.

21. Moy PK, Medina D, Shetty V, et al: Dental implant failure rates and associated risk factors. *Int J Oral Maxillofac Implants* 2005;20:569–577.

22. Heitz-Mayfield LJ, Huynh-Ba G: History of treated periodontitis and smoking as risks for implant therapy. *Int J Oral Maxillofac Implants* 2009;24 Suppl:39–68.

23. Sadowsky SJ, Bedrossian E: Evidenced-based criteria for differential treatment planning of implant restorations for the partially edentulous patient. *J Prosthodont* 2013;22: 319–329.

24. Bornstein MM, Cionca N, Mombelli A: Systemic conditions and treatments as risks for implant therapy. *Int J Oral Maxillofac Implants* 2009;24 Suppl:12–27.

25. Liddelow G, Klineberg I: Patient-related risk factors for implant therapy. A critique of pertinent literature. *Aust Dent J* 2011;56:417–426, quiz 41.

26. Friberg B, Jemt T, Lekholm U: Early failures in 4,641 consecutively placed Branemark dental implants: a study from stage 1 surgery to the connection of completed prostheses. *Int J Oral Maxillofac Implants* 1991;6:142–146.

27. Zitzmann NU, Marinello CP: Fixed or removable implant-supported restorations in the edentulous maxilla: literature review. *Pract Periodontics Aesthet Dent* 2000;12:599–608.

28. Weyant RJ, Burt BA: An assessment of survival rates and within-patient clustering of failures for endosseous oral implants. *J Dent Res* 1993;72:2–8.

29. Ekfeldt A, Christiansson U, Eriksson T, et al: A retrospective analysis of factors associated with multiple implant failures in maxillae. *Clin Oral Implants Res* 2001;12:462–467.

30. Zitzmann NU, Marinello CP: Treatment plan for restoring the edentulous maxilla with implant-supported restorations: removable overdenture versus fixed partial denture design. *J Prosthet Dent* 1999;82:188–196.

31. Eckert SE, Carr AB: Implant-retained maxillary overdentures. *Dent Clin North Am* 2004;48:585–601.

32. Mericske-Stern RD, Taylor TD, Belser U: Management of the edentulous patient. *Clin Oral Implants Res* 2000;11 Suppl 1: 108–125.

33. Taylor TD: Fixed implant rehabilitation for the edentulous maxilla. *Int J Oral Maxillofac Implants* 1991;6:329–337.

34. Sadowsky SJ: The implant-supported prosthesis for the edentulous arch: design considerations. *J Prosthet Dent* 1997;78: 28–33.

35. MacEntee MI, Walton JN: The economics of complete dentures and implant-related services: a framework for analysis and preliminary outcomes. *J Prosthet Dent* 1998; 79:24–30.

36. Jensen SS, Terheyden H: Bone augmentation procedures in localized defects in the alveolar ridge: clinical results with different bone grafts and bone-substitute materials. *Int J Oral Maxillofac Implants* 2009;24 Suppl:218–236.

37. Chiapasco M, Casentini P, Zaniboni M: Bone augmentation procedures in implant dentistry. *Int J Oral Maxillofac Implants* 2009;24 Suppl:237–259.

38. Johannsen A, Wikesjo U, Tellefsen G, et al: Patient attitudes and expectations of dental implant treatment—a questionnaire study. *Swed Dent J* 2012;36:7–14.

39. Chung WE, Rubenstein JE, Phillips KM, et al: Outcomes assessment of patients treated with osseointegrated dental implants at the University of Washington Graduate Prosthodontic Program, 1988 to 2000. *Int J Oral Maxillofac Implants* 2009;24:927–935.

40. Katsoulis J, Brunner A, Mericske-Stern R: Maintenance of implant-supported maxillary prostheses: a 2-year controlled clinical trial. *Int J Oral Maxillofac Implants* 2011;26:648–656.

41. Kim S, Lee YJ, Lee S, et al: Assessment of pain and anxiety following surgical placement of dental implants. *Int J Oral Maxillofac Implants* 2013;28:531–535.

42. Springer NC, Chang C, Fields HW, et al: Smile esthetics from the layperson's perspective. *Am J Orthod Dentofacial Orthop* 2011;139:e91–e101.

43. Thomason JM, Heydecke G, Feine JS, et al: How do patients perceive the benefit of reconstructive dentistry with regard to oral health-related quality of life and patient satisfaction? A systematic review. *Clin Oral Implants Res* 2007;18 Suppl 3: 168–188.

44. de Albuquerque Junior RF, Lund JP, Tang L, et al: Within-subject comparison of maxillary long-bar implant-retained prostheses with and without palatal coverage: patient-based outcomes. *Clin Oral Implants Res* 2000;11:555–565.

45. Allen PF, McMillan AS, Walshaw D: A patient-based assessment of implant-stabilized and conventional complete dentures. *J Prosthet Dent* 2001;85:141–147.

46. Zembic A, Wismeijer D: Patient-reported outcomes of maxillary implant-supported overdentures compared with conventional dentures. *Clin Oral Implants Res* 2014;25:441–450.

47. Visser A, Raghoebar GM, Meijer HJ, et al: Implant-retained maxillary overdentures on milled bar suprastructures: a 10-year follow-up of surgical and prosthetic care and aftercare. *Int J Prosthodont* 2009;22:181–192.

48. Heydecke G, Boudrias P, Awad MA, et al: Within-subject comparisons of maxillary fixed and removable implant prostheses: patient satisfaction and choice of prosthesis. *Clin Oral Implants Res* 2003;14:125–130.

49. Zou D, Wu Y, Huang W, Zhang Z, et al: A 5- to 8-year retrospective study comparing the clinical results of implant-supported telescopic crown versus bar overdentures in patients with edentulous maxillae. *Int J Oral Maxillofac Implants* 2013;28:1322–1330.

50. Slot W, Raghoebar GM, Vissink A, et al: Maxillary overdentures supported by four or six implants in the anterior region; 1-year results from a randomized controlled trial. *J Clin Periodontol* 2013;40:303–310.

51. Preciado A, Del Rio J, Lynch CD, et al: Impact of various screwed implant prostheses on oral health-related quality of life as measured with the QoLIP-10 and OHIP-14 scales: a cross-sectional study. *J Dent* 2013;41:1196–1207.

52. DeBoer J: Edentulous implants: overdenture versus fixed. *J Prosthet Dent* 1993;69:386–390.

53. Bryant SR, MacDonald-Jankowski D, et al: Does the type of implant prosthesis affect outcomes for the completely edentulous arch? *Int J Oral Maxillofac Implants* 2007;22 Suppl: 117–139.

54. Parel SM: Implants and overdentures: the osseointegrated approach with conventional and compromised applications. *Int J Oral Maxillofac Implants* 1986;1:93–99.

55. Drago C, Carpentieri J: Treatment of maxillary jaws with dental implants: guidelines for treatment. *J Prosthodont* 2011;20:336–347.

56. Kourkouta S: Implant therapy in the esthetic zone: smile line assessment. *Int J Periodontics Restorative Dent* 2011;31: 195–201.

57. Jensen OT, Adams MW, Cottam JR, et al: The All-on-4 shelf: maxilla. *J Oral Maxillofac Surg* 2010;68:2520–2527.

58. Bidra AS, Agar JR: A classification system of patients for esthetic fixed implant-supported prostheses in the edentulous maxilla. *Compend Contin Educ Dent* 2010;31:366–374.

59. Bidra AS, Agar JR, Parel SM: Management of patients with excessive gingival display for maxillary complete arch fixed implant-supported prostheses. *J Prosthet Dent* 2012; 108:324–331.

60. Jahanbin A, Pezeshkirad H: The effects of upper lip height on smile esthetics perception in normal occlusion and nonextraction, orthodontically treated females. *Indian J Dent Res* 2008;19:204–207.

61. Discacciati JA, Lemos de Souza E, Vasconcellos WA, et al: Increased vertical dimension of occlusion: signs, symptoms, diagnosis, treatment and options. *J Contemp Dent Pract* 2013;14:123–128.

62. Koller MM, Merlini L, Spandre G, et al: A comparative study of two methods for the orientation of the occlusal plane and the determination of the vertical dimension of occlusion in edentulous patients. *J Oral Rehabil* 1992;19:413–425.

63. Millet C, Jeannin C, Vincent B, et al: Report on the determination of occlusal vertical dimension and centric relation using swallowing in edentulous patients. *J Oral Rehabil* 2003; 30:1118–1122.

64. Loh PL, Chew CL: Interocclusal distance in patients with different skeletal patterns. *Singapore Dent J* 1995;20:4–7.

65. Miller CJ: The smile line as a guide to anterior esthetics. *Dent Clin North Am* 1989;33:157–164.

66. Pound E: Let/S/be your guide. *J Prosthet Dent* 1977;38:482–489.

67. Nissan J, Barnea E, Zeltzer C, et al: Relationship between occlusal plane determinants and craniofacial structures. *J Oral Rehabil* 2003;30:587–591.

68. Huynh-Ba G, Alexander P, Vierra MJ, et al: Using an existing denture to design a radiographic template for a two-implant mandibular overdenture. *J Prosthet Dent* 2013;109:53–56.

69. AbuJamra NF, Stavridakis MM, Miller RB: Evaluation of interarch space for implant restorations in edentulous patients: a laboratory technique. *J Prosthodont* 2000;9:102–105.

70. Phillips K, Wong KM: Vertical space requirement for the fixed-detachable, implant-supported prosthesis. *Compend Contin Educ Dent* 2002;23:750–756.

71. Phillips K, Wong KM: Space requirements for implant-retained bar-and-clip overdentures. *Compend Contin Educ Dent* 2001;22:516–522.

72. Desjardins RP: Prosthesis design for osseointegrated implants in the edentulous maxilla. *Int J Oral Maxillofac Implants* 1992;7:311–320.

73. Fajardo RS, Pruitt LA, Finzen FC, et al: The effect of E-glass fibers and acrylic resin thickness on fracture load in a simulated implant-supported overdenture prosthesis. *J Prosthet Dent* 2011;106:373–377.

74. Gray CF: Practice-based cone-beam computed tomography: a review. *Prim Dent Care* 2010;17:161–167.

75. Fortin T, Camby E, Alik M, Isidori M, et al: Panoramic images versus three-dimensional planning software for oral implant planning in atrophied posterior maxillary: a clinical radiological study. *Clin Implant Dent Relat Res* 2013;15:198–204.

76. Marquezan M, Osorio A, Sant'Anna E, et al: Does bone mineral density influence the primary stability of dental implants? A systematic review. *Clin Oral Implants Res* 2012;23:767–774.

77. Isoda K, Ayukawa Y, Tsukiyama Y, et al: Relationship between the bone density estimated by cone-beam computed tomography and the primary stability of dental implants. *Clin Oral Implants Res* 2012;23:832–836.

78. Fuster-Torres MA, Penarrocha-Diago M, Penarrocha-Oltra D, et al: Relationships between bone density values from cone beam computed tomography, maximum insertion torque, and resonance frequency analysis at implant placement: a pilot study. *Int J Oral Maxillofac Implants* 2011;26:1051–1056.

79. Del Fabbro M, Wallace SS, Testori T: Long-term implant survival in the grafted maxillary sinus: a systematic review. *Int J Periodontics Restorative Dent* 2013;33:773–783.

80. Jensen OT, Shulman LB, Block MS, et al: Report of the Sinus Consensus Conference of 1996. *Int J Oral Maxillofac Implants* 1998;13 Suppl:11–45.

81. Becktor JP, Isaksson S, Sennerby L: Survival analysis of endosseous implants in grafted and nongrafted edentulous maxillae. *Int J Oral Maxillofac Implants* 2004;19:107–115.

82. Wallace SS, Froum SJ: Effect of maxillary sinus augmentation on the survival of endosseous dental implants: a systematic review. *Ann Periodontol* 2003;8:328–343.

83. Testori T, Weinstein RL, Taschieri S, et al: Risk factor analysis following maxillary sinus augmentation: a retrospective multi-center study. *Int J Oral Maxillofac Implants* 2012;27:1170–1176.

84. Jokstad A: The evidence for endorsing the use of short dental implants remains inconclusive. *Evid Based Dent* 2011;12:99–101.

85. Stellingsma K, Raghoebar GM, Visser A, et al: The extremely resorbed mandible, 10-year results of a randomized controlled trial on 3 treatment strategies. *Clin Oral Implants Res* 2014;25:926–932.

86. Carr AB: Survival of short implants is improved with greater implant length, placement in the mandible compared with the maxilla, and in nonsmokers. *J Evid Based Dent Pract* 2012;12:18–191.

87. Esposito M, Grusovin MG, Rees J, et al: Interventions for replacing missing teeth: augmentation procedures of the maxillary sinus. *Cochrane Database Syst Rev* 2010; CD008397.

88. Blanes RJ, Bernard JP, Blanes ZM, et al: A 10-year prospective study of ITI dental implants placed in the posterior region. II: influence of the crown-to-implant ratio and different prosthetic treatment modalities on crestal bone loss. *Clin Oral Implants Res* 2007;18:707–714.

89. Anitua E, Pinas L, Orive G: Retrospective study of short and extra-short implants placed in posterior regions: influence of crown-to-implant ratio on marginal bone loss. *Clin Implant Dent Relat Res* 2013; doi: 10.1111/cid.12073.

90. Chen ST, Beagle J, Jensen SS, et al: Consensus statements and recommended clinical procedures regarding surgical techniques. *Int J Oral Maxillofac Implants* 2009;24 Suppl:272–278.

91. Balshi TJ, Wolfinger GJ, Slauch RW, et al: A retrospective comparison of implants in the pterygomaxillary region: implant placement with two-stage, single-stage, and guided surgery protocols. *Int J Oral Maxillofac Implants* 2013;28:184–189.

92. Candel E, Penarrocha D, Penarrocha M: Rehabilitation of the atrophic posterior maxilla with pterygoid implants: a review. *J Oral Implantol* 2012;38:461–466.

93. Yates JM, Brook IM, Patel RR, et al: Treatment of the edentulous atrophic maxilla using zygomatic implants: evaluation of survival rates over 5–10 years. *Int J Oral Maxillofac Surg* 2014;43:237–242.

94. Aparicio C, Ouazzani W, Garcia R, et al: A prospective clinical study on titanium implants in the zygomatic arch for prosthetic rehabilitation of the atrophic edentulous maxilla with a follow-up of 6 months to 5 years. *Clin Implant Dent Relat Res* 2006;8:114–122.

95. Bedrossian E: Rehabilitation of the edentulous maxilla with the zygoma concept: a 7-year prospective study. *Int J Oral Maxillofac Implants* 2010;25:1213–1221.

96. Att W, Bernhart J, Strub JR: Fixed rehabilitation of the edentulous maxilla: possibilities and clinical outcome. *J Oral Maxillofac Surg* 2009;67:60–73.

97. Monje A, Chan HL, Suarez F, et al: Marginal bone loss around tilted implants in comparison to straight implants: a meta-analysis. *Int J Oral Maxillofac Implants* 2012;27:1576–1583.

98. Francetti L, Corbella S, Taschieri S, et al: Medium- and long-term complications in full-arch rehabilitations supported by upright and tilted implants. *Clin Implant Dent Relat Res* 2013; doi: 10.1111/cid.12180.

99. Cavalli N, Barbaro B, Spasari D, et al: Tilted implants for full-arch rehabilitations in completely edentulous maxilla: a retrospective study. *Int J Dent* 2012;2012:180379.

100. Lambert PM, Morris HF, Ochi S: Positive effect of surgical experience with implants on second-stage implant survival. *J Oral Maxillofac Surg* 1997;55(12 Suppl 5):12–18.

101. Zoghbi SA, de Lima LA, Saraiva L, et al: Surgical experience influences 2-stage implant osseointegration. *J Oral Maxillofac Surg* 2011;69:2771–2776.

102. Krennmair G, Krainhofner M, Piehslinger E: Implant-supported maxillary overdentures retained with milled bars: maxillary anterior versus maxillary posterior concept—a retrospective study. *Int J Oral Maxillofac Implants* 2008;23: 343–352.

103. Tipton PA: The milled bar-retained removable bridge implant-supported prosthesis: a treatment alternative for the edentulous maxilla. *J Esthet Restor Dent* 2002;14:208–216.

104. Roccuzzo M, Bonino F, Gaudioso L, et al: What is the optimal number of implants for removable reconstructions? A systematic review on implant-supported overdentures. *Clin Oral Implants Res* 2012;23 Suppl 6:229–237.

105. Gotfredsen K, Wiskott A, Working Group 4: Consensus report—reconstructions on implants. The Third EAO Consensus Conference 2012. *Clin Oral Implants Res* 2012;23 Suppl 6:238–241.

106. Slot W, Raghoebar GM, Vissink A, et al: A systematic review of implant-supported maxillary overdentures after a mean observation period of at least 1 year. *J Clin Periodontol* 2010;37:98–110.

107. Kiener P, Oetterli M, Mericske E, et al: Effectiveness of maxillary overdentures supported by implants: maintenance and prosthetic complications. *Int J Prosthodont* 2001; 14:133–140.

108. Damghani S, Masri R, Driscoll CF, et al: The effect of number and distribution of unsplinted maxillary implants on the load transfer in implant-retained maxillary overdentures: an in vitro study. *J Prosthet Dent* 2012;107:358–365.

109. Stoumpis C, Kohal RJ: To splint or not to splint oral implants in the implant-supported overdenture therapy? A systematic literature review. *J Oral Rehabil* 2011;38:857–869.

110. Al-Ansari A: No difference between splinted and unsplinted implants to support overdentures. *Evid Based Dent* 2012;13: 54–55.

111. Osman RB, Payne AG, Ma S: Prosthodontic maintenance of maxillary implant overdentures: a systematic literature review. *Int J Prosthodont* 2012;25:381–391.

112. Cakarer S, Can T, Yaltirik M, et al: Complications associated with the ball, bar and Locator attachments for implant-supported overdentures. *Med Oral Patol Oral Cir Bucal* 2011;16: e953–e959.

113. Ferrigno N, Laureti M, Fanali S, et al: A long-term follow-up study of non-submerged ITI implants in the treatment of totally edentulous jaws. Part I: ten-year life table analysis of a prospective multicenter study with 1286 implants. *Clin Oral Implants Res* 2002;13:260–273.

114. Bueno-Samper A, Hernandez-Aliaga M, Calvo-Guirado JL: The implant-supported milled bar overdenture: a literature review. *Med Oral Patol Oral Cir Bucal* 2010;15: e375–e378.

115. Brudvik JS, Chigurupati K: The milled implant bar: an alternative to spark erosion. *J Can Dent Assoc* 2002;68:485–488.

116. Tolman DE, Laney WR: Tissue-integrated prosthesis complications. *Int J Oral Maxillofac Implants* 1992;7:477–484.

117. Paniz G, Stellini E, Meneghello R, et al: The precision of fit of cast and milled full-arch implant-supported restorations. *Int J Oral Maxillofac Implants* 2013;28:687–693.

118. Ortop A, Jemt T, Back T, et al: Comparisons of precision of fit between cast and CNC-milled titanium implant frameworks for the edentulous mandible. *Int J Prosthodont* 2003;16: 194–200.

119. Ortop A, Jemt T: CNC-milled titanium frameworks supported by implants in the edentulous jaw: a 10-year comparative clinical study. *Clin Implant Dent Relat Res* 2012;14:88–99.

120. Gobbato L, Avila-Ortiz G, Sohrabi K, et al: The effect of keratinized mucosa width on peri-implant health: a systematic review. *Int J Oral Maxillofac Implants* 2013;28:1536–1545.

121. Walton JN, MacEntee MI, Glick N: One-year prosthetic outcomes with implant overdentures: a randomized clinical trial. *Int J Oral Maxillofac Implants* 2002;17:391–398.

122. Payne AG, Tawse-Smith A, Thomson WM, et al: One-stage surgery and early loading of three implants for maxillary overdentures: a 1-year report. *Clin Implant Dent Relat Res* 2004;6:61–74.

123. Kumar S, Arora A, Yadav R: An alternative treatment of occlusal wear: cast metal occlusal surface. *Indian J Dent Res* 2012;23:279–282.

124. Livaditis JM, Livaditis GJ: The use of custom-milled zirconia teeth to address tooth abrasion in complete dentures: a clinical report. *J Prosthodont* 2013;22:208–213.

125. Mericske-Stern R, Oetterli M, Kiener P, et al: A follow-up study of maxillary implants supporting an overdenture: clinical and radiographic results. *Int J Oral Maxillofac Implants* 2002;17:678–686.

126. Kramer A, Weber H, Benzing U: Implant and prosthetic treatment of the edentulous maxilla using a bar-supported prosthesis. *Int J Oral Maxillofac Implants* 1992;7:251–255.

127. Stipho HD: Repair of acrylic resin denture base reinforced with glass fiber. *J Prosthet Dent* 1998;80:546–550.

128. Narva KK, Lassila LV, Vallittu PK: The static strength and modulus of fiber reinforced denture base polymer. *Dent Mater* 2005;21:421–428.

129. Schimmel M, Srinivasan M, Herrmann FR, et al: Loading protocols for implant-supported overdentures in the edentulous jaw: a systematic review and meta-analysis. *Int J Oral Maxillofac Implants* 2014;29 Suppl: 271–286.

130. Gallucci GO, Morton D, Weber HP: Loading protocols for dental implants in edentulous patients. *Int J Oral Maxillofac Implants* 2009;24 Suppl:132–146.

131. Strub JR, Jurdzik BA, Tuna T: Prognosis of immediately loaded implants and their restorations: a systematic literature review. *J Oral Rehabil* 2012;39:704–717.

132. Jemt T, Stenport V, Friberg B: Implant treatment with fixed prostheses in the edentulous maxilla. Part 1: implants and biologic response in two patient cohorts restored between

1986 and 1987 and 15 years later. *Int J Prosthodont* 2011; 24:345–355.

133. Jemt T, Stenport V: Implant treatment with fixed prostheses in the edentulous maxilla. Part 2: prosthetic technique and clinical maintenance in two patient cohorts restored between 1986 and 1987 and 15 years later. *Int J Prosthodont* 2011;24:356–362.

134. Bozini T, Petridis H, Garefis K, et al: A meta-analysis of prosthodontic complication rates of implant-supported fixed dental prostheses in edentulous patients after an observation period of at least 5 years. *Int J Oral Maxillofac Implants* 2011;26:304–318.

135. Heydecke G, Zwahlen M, Nicol A, et al: What is the optimal number of implants for fixed reconstructions: a systematic review. *Clin Oral Implants Res* 2012;23 Suppl 6:217–228.

136. Lambert FE, Weber HP, Susarla SM, et al: Descriptive analysis of implant and prosthodontic survival rates with fixed implant-supported rehabilitations in the edentulous maxilla. *J Periodontol* 2009;80:1220–1230.

137. Davis DM, Packer ME, Watson RM: Maintenance requirements of implant-supported fixed prostheses opposed by implant-supported fixed prostheses, natural teeth, or complete dentures: a 5-year retrospective study. *Int J Prosthodont* 2003;16:521–523.

138. Jemt T, Johansson J: Implant treatment in the edentulous maxillae: a 15-year follow-up study on 76 consecutive patients provided with fixed prostheses. *Clin Implant Dent Relat Res* 2006;8:61–69.

139. Ortorp A, Jemt T: Clinical experiences with laser-welded titanium frameworks supported by implants in the edentulous mandible: a 10-year follow-up study. *Clin Implant Dent Relat Res* 2006;8:198–209.

140. Drago C, Howell K: Concepts for designing and fabricating metal implant frameworks for hybrid implant prostheses. *J Prosthodont* 2012;21:413–424.

141. Stewart RB, Staab GH: Cross-sectional design and fatigue durability of cantilevered sections of fixed implant-supported prostheses. *J Prosthodont* 1995;4:188–194.

142. English CE: Critical A-P spread. *Implant Soc* 1990;1:2–3.

143. Carr AB, Laney WR: Maximum occlusal force levels in patients with osseointegrated oral implant prostheses and patients with complete dentures. *Int J Oral Maxillofac Implants* 1987;2:101–108.

144. Ucar Y, Brantley WA, Johnston WM, et al: Mechanical properties, fracture surface characterization, and microstructural analysis of six noble dental casting alloys. *J Prosthet Dent* 2011;105:394–402.

145. Malo P, de Araujo Nobre M, Borges J, et al: Retrievable metal ceramic implant-supported fixed prostheses with milled titanium frameworks and all-ceramic crowns: retrospective clinical study with up to 10 years of follow-up. *J Prosthodont* 2012;21:256–264.

146. Guess PC, Att W, Strub JR: Zirconia in fixed implant prosthodontics. *Clin Implant Dent Relat Res* 2012;14:633–645.

147. Hassel AJ, Shahin R, Kreuter A, et al: Rehabilitation of an edentulous mandible with an implant-supported fixed prosthesis using an all-ceramic framework: a case report. *Quintessence Int* 2008;39:421–426.

148. Rojas-Vizcaya F: Full zirconia fixed detachable implant-retained restorations manufactured from monolithic zirconia: clinical report after two years in service. *J Prosthodont* 2011;20:570–576.

149. Papaspyridakos P, Chen CJ, Chuang SK, et al: A systematic review of biologic and technical complications with fixed implant rehabilitations for edentulous patients. *Int J Oral Maxillofac Implants* 2012;27:102–110.

150. Attard NJ, Zarb GA: Long-term treatment outcomes in edentulous patients with implant-fixed prostheses: the Toronto study. *Int J Prosthodont* 2004;17:417–424.

151. Fischer K, Stenberg T: Prospective 10-year cohort study based on a randomized controlled trial (RCT) on implant-supported full-arch maxillary prostheses. Part 1: sandblasted and acid-etched implants and mucosal tissue. *Clin Implant Dent Relat Res* 2012;14:808–815.

152. Purcell BA, McGlumphy EA, Holloway JA, et al: Prosthetic complications in mandibular metal-resin implant-fixed complete dental prostheses: a 5- to 9-year analysis. *Int J Oral Maxillofac Implants* 2008;23:847–857.

153. Drago C, Gurney L: Maintenance of implant hybrid prostheses: clinical and laboratory procedures. *J Prosthodont* 2013;22:28–35.

154. Moffitt AR, Woody RD, Parel SM, et al: Failure modes with point loading of three commercially available denture teeth. *J Prosthodont* 2008;17:432–438.

155. Papaspyridakos P, Chen C-J, Chuang S-K, et al: Implant loading protocols for edentulous patients with fixed prostheses: a systematic review and meta-analysis. *Int J Oral Maxillofac Implants* 2014;29 Suppl:256–270.

156. Menini M, Signori A, Tealdo T, et al: Tilted implants in the immediate loading rehabilitation of the maxilla: a systematic review. *J Dent Res* 2012;91:821–827.

157. Patzelt SB, Bahat O, Reynolds MA, Strub JR: The All-on-Four treatment concept: a systematic review. *Clin Implant Dent Relat Res* 2013; doi: 10.1111/cid.12068.

158. Hinze M, Thalmair T, Bolz W, et al: Immediate loading of fixed provisional prostheses using four implants for the rehabilitation of the edentulous arch: a prospective clinical study. *Int J Oral Maxillofac Implants* 2010;25:1011–1018.

159. Browaeys H, Dierens M, Ruyffelaert C, et al: Ongoing crestal bone loss around implants subjected to computer-guided flapless surgery and immediate loading using the All-on-4 concept. *Clin Implant Dent Rel Res* 2014; doi: 10.1111/cid.12197.

160. Parel SM, Phillips WR: A risk assessment treatment planning protocol for the four implant immediately loaded maxilla: preliminary findings. *J Prosthet Dent* 2011;106:359–366.

161. Jivraj S, Chee W, Corrado P: Treatment planning of the edentulous maxilla. *Br Dent J* 2006;201:261–279.

162. Gallucci GO, Bernard JP, Belser UC: Treatment of completely edentulous patients with fixed implant-supported restorations: three consecutive cases of simultaneous immediate loading in

both maxilla and mandible. *Int J Periodontics Restorative Dent* 2005;25:27–37.

163. Schwartz-Arad D, Chaushu G: Full-arch restoration of the jaw with fixed ceramometal prosthesis. *Int J Oral Maxillofac Implants* 1998;13:819–825.

164. Streizel FP, Karmon B, Lorean A, et al: Implant-prosthetic rehabilitation of edentulous maxilla and mandible with immediately loaded implants: preliminary data from a retrospective study, considering time of implantation. *Int J Oral Maxillofac Implants* 2011;26:139–147.

165. Bragger U, Aeschlimann S, Burgin W, et al: Biological and technical complications and failures with fixed partial dentures (FPD) on implants and teeth after four to five years of function. *Clin Oral Implants Res* 2001;12:26–34.

166. Kinsel RP, Lin D: Retrospective analysis of porcelain fractures of metal ceramic crowns and fixed partial dentures supported by 729 implants in 152 patients: patient-specific and implant-specific predictors of ceramic failure. *J Prosthet Dent* 2009;101:388–394.

167. Salvi GE, Bragger U: Mechanical and technical risks in implant therapy. *Int J Oral Maxillofac Implants* 2009;24 Suppl: 69–85.

168. Klinge B, Meyle J: Post-implant tissue destruction. The Third EAO Consensus Conference 2012. *Clin Oral Implants Res* 2012;23 Suppl 6:108–110.

169. Pjetursson BE, Asgeirsson AG, Zwahlan M, et al: Improvements in implant dentistry over the last decade. Comparison of survival and complication rates in older and newer publications. *Int J Oral Maxillofac Implants* 2004;29 Suppl: 308–324.

170. Eckert SE, Choi YG, Sanchez AR, et al: Comparisons of dental implant systems quality of clinical evidence and prediction of 5-year survival. *Int J Oral Maxillofac Implants* 2005;20:406–415.

12

RELEVANT ANATOMIC AND BIOMECHANICAL STUDIES FOR IMPLANT POSSIBILITIES ON THE ATROPHIC MAXILLA: CRITICAL APPRAISAL AND LITERATURE REVIEW

PAULO HENRIQUE ORLATO ROSSETTI, DDS, MSC, PHD,[1] WELLINGTON CARDOSO BONACHELA, DDS, MSC, PHD,[2] AND LEYLHA MARIA NUNES ROSSETTI, DDS, MSC, PHD[3]

[1]Professor, Discipline of Prosthodontics and Implantology, Sagrado Coração University, Bauru, Sao PauloBrazil
[2]Associate Professor, Department of Prosthodontics, Bauru Dental School, Sao Paulo University, Bauru, São PauloBrazil
[3]Private Practice in Prosthodontics, Bauru, São PauloBrazil

Keywords

Atrophic; severely resorbed; maxilla; biomechanics; dental implants; review.

Correspondence

Paulo Henrique Orlato Rossetti, R. Dr. Servio T. C. Coube, 3–33 apto 21-B, 17012-632 Bauru, São Paulo, Brazil. E-mail: phrossetti@uol.com.br

Accepted August 14, 2009

Published in *Journal of Prosthodontics* August 2010; Vol. 19, Issue 6

doi: 10.1111/j.1532-849X.2010.00615.x

ABSTRACT

Purpose: The purpose of this review was to highlight anatomic and biomechanical aspects of atrophic maxillae for implant possibilities.

Materials and Methods: A MEDLINE electronic search of the years 1966 to 2009 was conducted with the keywords "atrophic," "resorbed," "edentulous," and "maxilla."

Results: Twenty papers presented the following findings: (1) previous use of a removable prosthesis is a risk factor for resorption, with flabby tissues related to the severity of resorption; (2) implants in the reconstructed maxilla (≤5 mm) and supporting overdentures had a higher risk for bone loss based on the worse peri-implant soft-tissue health observed; (3) bleeding on probing was found with pocket depths ≥5 mm in half of the zygomatic implants; (4) prevalence of bone septa is higher in atrophic maxillae, and changes on nasopalatine canal can reduce up to 44.4% of the full length of buccal bone plates; (5) female patients have less medullar bone quantity and connectivity than male patients; (6) transectioning of nutrient vessels is easier and accelerates resorption; (7) stress does not concentrate on maxillary sinus base cortical bone contiguous to trabecular bone; (8) splinted implants receive nine times less load than nonsplinted

Journal of Prosthodontics on Dental Implants, First Edition. Edited by Avinash S. Bidra and Stephen M. Parel.

implants even under oblique loading; (9) implant stability quotient (ISQ) values for implants ranged between 60 and 65; (10) in vivo force transfer to implants is similar between fixed prostheses and overdentures; (11) inclined implants generate better biomechanical responses; (12) masticatory efficiency

and bite forces improve in maxillectomized patients who receive obturators with milled bar attachments.

Conclusion: Sound implant-supported choices for an atrophic maxilla must be made with a thorough understanding of its anatomic and biomechanical factors.

The term atrophy is defined in the dictionary as "a wasting away; a diminution in the size of a cell, tissue, organ, or part."[1] According to Wolff's Law, "the bone remodels according to applied forces,"[2] and every time osseous function is modified, a definitive change on inner architecture and external configuration is seen.[3] The lack of stimuli (disuse atrophy) seen on maxillary arches after tooth extraction is more intense at the first year and continuous throughout life,[4] with many cases showing severe alveolar bone resorption in height and width. This phenomenon is variable, irreversible, and unpredictable, even for patients wearing immediate complete conventional prostheses.[5] Nowadays, most of the esthetic and functional deficiencies generated by bone atrophy have been supplemented with several implant-supported/retained modalities, accompanied or not by autogenous bone/biomaterial grafts.[6]

In this sense, knowledge of anatomic and biomechanical problems at the atrophic maxillary arches is fundamental for adequate treatment planning and success of these reconstructions. The aim of this review is to provide clinicians with solid scientific aspects for a thorough decision-making process.

MATERIALS AND METHODS

To verify relevant anatomic and biomechanical studies, a PubMed/MEDLINE electronic search was conducted within the years of 1966 to 2009. The keywords "atrophic," "resorbed," "edentulous," and "maxilla" were combined and resulted in 472 studies (atrophic AND maxilla), 189 studies (atrophic AND edentulous AND maxilla), and 41 studies (atrophic AND resorbed AND maxilla). The MESH terms "biomechanics," "atrophy," and "maxilla" generated one study. Citations on anatomic and biomechanical issues were manually checked throughout the texts by two examiners (LMNR, WCB). Both in vitro and in vivo data were included; animal trials were not found. For the first reviewed aspect, not all articles described the degree of atrophy according to a standard classification published in the literature. Also, no randomized controlled clinical trials were identified for the second reviewed aspect. Finally, only 20 references regarding anatomy (nine studies: one laboratorial; two case series; two clinical; three anatomic; one cadaveric sections) and biomechanical characteristics (11 studies: 3 clinical prospective;

1 clinical, short-term; 2 clinical, cross-sectional; 2 clinical, case series, 1 anatomic, cadaver sections, 2 laboratorial, cross-sectional) were selected. Details of these data (classification of atrophic maxillary state, study design, groups, results, and conclusions) are presented in Tables 12.1 and 12.2.

RESULTS

Anatomic Considerations—Extrinsic Morphology

The atrophic maxilla is composed of a residual alveolar ridge and a mucous tissue of varied resilience. These two components make up its extrinsic morphology. Variations in height are seen along the ridges and provide clinicians a previous idea of implant length. Orthopantomographic analysis (magnification rate 1:1.25) of 173 edentulous maxillae (90 men and 83 women, mean age: 60 years) showed the following mean height values: median line = 16 mm, first premolar region = 16.5 mm, and first molar region = 15.5 mm, distance from the inferior border of maxillary sinus to alveolar crest = 6.3 mm;[7] however, clinicians must remember that, even with such "enthusiastic" values, the degree of resorption at the alveolar ridge can also be severe. Another study showed previous use of a removable prosthesis was a risk factor for residual resorption (odds ratio = 2.4), as was the presence of a flabby tissue with the severity of resorption (odds ratio = 2.4); nevertheless, duration of edentulism in these patients was not a significant risk factor. When these 168 maxillae were compared to the panoramic radiographs of dentate patients, reductions in height at the anterior and posterior regions were of 18% and 11%, respectively.[8]

One of the first issues during treatment of maxillary atrophic arches is the achievement of adequate stability at the bone/implant interface. Fortunately, implant placement at posterior regions is not influenced by crest width, but related to the height of the ridges. After examining 47 histological sections, the authors verified that the height at the second premolar/first molar (M1) and at second molar (M2) regions ranged from 3.23 to 7.97 mm and 5.68 to 7.81 mm, respectively; however, it was observed that crest widths at 1 mm, 3 mm, 7 mm, and 10 mm above the top of the ridge (Cawood and Howell class VI) were for M1 and M2 regions, respectively, 3.31 and 4.42 mm, 6.86 and 6.45 mm, 14.07 and 10.2 mm, and zero.[9]

TABLE 12.1 Relevant Studies on Intrinsic and Extrinsic Anatomical Aspects for Implant Possibilities in the Atrophic Maxilla

Authors (Year)	Maxillary Atrophic Status	Design and Studied Parameters	Results	Conclusions
Güler et al (1995)[7]	Nonspecified	Laboratorial, retrospective - 173 edentulous patients (90 men, 83 women) - vertical height measurements at eight maxillary sites (median line, premolar, and molars), based on panoramic radiographs	The most inferior border of maxillary sinuses are located anterior to the first molar in 48.9% (men) and 55.4% (women)	Results can aid clinicians on treatment planning for implant location
Ulm et al (1995)[9]	Cawood and Howell	Retrospective, undecalcified anatomic sections - 36 complete and 11 partially edentulous patients - alveolar ridge height measurements - alveolar ridge widths from 1 mm, 7 mm, and 10 mm below alveolar ridge crest	For Cawood and Howell's class VI: height = 3.23 to 5.68 mm widths: (1 mm) = 3.31 to 4.42 mm (7 mm) = 14.07 to 10.22 mm (10 mm) = *	Bone widths in atrophic maxillae are efficient for implant placement
Xie et al (1997)[8]	Moderate resorption: ≤15% in height Severe resorption: >15% in height	Clinical, retrospective - 168 edentulous maxillae - panoramic radiographic analysis - parameters: history of edentulousness, use of previous dentures, use of complete denture, denture-bearing soft tissue lesions, dental status of opposing jaw, and oral hygiene habits	- bone height decreases of 12% and 18% on posterior and anterior regions, respectively - resorption not related to duration of edentulism, but to the quality of prosthesis - previous use of removable prostheses contributes to resorption (odds ratio = 2.4) - flabby tissue ridges related to severity of resorption (odds ratio = 2.4)	Influence of local resorption factors was more pronounced in the maxillary arches
Ulm et al (1999)[20]	Lekholm and Zarb	Retrospective - 134 available histological sections (29 women, 23 men) at lateral incisor, first premolar and molar tooth regions - parameters: volume, thickness, number, and trabecular separation; trabecular bone pattern factor	All analyzed parameters present reduced amounts at the first molar region	Women showed less bone quantity and trabecular connectivity than men
Solar et al (1999)[23]	Cawood and Howell	Retrospective: 18 anatomic sections (Cawood and Howell's classes II and III) - topography of posterior superior alveolar artery (PSAA) and related anastomosis; location of infraorbital artery (IOA) - distance between caudal main branches with the alveolar bone, as well as emergence of these arteries	- Eight cases of extraosseous arterial anastomosis - arterial lumen of PSAA and IOA are the same (1.6 mm)	Transectioning of important arterial communications accelerates resorption

(continued)

TABLE 12.1 (Continued)

Authors (Year)	Maxillary Atrophic Status	Design and Studied Parameters	Results	Conclusions
Kaptein et al (1999)[10]	Original bone height below maxillary sinus floor: <5 mm (severe atrophy) >5 mm or more	Clinical, prospective - Group I: sinus floor <5 mm (77 patients, 433 implants) - Group II: sinus floor ≥5 mm (11 patients, 37 implants) - maxillary sinus grafting with iliac crest bone and hydroxyapatite particles (3:1 ratio) - restorations: overdentures or fixed prostheses - parameters: probing depth, plaque, gingival, and bleeding indexes; keratinized mucosa	- probing depths and bleeding on probing frequently observed on Group I - significant increasing on peri-implant probing depth and gingival index of overdentures compared to fixed prostheses	Implants on reconstructed maxillae with overdentures had more risk of bone loss based on the worst soft tissue peri-implant observed condition
Al-Nawas et al (2004)[11]	Nonspecified (severe maxillary atrophy)	Case series, retrospective - 20 patients, 20 implants; 13 zygomatic fixtures (severe maxillary atrophy); and seven for tumor resection - microbiological analyses, DNA probes	- pathogens (4/20 implants) - bleeding on probing (9/20 implants); four positive microbiological findings - pockets ≥5 mm resulting in a 55% implant success rate	Soft tissue problems must be considered when zygomatic implants are an alternative for maxillary arches
Kim et al (2006)[18]	Nonspecified	Case series, prospective - 100 patients: 22% completely edentulous - 85 atrophic maxillary sinuses (42%) - septa height >2.5 mm - reformatted CTs: (field of view = 15 cm, 200 mA, 120 kV, sections 1 mm thick, scanning time = 1 s)	- septa prevalence (27 of 85) - lower septa height on atrophic maxillae - no differences on septa location - more frequency of primary septa on nonatrophic maxillae	- wide anatomic variations for all investigated parameters regardless of atrophic state - invaluable data to avoid complications on sinus augmentation procedures
Mardinger et al (2008)[19]	Lekholm and Zarb: Class A: control group Classes B to E: study group	Case series, retrospective - 207 Korean patients - mapping of shape, length, diameter (the nasopalatine canal) - mapping of residual alveolar ridge, buccal to the canal opening - reconstructed CTs	- funnel-shaped canal (56.6%) on type E ridges - canal lengths: from 10.7 mm (class A) to 9 mm (class E) - buccal bone plate: 44.4% less than its original length - regions anterior to the canal: 60% less than their original thicknesses	- the nasopalatine canal increases in all directions and after aging - the palatal opening is 32% enlarged and can occupy up to 58% of the alveolar width at potential sites for two central incisors implant placement

* According to Ulm et al, "In class 6 (extremely resorbed ridges), the measurements of width of the alveolar ridge at 10 mm below the ridge crest could not be made, as the alveolar ridges grouped in this class were markedly lower than 10 mm."

TABLE 12.2 Relevant Studies on Biomechanical Aspects for Implant Possibilities on the Atrophic Maxilla

Authors (Year)	Maxillary Atrophic Status	Design and Studied Parameters	Results	Conclusions
Mericske-Stern et al (2000)[35]	Nonspecified (the patient had a maxillary implant-supported overdenture)	Clinical, cross-sectional - one patient (49 years old) - five implants (3 years of use) - piezoelectric transducers - maximum bite force: centric occlusion and bite plane studies on overdenture (two bar designs) and fixed prostheses - selected chewing foods: bread, apples	- similar forces on both implant-supported prostheses - greater forces on posterior implants and along the long axis - vertical similar forces on food chewing	- similar force patterns for overdenture and fixed prostheses - overdenture's bar design did not influence force patterns
Duyck et al (2000)[36]	Nonspecified (patients wearing their prostheses with success for 0 to 12 years)	Clinical, cross-sectional - four patients (maxillary arch) - extensometers (20 registrations) - 50 N load - forces measured first on three to four implants and five to six implants later	- greater forces with reduced implant numbers - compressive forces on implants near application point	Higher bending moments with only three implants activated; more clinical research is necessary
Meyer et al (2001)[26]	- atrophic maxilla (8-mm height) - mean maxilla (12-mm height)	Laboratorial, cross-sectional - FEM mesh with 10,000 elements - bicortical fixation, two cortical bone modalities (2 mm and 0.5 mm) - 150 N axial loading	- stresses three times lower in the buccolingual direction - microstrains around implant neck: thick cortical (4000), lack of cortical (5000), reduced bone height (6000)	Supraphysiological bone deformations can be expected for implants in the atrophic maxillae
Fortin et al (2002)[37]	Bone height: 10 mm at posterior region	Clinical, prospective - immediate loading - 45 patients; 245 implants - 5-year follow-up - Marius bridge concept	- implant success rate: 97% - prosthesis success rate: 100% - few prosthetic failures without compromising overall patient well-being and prosthesis wear	Treatment type is effective and predictable; removable prosthesis can be considered a fixed type still providing lip support and adequate phonetics
Olsson et al (2003)[33]	Nonspecified. Lekholm and Zarb's classification for bone density	Clinical, case series - ten patients; 61 oxidized implants - RFA (resonance frequency analysis)	- bone loss (1.3 mm/year) - ISQ values: 60.1 and 62.8 after 4 months	Predictable immediate loading over six to eight implants in the atrophic maxilla; however, more longitudinal studies are necessary
Fukuda et al (2004)[39]	Nonspecified	Clinical, case series - seven maxillectomized patients (bone and sometimes muscle grafts); (some at HBO therapy) - parameters: masticatory function (questionnaire), biting capacity (pressure detector), speech (Hirose's score: 0 to 8 points); marginal bone loss (radiographs)	- improvements on masticatory function (77.1 points), biting capacity (317.9 N) and speech (mean of five points) - bone loss: 0.42 mm (first year), 0.61 mm (follow-up)	Obturator prostheses on milled bars are useful on oral rehabilitation of tumor resected, edentulous maxillary patients

(*continued*)

TABLE 12.2 (*Continued*)

Authors (Year)	Maxillary Atrophic Status	Design and Studied Parameters	Results	Conclusions
Hallman et al (2005)[32]	Cawood and Howell classes IV and V (posterior region); classes III and IV (anterior region)	Clinical, prospective follow-up - 20 patients, 108 implants - bovine and autogenous bone graft (80:20 ratio); implants placed 6 months after - RFA, CTs, and marginal bone loss	- implant survival rate: 86% - ISQ 66 for residual and grafted bones (after 3 years) - bone loss: 1.3 mm after 3 years - 71% of healthy maxillary sinuses according to CTs	Maxillary sinus grafting with a mixture of autogenous and bovine bone is a reliable procedure
Nomoto et al (2006)[28]	Nonspecified. Three-dimensional (3D) bone morphometric analysis	Laboratorial, cadaver model - 10 Japanese patients - micro-CT-based FEA - loads on first molar, corresponding alveolar region, and with implant placed	- stress around cortical bone only in the edentulous maxilla - stresses around implant similar to that found around first molar	A model simulating trabecular bone allows more precise evaluation on stress distribution
Sjöström et al (2007)[30]	Cawood and Howell	Clinical, prospective - 29 patients, iliac crest bone grafts - 192 implants inserted 6 to 8 months later - RFA (four times)	- premature failure (20 implants) - ISQs: 60 (abutment connection), 62.5 (after 6 months), and 61.8 (3 years of use with definitive prosthesis) - marginal bone loss (0.3 mm)	SQ values serve as risk indicators for implant loading on atrophic maxillae
Ujigawa et al (2007)[27]	Nonspecified (severely resorbed maxilla)	Laboratorial - CTs from a 68-year-old patient - mesh with 112,000 nodes for FEA - zygomatic implant splinted to the remaining infrastructure or not - applied loads: axial (150 N), lateral (50 N)	- nonsplinted implant: stress on the zygoma bone, median implant region, and implant - abutment junction - no stress on the alveolar bone of the splinted implant	The stress is supported by zygomatic bone, distributed along the infrazygomatic crest, and divided between the frontal and temporal processes of zygomatic bone
Veltri et al (2008)[31]	Cawood and Howell	Clinical, short-term - 12 patients: eight women, four men - 73 implants with surface treatment (Ø = 3.5 mm) - prostheses inserted 6 months later - RFA measurements - radiographic marginal bone loss	- implant success rate: 100% (1 year of function) - ISQs: 63 (implant placement), 60 (abutment connection), 61 (1 year later); bone loss: 0.3 mm (after 1 year of loading)	Narrow implants can be used to restore class IV atrophic maxillae as alternative to complex grafting techniques

Compared to the nongrafted ridges, the transplanted bone and the overlying soft tissues of atrophic maxillae show different quality, quantity, and topographic characteristics. During analysis of 470 implants placed in 88 patients with severe atrophy (maxillary sinus thickness less than 5 mm), bleeding was observed in 46.2% in the overdenture group and 38.6% in cases with fixed prostheses. Also, bleeding and greater pocket depths were observed in groups with less than 5 mm of the initial maxillary sinus floor height. The thickness of keratinized mucosa was similar in both groups.[10] Implants in the reconstructed maxilla and supporting overdentures had a higher risk for bone loss based on the worse peri-implant soft-tissue health observed.

In the same way, soft-tissue health assumes a particularly important role on zygomatic fixtures and their associated prostheses with transmucosal abutments. When 20 implants were inserted in 14 patients, colonization by periodontal pathogens was observed at four implants. Further, nine implants demonstrated bleeding on probing, four of these with positive microbiological findings; sites without bleeding present negative results ($p < 0.026$). At sites with bleeding, pocket probing depths ≥ 5 mm were found, indicating soft tissue problems and a success rate of only 55%.[11]

Over the years, some authors have categorized edentulous ridges (Atwood,[12] Fallschüssel[13]); however, two classifications are the most used: Cawood and Howell's classification,[14] which divides atrophic maxillae into four groups (class III = adequate height and width; class IV = knife-edge ridges, with adequate height, and inadequate width; class V = inadequate height and width; and class VI = depression found at ridges), and the Lekholm and Zarb classification,[15] which implies a quantitative and qualitative analysis of residual alveolar bones (type 1 = large homogenous cortical bone; type 2 = thick cortical layer surrounding a dense medullar bone; type 3 = thin cortical layer surrounding a dense medullar bone; type 4 = thin cortical layer surrounding a sparse medullar bone). Both classifications, however, are bi-dimensional representations and do not show the three-dimensionality of atrophic ridges and associated defects, now evidenced by modern cone-beam computerized tomography (CT) techniques.[16] Even so, most of the decision-making processes available in the literature were initially based on these classifications, and they still have their value for treatment planning.

Anatomic Considerations—Intrinsic Morphology

After tooth extraction, increased osteoclastic activity and bone resorption lead to coronal maxillary sinus floor expansion.[17] One study with reformatted CTs comparing the prevalence, height, location, and morphology of maxillary septa in 100 Korean patients (200 maxillary sinus in 41 women and 59 men), considered 85% of these sites atrophic (42.5% of patients). The prevalence of septa was significantly

higher in atrophic than nonatrophic maxillae (31.76% and 22.61%, respectively); however, no differences among distribution of septa (anterior, middle, and posterior maxillary sinuses) were found, regardless of degree of atrophy. Also, differences of septa height between atrophic (2.84 mm) and nonatrophic (4.19 mm) maxillae were statistically significant ($p < 0.05$).[18]

Progressive bone loss can also result in approximation of alveolar ridges and important anatomic structures (nasopalatine canal), preventing implant placement.[19] One study with 207 individuals verified these changes based on Lekholm and Zarb's classification (classes A to E). The canal length decreased from 10.7 mm (class A) to 9 mm (class E). The canal diameter increased as the resorption proceeded. The mean increase in diameter (classes B to E) was 1.8 mm (32%) at the palatal area and 0.7 mm at the nasal canal region. For the severely resorbed maxillae (classes C, D, and E) and when the canal was positioned over the ridge, 35.6% of the proposed site for the central incisor was occupied. The buccal bone plate lost almost 44.4% of its full length, reducing from 17.22 mm (class A) to 9.57 mm (class E) ($p < 0.01$). The buccal bony plate anterior to the canal lost 60% of its mean width and reduced from 6.4 mm (class A) to 2.6 mm (class E) ($p < 0.01$).

By means of histomorphometric studies, the trabecular pattern of atrophic edentulous maxillae was analyzed in 62 cadavers (29 women and 23 men) resulting in 156 sections with 5 mm of thickness, at the lateral incisor (I2), premolar (P1), and molar (M1) sites. When these sections were grouped according to Lekholm and Zarb's classification, types 1 and 2 were not found; for types 3 and 4, the following incidence values were seen (for men and women): (I2 = 82.61% and 82.76%; 17.39% and 17.24%), (P1 = 77.78% and 72.41%; 22.22% and 27.59%), and (M1 = 38.46% and 31.82%; 61.54% and 68.18%). Still, using 134 undecalcified sections of the same regions, the authors quantified the bone trabecular volume (I2 = 20.2 to 27.9%; P1 = 20.5 to 26.7%; M1 = 17.1 to 23.4%), mean trabecular thickness (I2 = 112 to 133 μm; P1 = 121 to 138 μm; M1 = 95 to 118 μm), mean trabecular number (I2 = 1.81 to 2.07 mm^{-1}; P1 = 1.68 to 1.91 mm^{-1}; 1.76 to 1.95 mm^{-1}), mean trabecular separation (I2 = 363 to 480 μm; P1 = 412 to 507 μm; M1 = 424 to 535 μm), as well as the trabecular bone pattern factor (TBPF) (I2 = −1.106 to 0.171 mm^{-1}; P1 = −0.562 to 0.450 mm^{-1}; M1 = −0.078 to 0.123 mm^{-1}). In most cases, the buccal and alveolar compartments were reduced, compared to the palatal ones. Women showed less medullar bone quantity and connectivity than men.[20]

One important aspect also observed in atrophic maxillae is that pneumatization at the sinus floor and continuous medullar bone loss result in a thin ridge at posterior regions; thus, nutrient vessels (arteries) to the alveolar process present a small-sized lumen, from a centromedullar to an exclusive mucoperiosteal origin. Thus, minimally invasive techniques avoiding too much bone exposition would prevent considerable resorption at host bone areas on healing.[21] Also, clinicians must observe two important communications: one between the infraorbital artery and the capillaries overlying the alveolar process, and the other between the infraorbital artery and the posterior superior alveolar artery inside the bony wall of the maxillary sinus.[22,23] For example, severing of these vessels that keep the regional blood flow during sinus lift or grafting procedures can lead to unexpected bone resorption and poor healing of the grafts.[24]

Biomechanics in the Atrophic Maxilla

Available studies on biomechanics were represented by finite element analysis (FEA), resonance frequency analysis (RFA), or strain-gauge/force transducer measurements. Even thus, the information is still scarce, with most studies represented by prospective or retrospective case series.

First, one must understand masticatory load distribution in totally dentate individuals: mandibular molars transmit load to the upper molars, where the lingual and the two buccal roots decompose the overall force vector to the cranial base. When FEA was performed based on CT models, the maxillary sinus showed the highest stress and deformation rates; also, similar findings were seen at the hard palate region and at the posterior bony portion of the nasal septa (vomer and perpendicular plate of ethmoid bone). In this way, bones lateral to the maxillary sinus underwent stress coming from buccal roots, as forces from the lingual roots are spread on the palatal septa complex (bones medial to the maxillary sinus).[25]

Under mechanical loading, FEA of implants inserted on normal and atrophic maxillae show supraphysiological bone strain at the implant surface on the latter. Stresses are more homogenous when more spongy bone is found. An atrophic ridge combined with inadequate bone quality generates up to 6000 microstrains at surface level. Here, less importance is given to the bone crest on the quality of dissipation stress and strains under mechanical cycling.[26]

Axial loading (150 N) on zygomatic implants splinted to conventional fixtures or not and lateral loading (50 N) at the palatal surface of suprastructures were conducted. The stresses concentrated around the alveolar bone in the splinted mode. On the other hand, the stresses are generated on the zygomatic bone, middle part of the fixture, and at the implant/abutment interface. First, the zygoma withstands the stresses from occlusal forces, which transfer them to the infrazygomatic crest, being divided at the frontal and temporal process of zygomatic bone in several directions.[27]

Micro-CT techniques were added to the FEA studies on atrophic alveolar maxillary ridges of ten adult cadavers (five dentate). Occlusal loads applied to the first molar region in the dentate model and at the corresponding alveolar ridge showed that in the former, the stress concentrated at the cortical bone and around the maxillary sinus floor adjacent to the trabecular bone of dental roots. In the latter, stress was found at the cortical bone of the alveolar ridge, but also on the inner trabecular bone; however, no stresses were observed at the cortical bone of the maxillary sinus floor adjacent to the trabecular bone. This cortical bone of the edentulous model only showed stresses when a cylindrical body 4 mm in diameter and 10 mm in length was modeled at this region.[28]

The bone/implant interface in the edentulous region can be protected by splinting of implants with a fixed prosthesis after surgery. This treatment modality is used most often and only recently confirmed by FEA. As expected, stresses around splinted implants are nine times lower than in non-splinted models, even when a simulated acrylic fixed prosthesis received 10° oblique loading of 300 N.[29]

On the other hand, Frequency Resonance Analysis is helpful to determine the moment of loading and to verify implant stability, mainly on treatment of atrophied maxilla with simultaneous bone grafts. These demonstrated good stability quotients after 3 years of implant loading. Twenty-five patients received 222 implants distributed according to Cawood and Howell's classification in the following way: class III = 17, class IV = 67, class V = 111, class VI = 25, no classification = 2. Implant Stability Quotient values showed statistically significant differences between abutment connection (60.2) and 6 months after loading (62.5), but these were not confirmed between 6 months and 3 years after loading (61.8). A multivariate logistic regression analysis indicated that factors such as gender (women) and implants at class VI before reconstruction significantly increased the risk of failure.[30] Preliminary results show that reduced diameter implants (3.5 mm) can be used with success on atrophic maxillae (Cawood and Howell's class IV) to avoid grafting procedures.[31] When implant-supported fixed prostheses were delivered after 6 months of healing, the implant survival rate was 100%, and bone loss registered around 0.3 mm; mean ISQ values were 63 (baseline), 60 (abutment connection), and 61 (1 year after loading). Also, the use of deproteinized bovine bone (autogenous bone + Bio-Oss, 20:80 ratio) after sinus lifting and implant loading (12 months) in atrophic maxillae generated ISQ values (65.6) very similar to non-grafted sites (67.4).[32] Finally, the use of surface-oxidized implants and definitive implant-supported prostheses generated values similar to those described above.[33]

Even in the resorbed maxilla, the bearing support area is two times greater than in the mandibular arch.[34] The use of piezoelectric force transducers revealed no differences on force transferring, regardless of prosthesis type (fixed or overdenture); however, magnitude of forces was higher in posterior implants, whereas on anterior implants, transversal forces reached up to 100% or more of axial forces during mastication. Although only one atrophic maxilla was used in this study, these values were confirmed 2 years later.[35] A reduced number of conventionally placed implants in the atrophic maxilla is not recommended, and force distribution only resolves when five to six implants are used;[36] however, the use of inclined implants along with a removable over-denture (Marius bridge) showed a 97% survival rate (five failures of 245) after 5 years, with ten related mechanical complications (one fracture of mesostructure, nine problems with attachments).[37]

One of the greatest difficulties is improving the biomechanical response in patients with tumor resections. One study showed that peri-implant resorption rate depends on implant location.[38] Conversely, when obturators are constructed with bar milled attachments, either masticatory efficiency (16 to 77 points) or bite force (317 N) is improved.[39] Another important situation is the edentulous state with cleft lip and palate defects, where experience and creativity are needed to achieve the desired prosthetic rehabilitation.[40]

DISCUSSION

In this review, important anatomic (morphological intrinsic and extrinsic) and biomechanical aspects on the atrophic maxilla were highlighted. The centripetal resorption pattern described in the maxillary arch makes bone the most precious source for facial and dental esthetics. In this way, every attempt to alleviate this condition is mandatory.

The use of a complete conventional maxillary prosthesis and a Kennedy class I removable denture in the mandibular arch is a common clinical finding, as is the presence of flabby tissues in the maxillary anterior and posterior regions, attributed to the mechanics of "combination syndrome."[41] Because both are considered risk factors influencing the severity of bone resorption, and not all patients can afford implant therapy, the clinician's role is to guarantee periodic denture base relining and to identify lack of adequate performance on prosthetic devices.

Factors related to the height of bone septa and changes on the nasopalatine canal reveal that these features can only be viewed in detail with modern CT techniques; thus, comprehensive interaction between clinicians and nuclear radiologists for a thorough bone evaluation is important, because presence and location of septa compromise maxillary sinus lifting procedures. The inclusion of considerable enlargement at the nasopalatine canal as a consequence of disuse atrophy is relevant. Also, these two anatomic changes mean a need for screening different populations to identify other possible characteristics related to the atrophic maxillae.

Although zygomatic implants have been considered an interesting resolution for atrophic maxillae, and the use of long transmucosal abutments is inevitable, the likelihood of bleeding on probing is increased. Further improvements on prosthesis design are necessary to reduce biological complications.

In the atrophic maxillae, stress does not concentrate on cortical bone at the maxillary sinus base continuous to trabecular bone. This constitutes an attempt for generating more accurate models with FEA studies based on bone micro-CT analysis. One possible indirect assumption here is that sinus floor pneumatization really has no opposing occlusal forces. Also, densitometric bone parameters used in this article were very similar to findings reported almost 10 years ago in another study[20] cited in this review.

ISQ values for implants placed in severely atrophic maxillae ranged from 60 to 65, which confirms the effect of splinting tested with finite element models to avoid bone damage evolution; however, these values did not diminish the risk of failures in Cawood and Howell's class VI. Even thus, successful application of narrow-diameter implants is possible in class IV cases. In addition, the use of inclined implants has been popularized in the atrophic maxilla, with good clinical survival rates already published.[42,43] Finally, the observation that prosthesis type (fixed or overdenture) does not influence in vivo force transfer can help clinicians decide for a more esthetic alternative when considerable lip support must be addressed. Surprisingly, biomechanics on the result of acquired maxillary atrophic deficiencies (tumor resection, cleft patients) remains an exciting but not totally explored area, given its implications on social behavior and quality of life; however, technological improvements on implant surfaces and macro/microdesigns will have a considerable impact here in the near future.

CONCLUSION

Clinicians must understand the possible anatomic and biomechanical implications of atrophic maxillary arches to prevent or avoid failures, as well as to meet patients' expectations based on sound choices of available biomaterials and technologies for implant-supported prostheses.

REFERENCES

1. The glossary of prosthodontic terms. *J Prosthet Dent* 2005; 94:10–92.
2. Wolff J: *The Laws of Bone Remodeling*. Berlin, Springer, 1986 (originally published in 1892).
3. Murray PDF: *Bones: A Study of the Development and Structure of the Vertebrate Skeleton*. Cambridge, Cambridge University Press, 1936.
4. Tallgren A: The continuing reduction of the residual alveolar ridges in complete denture wearers: a mixed longitudinal study covering 25 years. *J Prosthet Dent* 1972;27:120–132.
5. Bergman B, Carlsson GE: Clinical long-term study of complete denture wearers. *J Prosthet Dent* 1985;53:56–61.
6. Lundgren S, Sjöström M, Nystrom E, et al: Strategies in reconstruction of the atrophic maxilla with autogenous bone

grafts and endosseous implants. *Periodontol 2000* 2008;47: 143–161.

7. Güler AU, Sumer M, Sumer P, et al: The evaluation of vertical heights of maxillary and mandibular bones and the location of anatomic landmarks in panoramic radiographs of edentulous patients for implant dentistry. *J Oral Rehabil* 2005;32:741–746.

8. Xie Q, Narhi T, Nevalainen JM, et al: Oral status and prosthetic factors related to residual ridge resorption in elderly subjects. *Acta Odonto Scand* 1997;55:306–313.

9. Ulm CW, Solar P, Gsellmann B, et al: The edentulous maxillary alveolar process in the region of the maxillary sinus – a study of physical dimension. *Int J Oral Maxillofac Surg* 1995;24: 279–282.

10. Kaptein MLA, De Lange GL, Blijdorf PA: Peri-implant tissue health in reconstructed atrophic maxillae–report of 88 patients and 470 implants. *J Oral Rehabil* 1999;26:464–474.

11. Al-Nawas B, Wegener J, Bender C, et al: Critical soft tissue parameters of the zygomatic implant. *J Clin Periodontol* 2004;31:497–500.

12. Atwood DA: Reduction of residual ridges: a major oral disease entity. *J Prosthet Dent* 1971;26:266–279.

13. Fallschüssel GKH: Untersuchugen zur Anatomie des zahnlosen Oberkiefers. *Z Zahnärztl Implantol* 1986;41:64–72.

14. Cawood JI, Howell RA: A classification of edentulous jaws. *Int J Oral Maxillofac Surg* 1988;17:232–236.

15. Lekholm U, Zarb GA: Patient selection and preparation. In Brånemark P-I, Albrektsson T, Zarb GA (eds): *Tissue-Integrated Prostheses: Osseointegration in Clinical Dentistry*. Chicago, Quintessence, 1985, pp. 199–209.

16. Mupparapu M, Singer SR: Implant imaging for the dentist. *J Can Dent Assoc* 2004;70:32a–32g.

17. Watzek G: *Endosseous Implants: Scientific and Clinical Aspects*. Chicago, Quintessence, 1996.

18. Kim M-J, Jung U-W, Kin C-S, et al: Maxillary sinus septa; prevalence, height, location, and morphology. A reformatted computed tomography scan analysis. *J Periodontol* 2006;77: 903–908.

19. Mardinger O, Namani-Sadan N, Chaushu G, et al: Morphology changes of the nasopalatine canal related to dental implantation: a radiologic study in different degrees of absorbed maxillae. *J Periodontol* 2008;79:1659–1662.

20. Ulm C, Kneissel M, Schedle A, et al: Characteristic features of trabecular bone in edentulous maxillae. *Clin Oral Implants Res* 1999;10:459–467.

21. Bahat O: Treatment planning and placement of implants in the posterior maxilla. Report of 732 consecutive Nobelpharma implants. *Int J Oral Maxillofac Implants* 1993;8:151–161.

22. Solar P, Ulm C, Frey G, et al: A classification of the intra-osseous paths of the mental nerve. *Int J Oral Maxillofac Implants* 1994;9:339–344.

23. Solar P, Geyerhofer U, Traxler H, et al: Blood supply to the maxillary sinus relevant to sinus floor elevation procedures. *Clin Oral Implants Res* 1999;10:34–44.

24. Tepper G, Ulm C: Perfusion of compromised bone and implications for implant therapy. In Watzek G (ed): *Implants in Qualitatively Compromised Bone*. Chicago, Quintessence, 2004, pp. 43–54.

25. Hillowala R, Kanth H: The transmission of masticatory forces and nasal septum: structural comparison of the human skull and Gothic cathedral. *Cranio* 2007;25:166–171.

26. Meyer U, Vollmer D, Runte C, et al: Bone loading pattern around implants in average and atrophic edentulous maxillae: a finite-element analysis. *J Oral Maxillofac Surg* 2001; 29:100–105.

27. Ujigawa K, Kato Y, Kizu Y, et al: Three-dimensional finite elemental analysis of zygomatic implants in craniofacial structures. *Int J Oral Maxillofac Surg* 2007;36:620–625.

28. Nomoto S, Matsunaga S, Ide Y, et al: Stress distribution in maxillary alveolar ridge according to the finite element analysis using micro-CT. *Bull Tokyo Dent Coll* 2006;47:149–156.

29. Bergkvist G, Simonsson K, Rydberg K, et al: A finite element analysis of stress distribution in bone tissue surrounding uncoupled or splinted dental implants. *Clin Implant Dent Relat Clin Res* 2008;10:40–46.

30. Sjöström M, Sennerby L, Nilson H, et al: Reconstruction of the atrophic edentulous maxilla with free iliac crest grafts and implants: a 3-year report of a prospective clinical study. *Clin Implant Dent Relat Clin Res* 2007;9:46–59.

31. Veltri M, Ferrari M, Balleri P: One-year outcome of narrow diameter blasted implants for rehabilitation of maxillas with knife-edge resorption. *Clin Oral Implants Res* 2008; 19:1069–1073.

32. Hallman M, Sennerby L, Zetterqvist L, et al: A 3-year prospective follow-up study of implant-supported fixed prostheses in patients subjected to maxillary sinus floor augmentation with a 80:20 mixture of deproteinized bovine bone and autogenous bone. Clinical, radiographic and resonance frequency analysis. *Int J Oral Maxillofac Surg* 2005;34:273–280.

33. Olsson M, Urde G, Andersen JB, et al: Early loading of maxillary fixed cross-arch dental prostheses supported by six or eight oxidized titanium implants: results after 1 year of loading. Case series. *Clin Implant Dent Relat Res* 2003;5:S81–S86.

34. Zarb GA: Biomechanics of the edentulous state. In Zarb GA, Bolender CL (eds): *Prosthodontic Treatment for Edentulous Patients*. St. Louis, Mosby, 2004, pp. 8–29.

35. Mericske-Stern R, Venetz E, Fahrländer F, et al: In vivo force measurements on maxillary implants supporting a fixed prosthesis or an overdenture: a pilot study. *J Prosthet Dent* 2000;84: 535–547.

36. Duyck H, Vander Sloten J, De Cooman M, et al: Magnitude and distribution of occlusal forces on oral implants supporting fixed prosthesis: an in vivo study. *Clin Oral Implants Res* 2000; 11:465–475.

37. Fortin Y, Sullivan RM, Rangert B: The Marius implant bridge: surgical and prosthetic rehabilitation of the complete edentulous upper jaw with moderate to severe resorption: a 5-year retrospective clinical study. *Clin Implant Dent Relat Res* 2002;4:69–77.

38. Roumanas ED, Nishimura RD, Davis BK, et al: Clinical evaluation of implants retaining edentulous maxillary obturator prostheses. *J Prosthet Dent* 1997;77:184–190.

39. Fukuda M, Takahashi T, Nagai H, et al: Implant-supported edentulous maxillary obturators with milled bar attachments after maxillectomy. *J Oral Maxillofac Surg* 2004;62: 799–805.

40. Tuna SH, Peklan G, Buyukgural B: Rehabilitation of an edentulous cleft lip and palate patient with a soft palate defect using a bar-retained, implant-supported speech-aid prosthesis. A clinical report. *Cleft Pal Craniofac J* 2009;46:97–102.

41. Saunders TR, Gillis RE Jr, Desjardins RP: The maxillary complete denture opposing the mandibular bilateral distal extension. Partial denture treatment considerations. *J Prosthet Dent* 1979;41:124–128.

42. Maló P, Rangert B, Nobre M: All-on-4 immediate function concept with Brånemark system implants for completely edentulous maxillae: a 1 year retrospective clinical study. *Clin Implant Dental Relat Res* 2005;7(Suppl 1): 88–94.

43. Maló P, Nobre M, Lopes I: A new approach to rehabilitate the severely atrophic maxilla using extra-maxillary anchored implants in immediate function: a pilot study. *J Prosthet Dent* 2008;100:354–366.

13

A RETROSPECTIVE ANALYSIS OF 800 BRÅNEMARK SYSTEM IMPLANTS FOLLOWING THE ALL-ON-FOUR™ PROTOCOL

THOMAS J. BALSHI, DDS, PHD, FACP,[1] GLENN J. WOLFINGER, DMD, FACP,[2] ROBERT W. SLAUCH, BS,[3,4] AND STEPHEN F. BALSHI, MBE[5]

[1]Founder and Prosthodontist, PI Dental Center at the Institute for Facial Esthetics, Fort Washington, PA
[2]Prosthodontist, PI Dental Center at the Institute for Facial Esthetics, Fort Washington, PA
[3]Research Associate, PI Dental Center at the Institute for Facial Esthetics, Fort Washington, PA
[4]Dental Student, University of Maryland, Baltimore College of Dental Surgery, Baltimore, MD
[5]Director of Research, PI Dental Center at the Institute for Facial Esthetics; President, CM Prosthetics, Inc., Fort Washington, PA

The article is associated with the American College of Prosthodontists' journal-based continuing education program. It is accompanied by an online continuing education activity worth 1 credit. Please visit www.wileyhealthlearning.com/jopr to complete the activity and earn credit.

Keywords

Dental implant; tilted implant; osseointegration; maxilla; mandible; immediate loading.

Correspondence

Stephen Balshi, PI Dental Center at the Institute for Facial Esthetics, 467 Pennsylvania Ave., Ste. 201, Fort Washington, PA 19034. E-mail: balshi2@aol.com

The authors deny any conflicts of interest.

Accepted April 27, 2013

Published in *Journal of Prosthodontics* February 2014; Vol. 23, Issue 2

doi: 10.1111/jopr.12089

ABSTRACT

Purpose: The purpose of this study was to retrospectively evaluate implant survival rates in patients treated with the All-on-Four™ protocol according to edentulous jaws, gender, and implant orientation (tilted vs. axial).

Materials and Methods: All Brånemark System implants placed in patients following the All-on-Four™ protocol in a single private practice were separated into multiple classifications (maxilla vs. mandible; male vs. female; tilted vs. axial) by retrospective patient chart review. Inclusion criteria consisted of any Brånemark System implant placed with the All-on-Four™ protocol from the clinical inception (May 2005) until December 2011. Life tables were constructed to determine cumulative implant survival rates (CSR). The arches, genders, and implant orientations were statistically compared with ANOVA.

Results: One hundred fifty-two patients, comprising 200 arches (800 implants) from May 2005 until December 2011, were included in the study. Overall implant CSR was 97.3% (778 of 800). Two hundred eighty-nine of 300 maxillary implants and 489 of 500 mandibular implants survived, for CSRs of 96.3% and 97.8%, respectively. In male patients, 251 of 256 implants (98.1%) remain in function while 527 of 544 implants (96.9%) in female patients survived. Regarding implant orientation, 389 of 400 tilted implants and 389 of 400 axial implants osseointegrated, for identical CSRs of 97.3%. All comparisons were found to be statistically insignificant. The prosthesis survival rate was 99.0%.

Conclusions: The results from this study suggest that edentulous jaws, gender, and implant orientation are not significant parameters when formulating an All-on-Four[TM] treatment plan. The high CSRs for each variable analyzed demonstrate the All-on-Four[TM] treatment as a viable alternative to more extensive protocols for rehabilitating the edentulous maxilla or mandible.

Immediate loading of all-acrylic, implant-supported prostheses for maxillary and mandibular arches has been shown to provide numerous clinical advantages to patients and dentists.[1–6] Patients are able to receive fixed, full-arch restorations the same day as implant placement, providing esthetics, comfort, and limited function during the 3- to 6-month healing phase, all while achieving high implant survival rates.

Traditional treatment plans typically called for a large number of implants placed in fairly vertical positions throughout the entire arch.[7] However, the posterior maxilla and mandible may have several limitations associated with this approach. In the mandible, the inferior alveolar nerve and associated structures may provide minimal bone for implant anchorage or prevent the placement of implants distal to the mental foramina altogether. In the maxilla, it is not uncommon to see resorption in the posterior regions or enlargement of the sinuses.[8]

In the event that posterior implants could not be placed and to compensate for these biologic limitations, a lengthy cantilever distal to the terminal implant was typically needed to provide patients with adequate posterior dentitions; however, extensive posterior cantilevers are biomechanically unfavorable due to increased occlusal forces.[9–11] Alternative methods for the maxilla, such as sinus augmentations[12] or pterygomaxillary implants[13,14] have been used to establish adequate stability for posterior implants and decreased cantilevers. Sinus lifts often prolong treatment time in order for graft maturation to occur.

The introduction of tilted implants[8,15] has provided a significant alternative for restoration of maxillary and mandibular posterior segments without bone grafting. According to Krekmanov et al,[8] posterior tilting of distal implants will reduce cantilever lengths, broaden the prosthetic base, and improve implant-to-bone surface areas because longer implants can be used. In their study, tilted implants increased prosthesis length by an average of 6.6 mm in the mandible and 9.3 mm in the maxilla.[8] This resulted in better biomechanics.

The All-on-Four[TM] concept uses the simplicity of posterior tilted implants to create a full-arch restoration that can be less clinically invasive for patients. The concept was initially proposed in a 2003 study[16] as a treatment plan for mandibles, since immediate function had become widely accepted in that region. The design consisted of a fixed prosthesis supported by four endosseous implants: two axial implants in the anterior segment and one distal implant on each posterior segment tilted posteriorly. All implant apices are to engage cortical bone anterior to the mental foramina. The increased anterior/posterior spread[11] from the tilted implants generally provides first molar occlusion for patients with short cantilevered segments.

Edentulous maxillary jaws were initially thought to provide a significant challenge to the protocol, as maxillary bone is known to have decreased bone density, especially relative to mandibular bone.[16] However, Maló et al[17] demonstrated in 2005 that maxillary All-on-Four[TM] rehabilitations had a cumulative survival rate (CSR) of 97.6%, approximately 1% higher than their 2003 study in the mandible (96.7% CSR).[16] More recent studies[18,19] have further reinforced the viability of the All-on-Four[TM] protocol as a treatment alternative for both dental arches.

The purpose of this study was to retrospectively determine if there was a significant difference in implant survival rates relative to edentulous jaws, patient gender, and implant orientation following the All-on-Four protocol in a single private practice. Implant failures based on bone quality[20] and smoking habits were also measured. The null hypothesis for this study was there would be no significant differences relative to implant CSRs (outcome variable) in edentulous jaws, gender, and implant orientation.

MATERIALS AND METHODS

A retrospective chart review was performed for all patients who received Brånemark System implants (Nobel Biocare, Yorba Linda, CA) following the All-on-Four[TM] protocol in a single private practice (PI Dental Center, Fort Washington, PA). Data compilation was performed using an implant tracking database system (Implant Tracker; Hartford, CT).

As this research involved the study of existing records, and the records were made anonymous to the investigators, IRB approval was not sought. Inclusion criteria consisted of any implant placed in the practice in an All-on-Four™ treatment from May 2005 (the clinical inception of All-on-Four™) until December 2011. On the day of surgery, implants were placed and immediately loaded with all-acrylic resin, screw-retained interim prostheses (Teeth in a Day®). Approximately 3 months postsurgery, patients presented for definitive impressions, enabling the construction of highly accurate master casts used for the fabrication of the definitive prostheses. The definitive prostheses were delivered 4 to 8 weeks later.

Regarding failed implants, replacement implants were excluded from the study. A surviving (or osseointegrated) implant was defined as an implant that remained in function and had no clinical mobility or adverse symptoms at the time of definitive impressions. In contrast, an implant failure was defined as an implant that did not achieve osseointegration, as demonstrated by patients reporting pain or discomfort or by clinical mobility determined by the clinician. This resulted in eventual removal of the failed implant from the patient.

All implants were classified into three groups: maxillary vs. mandibular; male vs. female patients; and tilted (posterior) vs. axial (anterior). Separation into each group was conducted by reviewing postoperation radiographs and clinical notes. Life tables were constructed to determine the CSRs. MAN-OVA was performed in Microsoft Excel (Microsoft Inc., Redmond, WA) to compare the significance in the CSRs between the edentulous jaws, gender, and implant orientation groupings.

The number of failures based on implant type, bone quality, and smoking habits were also calculated. Bone quality was determined subjectively by the prosthodontist placing the implants, based on resistance to drilling and clinical experience. Bone quality was quantified by types 1 to 4 according to the Lekholm and Zarb[20] criteria. Smoking habits were recorded from the initial patient work-up.

RESULTS

One hundred fifty-two patients with 200 dental arches (800 implants) were included in this study. Of the Brånemark System implants placed following the All-on-Four™ protocol during the study period, 778 of the 800 implants successfully osseointegrated, resulting in a CSR of 97.3% (Table 13.1). Relative to edentulous jaw locations, 289 of the 300 (96.3%) maxillary implants placed remained in function (Table 13.2); mandibular implants had a survival rate of 97.8% (489 of 500, Table 13.3). Regarding gender, male patients had 251 of the 256 (98.1%) implants successfully osseointegrate (Table 13.4), and female patients had 527 of the 544 implants integrate (96.9%, Table 13.5). In the

TABLE 13.1   Master Life Table of Implants

Period	# of Implants	# of Failures	Survival Rate (%)	Cumulative Survival Rate (%)
0 to 3 months	800	12	98.5	98.5
3 to 6 months	776	4	99.6	98.0
6 to 9 months	737	1	99.9	97.9
9 to 12 months	660	5	99.3	97.3
1 year	588	0	100.0	97.3
2 years	375	0	100.0	97.3
3 years	168	0	100.0	97.3
4 years	93	0	100.0	97.3
5+ years	40	0	100.0	97.3

TABLE 13.2   Life Table for Implants in the Maxillary Arch

Period	# of Implants	# of Failures	Survival Rate (%)	Cumulative Survival Rate (%)
0 to 3 months	300	6	98.0	98.0
3 to 6 months	290	1	99.7	97.7
6 to 9 months	281	1	99.6	97.3
9 to 12 months	248	3	98.9	96.3
1 year	222	0	100.0	96.3
2 years	130	0	100.0	96.3
3 years	39	0	100.0	96.3
4 years	19	0	100.0	96.3
5+ years	8	0	100.0	96.3

TABLE 13.3   Life Table for Implants in the Mandibular Arch

Period	# of Implants	# of Failures	Survival Rate (%)	Cumulative Survival Rate (%)
0 to 3 months	500	6	98.8	98.8
3 to 6 months	486	3	99.4	98.2
6 to 9 months	456	0	100.0	98.2
9 to 12 months	412	2	99.5	97.8
1 year	366	0	100.0	97.8
2 years	245	0	100.0	97.8
3 years	129	0	100.0	97.8
4 years	74	0	100.0	97.8
5+ years	32	0	100.0	97.8

implant orientation groups, the tilted and axial implants had equal sample sizes ($n = 400$); CSRs both equaled 97.3% (Tables 13.6 and 13.7). The Mark III 4.0×15 mm implant had the highest failure rate (23.7%) of all specific implants used in the study (Table 13.8). Type 2 bone had the highest failure rate (4.1%) of all bone qualities (Table 13.9). Relative

TABLE 13.4   Life Table for Implants in Male Patients

Period	# of Implants	# of Failures	Survival Rate (%)	Cumulative Survival Rate (%)
0 to 3 months	256	3	98.8	98.8
3 to 6 months	241	2	99.2	98.1
6 to 9 months	223	0	100.0	98.1
9 to 12 months	203	0	100.0	98.1
1 year	178	0	100.0	98.1
2 years	100	0	100.0	98.1
3 years	40	0	100.0	98.1
4 years	16	0	100.0	98.1
5+ years	8	0	100.0	98.1

TABLE 13.5   Life Table for Implants in Female Patients

Period	# of Implants	# of Failures	Survival Rate (%)	Cumulative Survival Rate (%)
0 to 3 months	544	9	98.3	98.3
3 to 6 months	535	2	99.6	98.0
6 to 9 months	514	1	99.8	97.8
9 to 12 months	457	5	99.0	96.9
1 year	410	0	100.0	96.9
2 years	275	0	100.0	96.9
3 years	128	0	100.0	96.9
4 years	77	0	100.0	96.9
5+ years	32	0	100.0	96.9

TABLE 13.6   Life Table for Tilted Implants

Period	# of Implants	# of Failures	Survival Rate (%)	Cumulative Survival Rate (%)
0 to 3 months	400	6	98.5	98.5
3 to 6 months	388	3	99.2	97.8
6 to 9 months	368	1	99.7	97.5
9 to 12 months	329	1	99.7	97.3
1 year	294	0	100.0	97.3
2 years	188	0	100.0	97.3
3 years	85	0	100.0	97.3
4 years	47	0	100.0	97.3
5+ years	20	0	100.0	97.3

to smoking, eight implants failed in two patients who were documented as smokers (Table 13.10). The prosthesis survival rate was 99.0%. The CSR comparisons between dental arch, gender, and implant orientation were found to be statistically insignificant (MANOVA; $p > 0.05$). Examples of preoperation and postoperation radiographs are depicted in

TABLE 13.7   Life Table for Axial Implants

Period	# of Implants	# of Failures	Survival Rate (%)	Cumulative Survival Rate (%)
0 to 3 months	400	6	98.5	98.5
3 to 6 months	388	1	99.7	98.3
6 to 9 months	369	0	100.0	98.3
9 to 12 months	331	4	98.9	97.3
1 year	294	0	100.0	97.3
2 years	187	0	100.0	97.3
3 years	83	0	100.0	97.3
4 years	46	0	100.0	97.3
5+ years	20	0	100.0	97.3

TABLE 13.8   Number of Failures Based on Implant Dimension

Implant Dimension	Number of Failures	Failure Rate for Specific Implant Dimension (%)
Mk III 3.75×13 mm	2	6.3
Mk III 3.75×15 mm	1	1.6
Mk III 4.0×13 mm	1	4.5
Mk III 4.0×15 mm	3	23.7
Mk IV 4.0×10 mm	2	2.8
Mk IV 4.0×13 mm	2	2.0
Mk IV 4.0×15 mm	6	1.6
Mk IV 4.0×18 mm	5	3.2

TABLE 13.9   Number of Failures Based on Bone Quality

Bone Quality	Number of Implants in Bone Type	Number of Failures	Failure Percentage (%)
Type 1	25	1	4.0
Type 2	239	10	4.1
Type 3	479	11	2.3
Type 4	57	0	0.0

TABLE 13.10   Number of Failures Based on Smoking Status

Smoking Status	Number of Implants	Number of Failures	Failure Percentage (%)
Nonsmoker	668	14	2.1
Smoker	132	8	6.1

Figures 13.1 and 13.2. Figure 13.3 illustrates a radiograph following delivery of the definitive prostheses in the same patient.

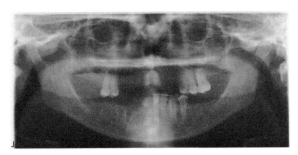

FIGURE 13.1 Preoperative panoramic radiograph of the patient elected for maxillary and mandibular All-on-Four™ implant rehabilitation.

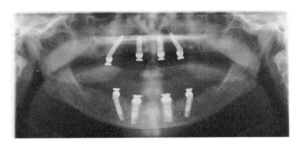

FIGURE 13.2 Postoperative panoramic radiograph following All-on-Four™ implant rehabilitation in the maxilla and mandible. The implants were immediately loaded with all-acrylic resin interim prostheses.

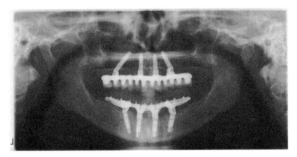

FIGURE 13.3 Panoramic radiograph following delivery of definitive prostheses for the maxilla and mandible. The maxillary CM prosthesis consists of a milled titanium framework with individual lithium disilicate crowns. The mandibular prosthesis is a milled titanium framework veneered with acrylic resin and denture teeth.

DISCUSSION

Immediate occlusal loading of edentulous jaws following the All-on-Four™ protocol has been demonstrated to provide patients with functional and esthetic screw-retained interim prostheses the same day of surgery.[5] Alternative protocols such as sinus augmentations are available to patients and may obtain the same definite treatment outcomes as the All-on-Four™ treatment protocols; however, these protocols require longer healing periods, and it may not be possible to employ an immediate loading protocol. The use of tilted implant placement protocols has allowed dental practitioners to use

the All-on-Four™ concept, which provides a viable alternative to restore dentitions in edentulous maxillae and mandibles. Due to the increased frequency of this protocol, as reported in multiple publications,[16–19,26] it is important to determine if specific variables such as dental arch, gender, or implant orientation produce any significant differences in the success of the procedure.

Regarding dental arches reconstructed with this specific protocol, this study found that the mandible produced a CSR 1.5% higher than (Table 13.3), but not statistically different relative to the maxilla (Table 13.2). The authors of this report suggest if cortical bone is present, implants may osseointegrate despite the arch rehabilitated. With gender, similar CSRs were obtained in male patients (98.1%) and female patients (96.9%); these results were also statistically insignificant.

Tilted and axial implants had identical CSRs (Tables 13.6 and 13.7). In a 2000 study,[8] axial implants had a lower CSR in the maxilla (90.2%) than tilted implants did (95.7%); however, the implants were not immediately loaded. The authors of this article mentioned that the increased contact between cortical bone and tilted implants may be the reason for the percentage difference. The same reason could account for the high CSR reported in the current study.

In a 2011 report by Butura et al,[18] tilted implants had a CSR of 99.8% and axial implants a CSR of 99.5% in the mandible. A study by Graves et al[19] in 2011 reported a CSR of 97.5% in the maxilla. In both studies, the surgical procedures for implant placement were similar, and all implants were immediately loaded with fixed all-acrylic resin screw-retained prostheses. The higher CSRs shown from these 2011 reports[18,19] and this current study, when compared to the original research conducted on tilted implants,[8] could be due to inception of the TiUnite[21,22] surface implant. Other possible explanations for the higher CSRs are related to immediate loading protocols and biomechanics: the splinting effect and cross-arch stabilization. The authors of the current study believe it is imperative that all implants be splinted together in the immediate loading protocol to distribute the forces throughout the entire arch. Cross-arch stabilization of immediately loaded implants limits micromotion to the individual implants. With optimal load distribution through splinting, single implants avoid overload that can lead to micromotion and prevent osseointegration. Relative to edentulous jaws, gender, and implant orientation results, it is suggested there are no biological or mechanical disadvantages regarding these variables when formulating an All-on-Four™ treatment plan when the aforementioned splinting condition exists.

At 3 months postsurgery, patients were scheduled for definitive impressions to enable fabrication of the definitive prostheses. Delivery of the definitive prosthesis typically occurred 1 to 2 months later (4 to 5 months postoperative). In this study, five implants (in two patients) failed in the 9- to 12-month timeframe after the definitive prostheses were already delivered; however, in both cases, all-acrylic resin definitive prostheses were used. The all-acrylic resin prosthesis was a cost-effective alternative to a metal framework for a definitive prosthesis as demonstrated by Malo et al.[26] Thus, a simple manipulation was achieved by removing the old abutment cylinders corresponding to the failed implant sites and adding additional acrylic resin to reposition the new implant orientations on the original prostheses. If this occurred with the definitive prosthesis containing a metal framework, the framework must be stripped, sectioned, and repositioned. The prosthesis survival rate for this study was 99.0%. Only two patients required a reversion back to a removable denture, due to all four implants failing to maintain osseointegration. In one of these, the patient (female, 41 years) presented herself with a periodontally compromised maxillary dentition. An All-on-Four[TM] fixed immediate prosthesis was the treatment plan presented and accepted by the patient to restore the maxillary dentition. Type 3 bone[20] was observed at the time of implant placement. Ten months after surgery, none of the four implants maintained osseointegration, suggesting there may be a systemic issue in the bone remodeling process. It was at this time that clinical mobility was noted for all implants. The patient was a heavy smoker and refused to quit, and continued to display poor oral hygiene, which may also have been possible mechanisms of implant failure.

In the other specific case, the patient (female, 45 years) presented with a chief complaint of a loose mandibular denture. The patient displayed unusual jaw and muscular movements that were considered a maladaptive response to the loose mandibular denture. After the implants were placed and the mandibular prosthesis was secured, the unusual jaw and muscular movements continued. The extreme occlusal and lateral forces caused micromotion to the immediately loaded prosthesis and prohibited osseointegration from occurring, leading to fibrous encapsulation. The patient was referred to a neurologist for evaluation and was later diagnosed with oromandibular dystonia. The patient never returned for replacement of the lost implants and prosthesis.

When implants fail in the All-on-Four[TM] protocol, tilted (posterior) implants are often more difficult to replace than axial (anterior) implants. For example, a mandibular receptor site more distal to the original site is likely to be anatomically challenging due to the location of the mental foramina; a receptor site more mesial will decrease the anterior/posterior spread. An implant site buccal or lingual to the original site may be acceptable if there is sufficient alveolar ridge width for implant placement. In the maxilla, similar challenges exist for the tilted (posterior) implants relative to the anterior wall of the maxillary sinus. In both dental arches, axial implants placed in the anterior segments have more freedom for clinicians to move the new implant sites mesial or distal when compared to previous sites.

Prior research[9,23–25] has shown protocols that use pterygomaxillary implants or a large number of implants have success rates well into the 90% range; however, factors such as the amount of occlusal surface areas differ when comparing the All-on-Four[TM] concept to previous concepts. Due to their ability to provide posterior maxillary support, pterygomaxillary implants typically provide patients with second molar occlusion with no distal cantilevers being needed. The All-on-Four[TM] method typically provides first molar occlusion, often with the use of a distal cantilever.

The high overall CSR for the All-on-Four[TM] concept (97.3%, Table 13.1) in this study demonstrates similar success rates when compared with these alternative protocols. The data in this study suggest that the All-on-Four[TM] protocol as described is a treatment plan that produces similar, if not higher, success rates and allows clinicians to achieve the satisfactory immediate functional and esthetic outcomes. There are also great advantages afforded to patients in terms of postoperative comfort and decrease in overall treatment time.

CONCLUSION

The All-on-Four[TM] concept provides a predictable method to restore edentulous jaws. The high implant survival rates relative to edentulous jaws, patient gender, and implant orientation when following the All-on-Four[TM] protocol suggests that the procedure is a viable alternative to restore dentitions for edentulous patients.

ACKNOWLEDGMENT

The authors would like to thank Chris Raines for her assistance in data collection using Implant Tracker; the staff of the PI Dental Center for their kind and gentle treatment of the patients; and Dr. Brian Wilson and Mr. Dan Delaney for their support in the administration of general anesthetics, when needed.

REFERENCES

1. Zarb GA, Zarb FL, Schmitt A: Osseointegrated implants for partially edentulous patients. *Dent Clin North Am* 1987;31:457–472.
2. Balshi TJ, Wolfinger GJ: Immediate loading of Brånemark implants in edentulous mandibles. A preliminary report. *Implant Dent* 1997;6:83–88.
3. Schnitman PA, Wohrle PS, Rubenstein JE, et al: Ten-year results for Brånemark implants immediately loaded with fixed prostheses at implant placement. *Int J Oral Maxillofac Implants* 1997;2:495–503.

4. Tarnow D, Emtiaz S, Classi A: Immediate loading of threaded implants at stage I surgery in edentulous arches: ten consecutive case reports with 1–5 year data. *Int J Oral Maxillofac Implants* 1997;12:319–324.

5. Balshi TJ, Wolfinger GJ: Teeth in a day. *Implant Dent* 2001;10:231–233.

6. Randow K, Ericsson I, Nilner K, et al: Immediate functional loading of Brånemark dental implants: an 18-month clinical follow-up study. *Clin Oral Impl Res* 1999;110:8–15.

7. Block MS, Winder JS: Method for insuring parallelism of implants placed simultaneously with maxillary sinus bone grafts. *J Oral Maxillofac Surg* 1991;49:435–437.

8. Krekmanov L, Kahn M, Rangert B, et al: Tilting of posterior mandibular and maxillary implants for improved prosthesis support. *Int J Oral Maxillofac Implants* 2000;15:405–414.

9. Bahat O: Brånemark system implants in the posterior maxilla: clinical study of 660 implants followed for 5 to 12 years. *Int J Oral and Maxillofac Implants* 2000;15:646–653.

10. Rangert B, Jemt T, Jörnéus I: Forces and moments on Brånemark implants. *Int J Oral Maxillofac Implants* 1989;4:241–247.

11. English C: Biomechanical concerns with fixed partial dentures involving implants. *Implant Dent* 1993;2:221–242.

12. Balshi TJ: Preventing and resolving complications with osseointegrated implants. *Dent Clinics North Am* 1989;33:821–868.

13. Tulasne JF: Osseointegrated fixtures in the pterygoid region. In Worthington P, Brånemark PI (eds): *Advanced Osseointegration Surgery, Applications in the Maxillofacial Region*. Chicago, Quintessence, 1992, pp. 182–188.

14. Graves SL: The pterygoid plate implant. A solution for restoring the posterior maxilla. *Int J Periodont Rest Dent* 1994;14:512–523.

15. Aparicio C, Arevalo X, Ouzzani W, et al: A retrospective clinical and radiographic evaluation of tilted implants used in the treatment of the severely resorbed maxilla. *Appl Osseo Res* 2000;3:17–21.

16. Maló P, Rangert B, Nobre M: "All-on-4" immediate-function concept with Brånemark system implants for completely edentulous mandibles: a retrospective clinical study. *Clin Implant Dent Relat Res* 2003;5 Suppl 1:2–9.

17. Maló P, Rangert B, Nobre M: "All-on-4" immediate-function concept of Brånemark system implants for completely edentulous maxilla: a 1-year retrospective clinical study. *Clin Implant Dent Relat Res* 2005;7 Suppl 1:S88–S94.

18. Butura C, Galindo D, Jensen O: Mandibular all-on-four therapy using angled implant: a three year clinical study of 857 implants in 219 jaws. *Oral Maxillofac Surg Clin North Am* 2011;23:289–300.

19. Graves S, Mahler BA, Javid D, et al: Maxillary all-on-four therapy using angled implants: a 16 month clinical study of 1110 implants in 276 jaws. *Dent Clin North Am* 2011;55:779–794.

20. Lekholm U, Zarb G: Patient selection and preparation. In Brånemark P-I, Zarb G, Albrektsson T (eds): *Tissue-Integrated Prostheses: Osseointegration in Clinical Density*. Chicago, Quintessence, 1985, pp. 199–220.

21. Bahat O: Technique for placement of oxidized titanium implants in compromised maxillary bone: prospective study of 290 implants in 126 consecutive patients followed for a minimum of 3 years after loading. *Int J Oral Maxillofac Implants* 2009;24:325–334.

22. Balshi SF, Wolfinger GJ, Balshi TJ: Analysis of 164 titanium oxide-surface implants in completely edentulous arches for fixed prosthesis anchorage using the pterygomaxillary region. *Int J Oral Maxillofac Implants* 2005;20:946–952.

23. Kinsel RP, Liss M: Retrospective analysis of 56 edentulous dental arches restored with 344 single-stage implants using an immediate loading fixed provisional protocol: statistical predictors of implant failure. *Int J Oral Maxillofac Implants* 2007;22:823–830.

24. Degidi M, Piattelli A: A 7-year follow-up of 93 immediately loaded titanium dental implants. *J Oral Implantol* 2005;1:25–31.

25. Balshi TJ, Wolfinger GJ, Balshi SF: Analysis of 356 pterygomaxillary implants in edentulous arches for fixed prosthesis anchorage. *Int J Oral Maxillofac Implants* 1999;14:398–406.

26. Malo P, de Araujo Nobre M, Lopes A, et al: "All-on-4" immediate-function concept for completely edentulous maxillae: a clinical report on the medium (3 years) and long-term (5 years) outcomes. *Clin Implant Dent Relat Res* 2012;14 Supp 1:e139–e150.

14

PRACTICE-BASED EVIDENCE FROM 29-YEAR OUTCOME ANALYSIS OF MANAGEMENT OF THE EDENTULOUS JAW USING OSSEOINTEGRATED DENTAL IMPLANTS

Matilda Dhima, DMD, MS,[1] Vladimira Paulusova, MD,[2] Christine Lohse, MS,[3] Thomas J. Salinas, DDS,[4] and Alan B. Carr, DMD, MS[5]

[1]Assistant Professor, Mayo Clinic College of Medicine and Chief Resident, Prosthodontics and Maxillofacial Prosthetics, Department of Dental Specialties, Division of Prosthetic and Esthetic Dentistry, Mayo Clinic, Rochester, MN

[2]Assistant Professor, Department of Dentistry, Faculty of Medicine and University Hospital in Hradec Králové, Charles University, Prague, Czech Republic

[3]Statistician, Department of Biostatistics, Mayo Clinic, Rochester, MN

[4]Professor, Mayo Clinic College of Medicine and Consultant, Department of Dental Specialties, Division of Prosthetic and Esthetic Dentistry, Mayo Clinic, Rochester, MN

[5]Professor, Mayo Clinic College of Medicine and Consultant, Chair, Department of Dental Specialties, Division of Prosthetic and Esthetic Dentistry, Mayo Clinic, Rochester, MN

Keywords

Edentulous jaw; dental implants; outcome analysis; practice-based evidence; hybrid; implant-retained dental prosthesis; complications; follow-up; management.

Correspondence

Alan B. Carr, DMD, MS, Mayo Clinic 200 1st St. SW, Rochester, MN 55905. E-mail: carr.alan@mayo.edu

The findings of this manuscript were presented at the American College of Prosthodontists Annual Session, Baltimore, Maryland, 2012.

The authors deny any conflicts of interest.

Accepted April 27, 2013

Published in *Journal of Prosthodontics* April 2014; Vol. 23, Issue 3

doi: 10.1111/jopr.12084

ABSTRACT

Purpose: The aim of this retrospective study was to summarize practice-based evidence associated with long-term outcomes (>20 years) in the management of edentulous patients. The patient population was managed with implant-supported prostheses, following the original osseointegration protocol, provided over the period from 1983 to 1991 in the group prosthodontics practice at the Mayo Clinic. The data are an example of practice quality assurance monitoring and are used to refine care delivery when needed and to provide information regarding expected outcomes in a shared decision-making interaction with prospective patients.

Materials and Methods: Two hundred and sixty four patients with at least one edentulous jaw were identified. Of these, 255 completed their care and follow-up at the Mayo Clinic (209 mandible only, 35 maxilla only, 11 mandible and maxilla). Prosthodontic outcomes categorized as anticipated or unanticipated prosthetic and biologic events and the respective interventions required for each were recorded to assess follow-up event dynamics for this care modality.

Results: The mean duration of follow-up for 190 of the 255 patients (65 died at a mean follow-up of 12.6 years) was 13.0 years (median 13.6; range 0.3 to 28). At least one prosthetic event was experienced by 148 patients (58%), and 81 (32%) experienced at least one biologic event. Overall, patients experienced 3.8 times more prosthetic events than biologic events. Twenty-four (9%) patients experienced 35 implant failures. Overall survival rates at 20 years were 86% for prostheses, 15% survived free of any event, and 92% experienced survival free of implant failure (95% confidence interval).

Conclusion: Anticipated and unanticipated prosthetic events occur throughout the life of the hybrid prosthesis. Prosthetic events significantly surpass (four times more) biologic events and occur significantly later in the follow-up. For this patient group, 8.6% (22/255) had implant-supported prostheses remade during follow-up in this patient population. These findings support the recommendation that prosthodontic care for missing teeth be thought of in a "chronic condition" context, recognizing that long-term outcome monitoring to provide realistic care expectations is important for demonstrating care value in oral health promotion.

Management of tooth loss over the past three decades has grown in scope due to the demonstrated predictability of dental implants. The original introduction of dental implants to North America demonstrated a predictable application for the edentulous jaw,[1] and similar clinical application began across the United States and Canada as a result.[2,3] Conscientious clinicians, using a shared decision-making[4] approach in consultation (i.e., informing patients as to the difference between and results of options available to them), have provided edentulous patients evidence as to benefit and harm based on published reports that now reach three decades.[5]

Meaningful decision making with patients seeking prosthodontic care involves sharing clinical outcome evidence that reflects the patient perspective of the care provided and is associated with a period of time that has significance relative to the care expectations of patients.[6] For the permanent condition "tooth loss," the expectation of replacements providing adequate performance for an extended period of time is understandable. In this long-term health-care context, tooth loss is similar to other chronic conditions in medicine and requires long-term management[7] of time-dependent events, which are often unique to the selected prosthetic management option.[8] This perspective suggests that outcome measures discussed with patients should reflect meaning from a patient perspective over a period of time that captures time-dependent differences of value to shared decision-making needs.[9]

Much research has been reported from clinical trials related to implant outcomes.[10-12] The applicability of clinical trial-based evidence to practice has been the subject of many reports.[13,14] Expressed concerns over trials in general and those involving "procedural specialties"[15] include issues of generalizability, the use of surrogate outcomes, and short-term outcome applicability or meaningfulness.[16] Evidence obtained from practice settings that provide care outcomes of

importance to patients can add valuable insight to providers interested in monitoring quality and patients interested in hearing about care expectations. Care outcomes from practice, termed practice-based evidence (PBE [16]) is complementary to trial-based evidence (complementary in that trial evidence demonstrates which treatment is effective; practice evidence demonstrates what results are observed when an effective treatment is provided), as it addresses evidence needs when trials are not performed or when care outcomes are needed for long-term chronic conditions.

This report provides practice evidence for the management of edentulism using cantilevered fixed implant prostheses for patients presenting to the Mayo Clinic from 1983 to 1991. The report provides outcome data for prosthesis survival and biological and technical outcomes for original osseointegrated surgical and prosthetic protocols, and represents PBE over a period of care of up to 29 years.

MATERIALS AND METHODS

A retrospective cohort was identified of all patients receiving edentulous implant care from 1983 to 1991. Appropriate institutional review board approval was obtained. The cohort comprised 308 patients with at least one edentulous jaw receiving an implant-supported prosthesis following the original Brånemark protocol.[17,18] Complete records review (electronic and paper) resulted in 28 patients being excluded due to incomplete or missing documentation, and 15 patients excluded due to written patient requests on file for their records not to be used for research.

The remaining 265 patient records were reviewed, and data were sought from diagnostic, treatment, and follow-up phases. Data were abstracted by two clinicians familiar with the record environment and the data "exposures" sought.

TABLE 14.1   Characteristics of Data Collected

Patient characteristics	Age
	Gender
	Geographical identity
	Living status
	Smoking history
	Medical comorbidities
Clinical characteristics	Implant dates by stage
	Prosthesis type
	Prosthesis placement date
	Opposing dentition
Event(s) characteristics	Event type/date
	Event interventions/number/date
	Visits to last appointment

TABLE 14.2   Description of Anticipated and Unanticipated Prosthetic and Biologic Events

Prosthetic Events	
Anticipated	Unanticipated
Lip biting	Fractured gold screw
Change of opposing dentition	Loose abutment
Loose opposing denture	Fractured abutment screw
Lost composite filling	Fractured multiple abutment screws
Difficulty cleaning under prosthesis	Prosthesis fracture
Loose opposing overdenture	Broken opposing denture
Loose O rings	Fractured acrylic base
Tooth broken opposing partial denture	Distorted implant platform
Lost gold matrix	Removal of failed implant
Prosthesis tooth fracture	
Prosthesis tooth wear	
Tooth broken on opposing denture	
Loose gold screw	

Biologic Events	
Anticipated	Unanticipated
Plaque/calculus	Periapical radiolucency
Hyperplasia	Infection
Tingling when flossing	Mobile implant
Paresthesia	Benign/malignant process

All events types were collected and categorized. Anticipated/unanticipated designations were chosen to assist clarification of recall dynamics. An event associated with continued functional performance and reversible return to biological health is considered as less disruptive to follow-up, which is anticipated. An event that leads to harm with function and is irreversible biologically would be more demanding at follow-up, both an unanticipated and undesirable outcome.

Initial abstraction efforts were formally reviewed by duplicating abstraction for 12 charts to assure completeness and accuracy. All data were collected on a secure Microsoft Excel 2010 file.

Data abstracted included both patient and clinical characteristics and event-related data (Table 14.1), following event reporting designations used in clinical-trial monitoring for human protection.[19] Prosthetic and biological outcome events are categorized as anticipated (when prosthetically functional; biologically reversible) or unanticipated (when prosthetically harmful with continued function; biologically irreversible and requiring care) (Table 14.2).

Overall survival, survival free of event, and survival free of implant failure were estimated using the Kaplan-Meier method. Overall survival was designated by prosthesis presence in the mouth with or without anticipated events. Survival "free of event" was defined as prosthesis present and with no record of any event(s). The duration of follow-up for overall survival was calculated from the date of implant placement to the date of patient death or last check-up. The duration of survival free of event was calculated from the date of implant to the date of the first event or last check-up. The duration of survival free of implant failure was calculated from the date of implant to the date of first implant failure or last follow-up. All statistical analyses were performed using the SAS software package (SAS Institute, Cary, NC).

RESULTS

The mean duration of follow-up for 190 of the 255 patients (65 died at a mean follow-up of 12.6 years) was 13.0 years (median 13.6; range 0.3 to 28). The majority of the 255 patients (97%) underwent surgery and prosthesis placement at Mayo Clinic, while 9 (3%) had their prosthesis fabricated

elsewhere. Relative to age, gender, and arch restored, there were no differences between patient groups. Regarding residence, 78% (7 of 9) of the patients restored elsewhere were National residents, compared to 44% National residents in the Mayo-treated cohort (Table 14.3). Single-arch prostheses were provided the majority of the time (209 mandibular, 35 maxillary), and 11 patients received both mandibular and maxillary prostheses. The 255 patients received 1325 implants, 1089 in the mandible and 236 in the maxilla.

The average age of cohort patients was 56.4 years [68 (27%) less than 50 years of age, 83 (33%) between 50 and 60 years of age, 104 (41%) over 60 years of age] at the time of implant placement. In this group of implant patients, these patients were largely existing denture wearers with a history of maladaptation to removable prostheses. Patients were followed an average of 11.8 years from the time of implant placement to last check-up [140 (53%) followed over

TABLE 14.3 Summary of Patient Specific Features

Feature (n = 255 Completed Rehabilitations)	Mean (Range)
Age at first implant in years	56.4 (9–82)
Years from first implant to last check-up	11.8 (0.0–27.9)
Overall number of visits	23.8 (0–113)
Number of visits per year	4.3 (0–69)
Sex	N (%)
Female	190 (75)
Male	65 (25)
Residence	
National	111 (44)
Local	84 (33)
Regional	53 (21)
International	7 (3)
Arch restored	
Mandible	209 (82)
Maxilla	35 (14)
Both mandible and maxilla	11 (4)
Prosthetic design	
Metal acrylic	229 (90)
Spark erosion	8 (3)
Bar with RPD	7 (3)
Metal ceramic	3 (1)
Bar milled/OD	1 (<1)
Metal acrylic—switch to spark erosion	4 (2)
Metal acrylic—switch to bar with RPD	2 (1)
Metal acrylic—switch to metal ceramic	1 (<1)
Smoker	82 (32)
Cardiovascular disease	136 (53)
Osteoporosis	59 (23)
GERD	28 (11)
Hypertension	185 (73)
Hyperlipidemia	164 (64)
Carcinoma	34 (13)

Feature (n = 9 Prostheses Placed Elsewhere)	Mean (Median; Range)
Age at first implant in years	60.6 (61; 43–81)
Years from first implant to last check-up	0.5 (0.5; 0.0–1.1)
Sex	N (%)
Female	6 (67)
Male	3 (33)
Residence	
National	7 (78)
Regional	2 (22)
Arch restored	
Mandible	7 (78)
Maxilla	1 (11)
Both mandible and maxilla	1 (11)
Prosthetic design	
Metal acrylic	2 (22)
Spark erosion	1 (11)
Unknown	6 (67)

Local: State of Minnesota.
Regional: North Dakota, South Dakota, Nebraska, Wisconsin, Iowa.
National: United States of America excluding local and regional.
International: Outside the United States of America.

10 years, 96 (36%) followed over 15 years, and 58 (23%) followed over 20 years]. Patients returned for an average of five visits per year after prosthesis placement.

Overview of Prosthesis Survival

Overall prosthesis survival rates at 5, 10, 15, and 20 years following the date of implant reveal a 20-year survival rate of 86% (Fig 14.1). Survival free of prosthetic or biologic events for the same time intervals reveals 51% at 5 years and 11% at 20 years (Fig 14.2). Prosthesis survival free of any prosthetic events is shown in Figure 14.3. Survival free of implant failure rates for the same time intervals reveals that at 20 years, 12% of the prostheses had experienced implant failure (Fig 14.4). Of the prostheses, 15% survived free of any event, and 92% experienced survival free of implant failure (95% confidence interval).

Twenty two of the cohort patients (8.6%) had a prosthesis remake. The timing of the remakes ranged from 1.2 to 25.6 years following the date of implant insertion (mean 9.6 years). The most common reason for a prosthesis remake was due to prosthetic events, and was often related to repeated events suggesting the need for improved prosthesis-implant fit.

Overview of Events

A summary of prosthetic and biologic events, both those anticipated and unanticipated, is shown in Table 14.4. There were over three times as many prosthetic events as biologic events in this patient group. Regarding the prosthetic events, unanticipated events occurred more commonly, they required fewer than two visits on average to resolve, and were seen from year 1 through year 26 of follow-up (mean 7.6 years from implant placement). Regarding biologic events, anticipated events occurred more than twice as frequently as unanticipated events, both types were resolved in two or fewer visits, and each type was seen sooner, on average, than prosthetic events.

The mean number of prosthetic events observed per patient was two times more than the mean number of biologic events observed per patient (4.3 and 2.1, respectively). The mean number of unanticipated prosthetic events observed per patient was 4, while the mean number of unanticipated biologic events observed per patient was 1.5.

On average, the first anticipated prosthetic events occurred 10.5 years after implant placement and significantly later than the first anticipated biologic event, which occurred 4.1 years after implant placement (Table 14.4). The mean number of visits to address anticipated prosthetic events were 2.8 (range 1 to 8) with 43% of them addressed in one visit. The mean number of visits to address anticipated biologic events was 1.4 (range 1 to 9) with 72% of them addressed in one visit (Table 14.4).

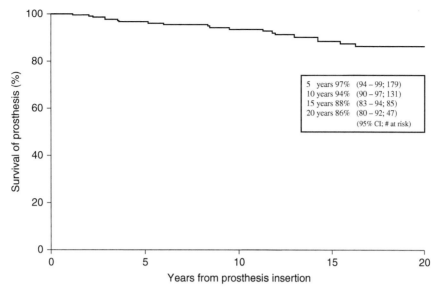

FIGURE 14.1 Overall prosthesis survival.

Table 14.5 summarizes events at the patient level. Over one-third of the patients experienced no prosthetic or biologic events over the period of follow-up. Nearly one-fourth of the patients experienced both types of events, one-third experienced only prosthetic events, and less than one-tenth experienced only biologic events. Well over half (58%) experienced at least one prosthetic event, and for the patients with at least one event (i.e., at least one prosthetic or biologic event) the mean time to their first event was approximately 5 years.

Most Common Prosthetic and Biologic Events

Table 14.6 shows fractured screws and abutments were the top two prosthetic events observed; occurring at the 6- to 7-year mean time period and requiring a single visit to address more than 85% of the time. The third most common prosthetic event observed, wear, occurred at a much later mean time period (14 years) and, as would be expected, required more visits to address. The most frequent prosthetic event was fracture of a single gold screw, which on

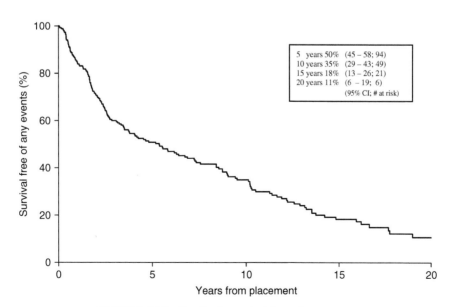

FIGURE 14.2 Prosthesis survival free of any events.

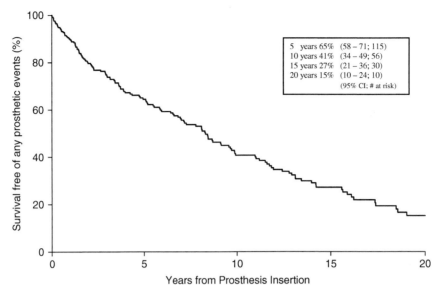

FIGURE 14.3   Prosthesis survival free of any prosthetic events.

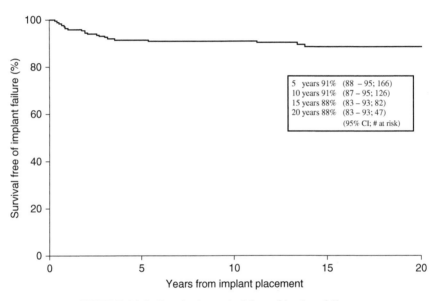

FIGURE 14.4   Prosthesis survival free of implant failure.

TABLE 14.4   Summary of Anticipated and Unanticipated Events and Visits to Address Events

			Visits to Resolve Event	Visits to Resolve Event N (%)		
	N	Years from Implant Placement Mean (Range)*	N	1	2	>2
Prosthetic	643					
Anticipated	251	10.5 (0.4–25.3)	2.8 (1–8)	107 (43)	40 (16)	104 (41)
Unanticipated	392	7.6 (0.3–26.0)	1.7 (1–12)	312 (80)	27 (7)	53 (14)
Biologic	169					
Anticipated	117	4.1 (0.3–21.3)	1.4 (1–9)	85 (72)	27 (23)	5 (4)
Unanticipated	52	5.0 (0.1–19.5)	2.1 (1–8)	18 (35)	23 (44)	11 (21)

*All values are listed for sample sizes ≤3.

TABLE 14.5 Summary of Patient Experiences with Events

Event Type	Patients N (%) N$_{total}$ = 255	Years from Implant Placement to the First Event Mean (Range)
At least one prosthetic	148 (58)	4.9 (2.6; 17 days to 26.0 years)
At least one biologic	81 (32)	
Only prosthetic	86 (34)	
Only biologic	19 (7)	
Prosthetic and biologic	62 (24)	
None	88 (35)	

average occurred 7.4 years after prosthesis insertion. The most frequent biologic event was peri-implant soft tissue hyperplasia, which on average occurred 3.3 years after implant placement.

Implant Failures

Fewer than 10% of the patients experienced 35 implant failures over the course of the observation period. Ten failures occurred less than 1 year after implant placement, with the remaining 25 implant failures occurring in patients a mean of 4.7 years (range 1 to 13.1) after implant placement. Nineteen of the implant failures occurred in the mandible and 16 in the maxilla.

This failure cohort also experienced mostly unanticipated prosthetic events. Of particular note for this edentulous population is the finding that opposing dentition type did not have a statistically significant impact on implant failure or time of failure. For the group, 60% had an opposing complete denture, and 31% had natural opposing dentition.

DISCUSSION

The evidence-based history in prosthodontics is longstanding. It began with a formal scholarly exposure to the principles involved at McMaster University in the early 1990s, followed by educational workshops targeting dissemination of these principles to residency directors and educators, and included publication of prosthodontic-specific evidence-based learning and practice aids modeled after those originally published in medicine.[20]

Since that time, progress has been made in the understanding of clinical evidence and its application to the clinical encounter of patient care. Yet clinical trial reports consistently fall short of providing outcomes that delineate long-term expectations that patients and providers use to understand complex care decisions in prosthodontics.[21] This does not mean that evidence-based efforts are not worthwhile, but does suggest the need to consider defining best practice using evidence complementary to trial-based evidence and doing so with careful understanding as to how much confidence we can infer from evidence sources to our unique situations.[13] This article suggests that evidence from practice, systematically collected and studied by conscientious practitioners, should be considered.

Long-Term Practice Outcome Data

The data in this report represent outcomes from a time frame of care beginning 29 years ago; it serves as an example of a database maintenance report used as part of practice monitoring, and its specific use will be to (1) guide decisions regarding scheduling of maintenance visits, and (2) inform shared decision-making discussions with patients in a group prosthodontic practice. The practice scope requires database use to systematically monitor care quality, and for the chronic condition of missing teeth, doing so allows identification of time-dependent influences on the clinical course, categorized as clinical outcomes. Such a systematic monitoring,

TABLE 14.6 The Three Most Common Prosthetic and Biologic Events and How They Were Addressed

Event	Top 3	N (%)	Years from Implant Placement to the First Event Mean (Range)	Visits to Address N	Visits to Address N (%)		
					1 Visit	2 Visits	>2 Visits
Prosthetic N = 643	Fractured screw	113 (18)	7.4 (0.6–25.5)	1.4 (1–9)	100 (89)	4 (4)	9 (8)
	Fractured abutment	73 (11)	6.4 (0.9–25.5)	1.3 (1–5)	64 (88)	3 (4)	6 (8)
	Wear	63 (8)	13.9 (2.3–23.2)	4.6 (1–8)	5 (8)	4 (6)	56 (86)
Biologic N = 169	Hyperplasia	97 (57)	3.3 (0.3–15.4)	1.4 (1–9)	68 (70)	25 (26)	4 (4)
	Mobile implant	23 (14)	3.4 (0.1–13.4)	1.7 (1–4)	11 (48)	10 (43)	2 (9)
	Infection	15 (9)	6.3 (0.2–19.5)	2.2 (1–5)	3 (20)	8 (53)	4 (27)

analyzing, and responding to outcomes of care with a quality target in mind is a longstanding goal of outcomes research.[22]

Outcomes Research

Outcomes research has meant various things to different groups over the past few decades. Lee et al share a historical perspective of this confusing field and summarize current understanding of outcomes research as being concerned with improving clinical practice as applied to patients treated outside clinical trials.[23] Specific to the field of prosthodontics, outcomes are the consequences of management decisions for missing and defective teeth, made at the individual patient level, involving multiple factors of importance to the patient and, based on the clinical findings, the clinician. A fundamental principle involved in the patient-provider interaction is that the patient elects to pursue care for self-defined reasons.[24] Therefore, in shared decision-making discussions, all factors important to a management decision must have value to the individual electing the intervention.[9] Consequently, pertinent outcomes should be identified as consistent with patient expectations, helpful to providers in quality assurance (QA) monitoring relative to meeting treatment targets, and providing data for summary and sharing with patients considering care. When outcomes directly address common patient concerns regarding expectations, options, benefit and risk, and self-care they directly inform best practices (Table 14.7).

Outcome Comparison

It is important to view the evidence in this report against previous reports. Favorable long-term outcomes have been shown for edentulous patients treated using a two-stage

TABLE 14.7   Summary of Patient-Centered Questions for Informed Healthcare Decisions as Suggested by the Patient-Centered Outcomes Research Institute. Available Online at http://www.pcori.org/research-we-support/pcor/ *

Patient Centered Questions to Ask
1 "Given my personal characteristics, conditions and preferences, what should I expect will happen to me?"
2 "What are my options and what are the potential benefits and harms of those options?"
3 "What can I do to improve the outcomes that are most important to me?"
4 "How can clinicians and the care delivery systems they work in help me make the best decisions about my health and healthcare?"

*Last accessed on February 9, 2013.

surgical protocol, machined titanium implants, and implant-supported cantilevered prostheses at the abutment level.[11,12,18] Several articles have also reported implant and prosthetic component performance events such as loose and fractured screws, prosthesis superstructure wear and fracture, alteration of opposing dentition, and even the need for prosthesis replacement.[18,25–28] Reports of prosthesis maintenance needs and the impact of implant failures on long-term care are important, yet when reports are limited in patient sample size and length of follow-up,[12,18] and when concern exists as to how applicable the outcomes are to an individual practice, it is difficult to know with surety if practice change is required. This overall prosthesis survival of 86% at 20 years is similar to the lower limit of previous reports in the literature, which ranged from 84% to 34%[12] to 100%.[11] Material fatigue of superstructure and first-generation implant components contributed to the events observed. Unlike other studies that showed minimal prosthetic events,[10,11] this study reveals significantly more prosthetic events than biologic events. Furthermore, prosthetic events occurred significantly later than biologic events. The anticipated prosthetic events occurred on average more than 10 years after initial treatment, while unanticipated prosthetic events occurred on average almost 8 years after initial treatment. As suggested in the literature,[10–12,17] time-dependent outcomes are critical to understand from a prosthetic maintenance perspective. The comparative difference between event types (four times more prosthetic events than biologic events) is not in agreement with previous reports, which described minimal screw fractures, screw loosening, wear, and loss of access fillings. Prosthesis tooth wear was the third most common event with 65 (10%) patients, consistent with previous literature[12] when differences in the size of the patient population were taken into account (308 patients in this study vs. 45 to 58 patients). An early study[10] showed that, on average, a patient received 2.27 implant-retained prostheses (range 1 to 4), more than reported in this study.

Population Characteristics

The population in this report represents approximately six times more patients than similar patient populations reviewed in the literature. Regarding the comparability of patients, the patients in this cohort included all patients from implant care inception through 1991. No selection bias is expected, and all data are part of the current clinical outcome database used prospectively. The inclusion of a large portion of patients who travel some distance for care (44% National patients) is unique, yet follow-up remains robust, as 140 (53%) patients have been followed for 10 years, 96 (36%) for more than 15 years, and 58 (23%) for more than 20 years.

Events

With 75% of this patient population still living after 30 years of initial treatment, the data reveal that time-dependent events become more frequent. Also, biologic events reflect a remarkable biological tolerance over time.[29] Although the majority of the prosthetic events could be addressed in one or two visits, visits ranged from 1 to 9. This information is valuable for describing potential long-term care needs, and financial and maintenance expectations associated with such treatment. One in three patients experienced no events during follow-up; one of four experienced both a biological and prosthetic event; 58% had at least one prosthetic event.

Prosthetic events were felt to be related to cantilever constructions and are not unexpected, given previous reports.[30,31] Screw loosening related to the prosthetic screw is known to have a design safety feature of this original system, placing the most "at-risk" component in a retrievable location. The data support the finding that prosthetic events were managed in timely manner on average.

Biologic events can be characterized as low in severity, resolved in a timely manner, and when involving a failure of an implant, this did not always detract from prosthesis function. Regarding implant failure, approximately one out of three (10/35) failed in the first year, and failure was not associated with opposing dentition type. This implant survival finding of 88% (83 to 93, 95% CI) at 20 years is consistent with other studies of a similar patient population.[10-12]

Prosthesis-Specific Survival

The findings of this report suggest that patients considering similar care have a very good chance (86%) that at 20 years they will have a functioning prosthesis. When we found the need to remake a prosthesis, it occurred infrequently (22 of 255 patients) and at varying times after the original prosthesis (from 1.2 to 25.6 years). This outcome compares very favorably with conventional fixed prostheses, where one systematic review describes an 89% 10-year survival estimate.[32]

Practice Application

As this practice evolves, we are faced with considering what key findings from this time period can best inform current and future care. The patient population in this report is more homogeneous than edentulous patients seen in the last 5 to 10 years. In 1983 when this treatment approach was implemented, presenting patients had been edentulous for several years and were considered for care based on presentation with significant residual alveolar ridge resorption and attendant maladaptation to conventional prostheses. This type of patient with such significant residual ridge resorption resulted in a significantly large restorative space to accommodate implant and prosthetic components for resin to metal prostheses. On the contrary, current populations being managed with implant-supported prostheses also include patients who received elective extractions, creating situations with potentially limited restorative space. This situation more often requires consideration of strategically prescribed terminal implants, which reduces or eliminates cantilever influences.

CONCLUSION

This report of practice-based outcome evidence from a 29-year follow-up period of implant prostheses provides long-term data useful for practice QA and shared decision-making patient discussions.

The clinical events associated with patient follow-up visits revealed the following:

1. Overall prosthesis survival at 20 years was 86%.
2. Prosthetic events occur significantly later and more frequently than biologic events.
3. The most common prosthetic event was fractured gold screws, and the most common biologic event was hyperplasia.

These findings support the suggestion that prosthodontic care for edentulism be managed within a "chronic condition" context for a more realistic understanding of maintenance expectations for patients and providers.

ACKNOWLEDGMENTS

The authors acknowledge the contributions to the clinical work reviewed in this report from all consultants, residents, and allied staff providing patient care within the Department of Dental Specialties at Mayo Clinic since 1983.

REFERENCES

1. Branemark PI, Adell R, Albrektsson T, et al: Osseointegrated titanium fixtures in the treatment of edentulousness. *Biomaterials* 1983;4:25–28.
2. Laney WR, Tolman DE, Keller EE, et al: Dental implants: tissue-integrated prosthesis utilizing the osseointegration concept. *Mayo Clin Proc* 1986;61:91–97.
3. Cox JF, Zarb GA: The longitudinal clinical efficacy of osseointegrated dental implants: a 3-year report. *Int J Oral Maxillofac Implants* 1987;2:91–100.
4. Legare F, Ratte S, Stacey D, et al: Interventions for improving the adoption of shared decision making by healthcare professionals. *Cochrane Database Syst Rev* 2010;CD006732.

5. Branemark PI, Albrektsson T: Titanium implants permanently penetrating human skin. *Scand J Plast Reconstr Surg* 1982;16:17–21.

6. Cronin M, Meaney S, Jepson NJ, et al: A qualitative study of trends in patient preferences for the management of the partially dentate state. *Gerodontology* 2009;26:137–142.

7. Griffin S, Kinmonth AL: Diabetes care: the effectiveness of systems for routine surveillance for people with diabetes. *Cochrane Database Syst Rev* 2000:CD000541.

8. Carr AB: Effect of prosthetic remedial treatments on the oral health status of individuals and populations. *Int J Prosthodont* 2003;16(Suppl):55–58.

9. Carr AB: Successful long-term treatment outcomes in the field of osseointegrated implants: prosthodontic determinants. *Int J Prosthodont* 1998;11:502–512.

10. Attard NJ, Zarb GA: Long-term treatment outcomes in edentulous patients with implant-fixed prostheses: the Toronto study. *Int J Prosthodont* 2004;17:417–424.

11. Ekelund JA, Lindquist LW, Carlsson GE, et al: Implant treatment in the edentulous mandible: a prospective study on Branemark system implants over more than 20 years. *Int J Prosthodont* 2003;16:602–608.

12. Astrand P, Ahlqvist J, Gunne J, et al: Implant treatment of patients with edentulous jaws: a 20-year follow-up. *Clin Implant Dent Relat Res* 2008;10:207–217.

13. Feinstein AR, Horwitz RI: Problems in the "evidence" of "evidence-based medicine". *Am J Med* 1997;103:529–535.

14. Berwick DM: Broadening the view of evidence-based medicine. *Qual Saf Health Care* 2005;14:315–316.

15. Cook JA: The challenges faced in the design, conduct and analysis of surgical randomised controlled trials. *Trials* 2009;10:9.

16. Pincus T, Sokka T: Evidence-based practice and practice-based evidence. *Nat Clin Pract Rheumatol* 2006;2:114–115.

17. Adell R, Lekholm U, Rockler B, et al: A 15-year study of osseointegrated implants in the treatment of the edentulous jaw. *Int J Oral Maxillofac Surg* 1981;10:387–416.

18. Attard NJ, Zarb GA: Long-term treatment outcomes in edentulous patients with implant overdentures: the Toronto study. *Int J Prosthodont* 2004;17:425–433.

19. Office for Human Research Protections (OHRP): Draft guidance on reporting and reviewing adverse events and unanticipated problems involving risks to subjects or others. OHRP, 2005. Available online at http://www.hhs.gov/ohrp/archive/rfc/aerg.html. Last accessed on February 9, 2013.

20. McGivney GP: Evidence-based dentistry article series. *J Prosthet Dent* 2000;83:11–12.

21. Abt E, Carr AB, Worthington HV: Interventions for replacing missing teeth: partially absent dentition. *Cochrane Database Syst Rev* 2012;2:CD003814.

22. AHRQ Outcomes Research Fact Sheet: AHRQ Publication No. 00-P011, March 2000. Rockville, MD, Agency for Healthcare Research and Quality. Available online at http://www.ahrq.gov/clinic/outfact.htm. Last accessed on February 9, 2013.

23. Lee SJ, Earle CC, Weeks JC: Outcomes research in oncology: history, conceptual framework, and trends in the literature. *J Natl Cancer Inst* 2000;92:195–204.

24. Davies AR: Patient defined outcomes. *Qual Health Care* 1994;3(Suppl):6–9.

25. Henry PJ, Bower RC, Wall CD: Rehabilitation of the edentulous mandible with osseointegrated dental implants: 10 year follow-up. *Aust Dent J* 1995;40:1–9.

26. Carlsson GE, Lindquist LW, Jemt T: Long-term marginal periimplant bone loss in edentulous patients. *Int J Prosthodont* 2000;13:295–302.

27. Snauwaert K, Duyck J, van Steenberghe D, et al: Time dependent failure rate and marginal bone loss of implant supported prostheses: a 15-year follow-up study. *Clin Oral Investig* 2000;4:13–20.

28. Ferrigno N, Laureti M, Fanali S, et al: A long-term follow-up study of non-submerged ITI implants in the treatment of totally edentulous jaws. Part I: ten-year life table analysis of a prospective multicenter study with 1286 implants. *Clin Oral Implants Res* 2002;13:260–273.

29. Koka S, Zarb G: On osseointegration: the healing adaptation principle in the context of osseosufficiency, osseoseparation, and dental implant failure. *Int J Prosthodont* 2012;25:48–52.

30. Zurdo J, Romao C, Wennstrom JL: Survival and complication rates of implant-supported fixed partial dentures with cantilevers: a systematic review. *Clin Oral Implants Res* 2009; 20(Suppl 4):59–66.

31. Aglietta M, Siciliano VI, Zwahlen M, et al: A systematic review of the survival and complication rates of implant supported fixed dental prostheses with cantilever extensions after an observation period of at least 5 years. *Clin Oral Implants Res* 2009;20:441–451.

32. Jokstad A: After 10 years seven out of ten fixed dental prostheses (FDP) remain intact and nine out of ten FDPs remain in function following biological and technical complications that have been repaired. *J Evid Based Dent Pract* 2010;10:39–40.

15

DOUBLE FULL-ARCH VERSUS SINGLE FULL-ARCH, FOUR IMPLANT-SUPPORTED REHABILITATIONS: A RETROSPECTIVE, 5-YEAR COHORT STUDY

Paulo Maló, DDS, PHD,[1] Miguel De Araújo Nobre, RDH, MSC EPI,[2] Armando Lopes, DDS, MSC,[1] AND Rolando Rodrigues, DDS[3]

[1]Oral Surgery Department, Maló Clinic, Lisbon, Portugal
[2]Research and Development Department, Maló Clinic, Lisbon, Portugal
[3]Prosthodontics Department, Maló Clinic, Lisbon, Portugal

Keywords
Dental implants; immediate function; All-on-4.

Correspondence
Paulo Maló, Maló Clinic, Avenida dos Combatentes, 43, 9° C, Ed. Green Park, 1600-042 Lisbon, Portugal. E-mail: research@maloclinics.com

This study was funded by a grant from Nobel Biocare Services AG (grant no. 2012-1103). Professor Paulo Maló is currently a consultant for Nobel Biocare AB.

Accepted June 10, 2014

Published in *Journal of Prosthodontics* online October 1, 2014

doi: 10.1111/jopr.12228

ABSTRACT

Purpose: To report the 5-year outcome of the All-on-4 treatment concept comparing double full-arch (G1) and single-arch (G2) groups.

Materials and Methods: This retrospective cohort study included 110 patients (68 women and 42 men, average age of 55.5 years) with 440 NobelSpeedy groovy implants. One hundred sixty-five full-arch, fixed, immediately loaded prostheses in both jaws were followed for 5 years. G1 consisted of 55 patients with double-arch rehabilitations occluded with implant-supported fixed prostheses, and G2 consisted of 55 patients with maxillary single-arch rehabilitations or mandibular single-arch rehabilitations occluded with natural teeth or removable prostheses. The groups were matched for age (±6 years) and gender. Primary outcome measures were cumulative prosthetic (both interim and definitive) and implant survival (Kaplan-Meier product limit estimator). Secondary outcome measures were marginal bone levels at 5 years (through periapical radiographs and using the patient as unit of analysis) and the incidence of mechanical and biological complications. Differences in survival curves (log-rank test), marginal bone level (Mann-Whitney U test), and complications (chi-square test) were compared inferentially between the two groups using the patient as unit of analysis with significance level set at $p \leq 0.05$.

Results: No dropouts occurred. Prosthetic survival was 100%. Five patients lost 5 implants (G1: $n = 3$; G2: $n = 2$) before 1 year, rendering an estimated cumulative survival rate of 95.5% (G1: 94.5%; G2: 96.4%; Kaplan-Meier, $p = 0.645$, nonsignificant). The average (SD) marginal bone level was 1.56 mm (0.89) at 5 years [G1: 1.45 mm (0.77); G2: 1.67 mm (0.99); $p = 0.414$]. The incidence rate of mechanical complications (in both interim and definitive prostheses) was 0.16 and 0.13 for G1 and G2, respectively ($p = 0.032$). The incidence rate of biological complications was 0.06 and 0.05 for G1 and G2, respectively ($p = 0.669$).

Conclusions: Based on the results, rehabilitating double- or single-arch edentulous patients did not yield significant differences on survival curves. The incidence of mechanical complications was significantly higher for double-arch rehabilitated patients but nevertheless, these mechanical complications did not affect the long-term survival of either the prostheses or the implants.

The success of an edentulous rehabilitation is dependent on the development of shared goals for both the patient and the clinical team. New and improved treatment procedures, such as the continuous development of dental implant therapies, the evaluation of issues concerning prosthetic function, and prosthesis quality, are necessary to successfully rehabilitate the edentulous patient.[1] The use of removable prosthetics frequently leads to mucosal irritation, under-extension of the denture bases, incorrect jaw relationships, incorrect occlusal vertical dimension, and inadequate posterior palatal seal.[2] Some pathological manifestations of denture use include stomatitis, traumatic ulcers, irritation-induced hyperplasia, altered taste perception, burning mouth syndrome, and gagging. Some rehabilitation therapies do not replace dimensional changes of the lower third of the face caused by continued resorption of the mandibular alveolar bone, which causes greater difficulties for denture construction: overall, removable dentures do not obtain the physiological, psychological, and social complete satisfaction of the individual who needs full-arch rehabilitation.[3] Oral implant placement may prevent the continued resorption of bone and has been associated with increased mandibular bone height distal to the implant location.[4,5] High success rates have been reported when rehabilitating completely edentulous patients using four or more implants, and in the late 1990s, various authors published clinical reports regarding the possibility of early or immediate loading of implants with fixed provisional full-arch restorations.[6-8]

In 2003, Maló et al[9] introduced the All-on-4 treatment concept. This protocol requires the placement of four interforaminal implants in the mandible, with the distal implants tilted distally by 30° to achieve a more favorable distribution of implants, thereby minimizing cantilever extensions that could jeopardize osseointegration of the distal implants.[10]

Immediate loading in the edentulous maxilla is perceived as a greater challenge than in the mandible, mostly due to the lower bone density in this jaw. Furthermore, implant anchorage in the totally edentulous maxilla is often restricted because of bone resorption, a frequent condition in the posterior regions of the jaws where bone grafting is often indicated. Implant tilting has been shown to be a good alternative to bone grafting in the maxilla, as indicated in the clinical results of several studies.[11-13] By tilting the posterior implant, a more posterior implant position can be reached, reducing the cantilever compared to axially placed implants. Cantilever extensions seem to be associated with a decreased prosthetic survival rate.[14-16] Tilting the posterior implant can also provide improved implant anchorage by engaging the apex of the implants with the cortical bone of the anterior wall of the sinus and the nasal fossae.[17]

The use of four implants in the maxilla is supported by results from short- and long-term clinical studies.[12,13,17-19] Good clinical outcomes from studies using protocols in which four implants were placed to support a full-arch prosthesis indicate that the placement of additional implants may not be necessary for successful implant treatment of edentulous jaws.[19,20]

More recently, several authors have noted that the use of the All-on-4 treatment concept with a 30° inclination of the distal implants reduced the maximum stress in the distal crestal bone,[21,22] with no difference in marginal bone resorption between tilted and straight implants.[23] Furthermore, other authors[24] reported no significant differences in loading parameters when comparing the use of more implants, demonstrating the importance of conceding enough space between implants.

The implant surgical protocol may influence the outcome of full-arch rehabilitation in the long-term, as can the size of cantilever, bar material, and type of bone.[25] A recent systematic review[26] stated that biologic and technical complications occur continuously over time as a result of fatigue and stress.

Fazi et al[10] reported that when comparing several implant numbers and positions, the use of the All-on-4 treatment concept not only reduced load bearing from bone, but also from implants and frameworks. Rehabilitating the completely edentulous patient is still a challenge. The rate for absence of complications in prosthetic full-arch rehabilitations is less than 30% at 5 years and 8% at 10 years,[26] with the most common complications being peri-implant bone loss, screw fracture, hypertrophy or hyperplasia of the soft tissue around the rehabilitation, and chipping or fracture of the veneering material, which requires repair, maintenance, time, and cost to both the clinician and patient.

The biomechanics of double full-arch edentulism and the effect of an implant-supported fixed prosthesis as opposing dentition is not known to a great extent, with few clinical studies addressing this issue.[6,8,27,28] It may be that an implant rehabilitation as opposing dentition constitutes a risk factor for late implant loss.[27] Studies addressing this finding in immediate function implants are nonexistent.

The aim of this retrospective cohort study was to compare the outcome of double full-arch versus single full-arch rehabilitations in long-term outcome. This study aimed to determine the influence of opposing dentition on the treatment outcome of immediate implant-supported fixed prostheses for rehabilitation of completely edentulous jaws. The null hypothesis was that there is no difference in the long-term outcome of implant-supported fixed rehabilitations, regardless of the opposing dentition.

MATERIALS AND METHODS

This article was written following Strengthening the Reporting of Observational Studies in Epidemiology (STROBE) guidelines.[29] This retrospective cohort study was performed at a private rehabilitation center (Malo Clinic, Lisbon, Portugal). This study was approved by an independent ethical committee (Ethical Committee for Health; Authorization no. 014/2010). The inclusion criterion was edentulous arches, or arches with hopeless teeth, in need of fixed implant restorations as requested by the patient. As exclusion criteria, patients presenting with emotional instability, and patients who were not followed at the rehabilitation center were excluded from the study. From January 2004 to December 2006, a total of 149 patients were rehabilitated with full-arch rehabilitations according to the All-on-4 treatment concept (Nobel Biocare, Göteborg, Sweden) in both jaws on the same day, and 311 were rehabilitated with one full-arch rehabilitation according to the All-on-4 treatment concept (maxilla: 153; mandible: 158). Fifty-five patients were randomly selected from the double full-arch rehabilitations

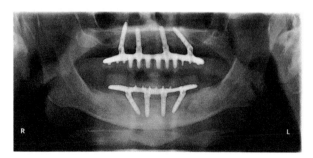

FIGURE 15.1 Orthopantomography of a double full-arch All-on-4 rehabilitation.

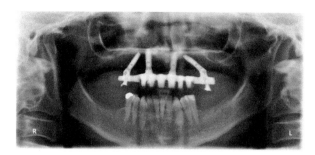

FIGURE 15.2 Orthopantomography of a maxillary single full-arch All-on-4 rehabilitation.

(Group 1 [G1]; Fig 15.1) using a random sequence generator. The patients with single full-arch were selected based on the absence of an opposing dentition containing implant-supported fixed prostheses, and matching for age (±6 years of a double full-arch patient) and gender with patients from G1. Of the 169 patients with single full-arch rehabilitation who qualified in the matching procedure, 55 were randomly selected (group 2 [G2], 26 maxillae and 29 mandibles; Figs 15.2 and 15.3), resulting in a total of 110 patients (68 women and 42 men; average age = 55.5 years old [standard deviation: 8.9 years]; range: 38 to 80 years old) having received a total of 660 NobelSpeedy implants (Nobel Biocare AB, Gothenburg, Sweden). As opposing dentition, patients from G1 presented an implant-supported fixed prosthesis ($n = 55$), while in G2 there were 35 patients with natural teeth, and 20 had a removable prosthesis.

Sample Size Calculation

The sample size calculation was performed using a software program (Power and Sample Size Calculations, version 3.0.34, Dupont WD and Plummer WD Jr, Department of Biostatistics, Vanderbilt University, Nashville, TN). The authors planned a study with one control per experimental subject, an accrual interval of 6 time units (1 year = 1 time unit), and additional follow-up after the accrual interval of 3 time units. Prior data indicated that the median survival time on the control treatment was 6 time units.[13,30] If the true median survival times on the control and experimental treatments are 6 and 3 time units, respectively, it was deemed

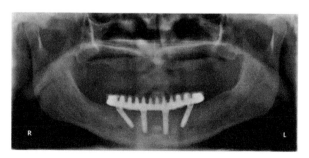

FIGURE 15.3 Orthopantomography of a mandibular single full-arch All-on-4 rehabilitation.

necessary to include 55 experimental subjects and 55 control subjects to be able to reject the null hypothesis that the experimental and control survival curves are equal with probability (power) 0.8. The type I error probability associated with this test of this null hypothesis was 0.05.

Surgical Protocol

The patients' medical histories were reviewed, together with clinical observation (treatment planning) and complementary radiographic exams with an orthopantomography (for bone height evaluation) and computerized tomography scan (for bone volume and evaluation of anatomical structures evaluation such as the dental nerve). The surgical procedures were described in previous reports following the All-on-4 treatment concept.[13,30]

Immediate Provisional Prosthetic Protocol

Implant-supported fixed prostheses of high-density acrylic resin (PalaXpress Ultra; Heraeus Kulzer GmbH, Hanau, Germany) with titanium cylinders (Nobel Biocare AB) were manufactured at the dental laboratory and inserted on the same day (G1: 110; G2: 55). Anterior occlusal contacts and canine guidance during lateral movements were preferred in the interim prosthesis. No cantilevers were used in the interim prostheses. The emergence positions of the screw-access holes at the posterior implants of the prostheses were normally at the level of the second premolar, and the prostheses were designed to hold a minimum of 10 teeth due to the favorable position achieved by the posterior tilting of the distal implants.

Final Prosthetic Protocol

Considering patient desires, a metal ceramic implant-supported fixed prosthesis with a titanium framework and all-ceramic crowns (Procera Ti framework, Procera crowns, NobelRondo ceramics; Nobel Biocare AB), or a metal-acrylic resin implant-supported fixed prosthesis with a Ti framework (Procera Ti framework) and acrylic resin prosthetic teeth (Heraeus Kulzer GmbH) was used to replace the interim prosthesis. In this definitive prosthesis, the occlusion mimicked natural dentition. The definitive prosthesis was typically delivered 6 months postsurgically.

Outcome Measures

Primary outcome measure was prosthetic survival and implant survival. Prosthetic survival (both interim and definitive) was based on function, with the necessity of removing the prostheses classified as failure. Implant survival was based on the Malo Clinic survival criteria:[13] (1) implant fulfilled its purported function as support for

reconstruction; (2) it was stable when individually and manually tested; (3) no signs of persistent infection observed; (4) no radiolucent areas around the implants; (5) demonstrated a good esthetic outcome in the rehabilitation; and (6) allowed the construction of an implant-supported fixed prosthesis that provided patient comfort and good hygienic maintenance. The implants removed were classified as failures. Secondary outcome measures were marginal bone level, biological complications (peri-implant pathology; fistulae formation, abscess formation), and mechanical complications (loosening or fracture of any prosthetic component).

Marginal Bone Level

Periapical radiographs were made using the parallel technique with a film holder (Super-bite; Hawe-Neos, Bioggio, Switzerland). The holder's position was adjusted manually for an estimated orthogonal film position. A blinded operator examined all radiographs of the implants for marginal bone level. Each periapical radiograph was scanned at 300 dpi with a scanner (HP Scanjet 4890; HP Portugal, Paço de Arcos, Portugal), and the marginal bone level was assessed with image analysis software (Image J version 1.40g for Windows; National Institutes of Health, Bethesda, MD). The reference point for the reading was the implant platform (the horizontal interface between the implant and the abutment), and marginal bone level was measured to the first contact between implant and bone. The radiographs were accepted or rejected for evaluation based on the clarity of the implant threads: a clear thread guarantees both sharpness and an orthogonal direction of the radiographic beam toward the implant axis. Calibration of the radiographs was performed using the implants' platform diameter. The marginal bone levels, evaluated on periapical radiographs, were registered at 5 years of follow-up. The bone levels were averaged per patient and presented using the rehabilitation as unit of analysis.

Statistical Analysis

Patient-related survival (using the patient as unit of analysis and considering the first incidence of implant failure) was computed using the Kaplan-Meier product limit estimator (SPSS 17.0; SPSS Inc., Chicago, IL) with comparison of survival curves between groups through the log-rank test. The incidence of mechanical and biological complications, systemic compromises, smoking habits, and bruxism between both groups was analyzed by the chi-square test. The marginal bone levels were compared between the two groups using the Mann-Whitney test after testing the variable for normality through the Kolmogorov-Smirnov test. The level of significance was 0.05. Statistics were computed using the Statistical Package for Social Science (SPSS 17.0).

TABLE 15.1 Implant Survival of the Completely Edentulous Rehabilitations Using the Rehabilitation as Unit of Analysis (Kaplan-Meier Product Limit Estimator)

Time (Months)	Status (0 = Nonfailure; 1 = Failure[a])	Cumulative Proportion Surviving at the Time		No. of Cumulative Events	No. of Patients at Risk
		Estimate	Std. Error		
		Overall Rehabilitations			
0	0	–	–	0	110
3	2	0.982	0.013	2	108
6	1	0.973	0.016	3	107
7	1	0.964	0.010	4	106
10	1	0.955	0.020	5	105
12	0	–	–	5	105
24	0	–	–	5	105
36	0	–	–	5	105
48	0	–	–	5	105
60	0	–	–	5	105

[a]Failure was defined as the first implant to fail in one patient.

RESULTS

A total of 26 patients presented at least one systemic condition (G1: 11 patients; G2: 15 patients, $p = 0.369$); 33 patients were smokers (G1: 19 patients; G2: 14 patients, $p = 0.298$), and 37 patients were suspected to be heavy bruxers (G1: 22 patients; G2: 15 patients, $p = 0.158$). No dropouts occurred in this study, and the patients were followed for 5 years. Five patients lost five implants (G1: 3 patients; G2: 2 patients), rendering an estimated survival rate of 95.5% (Kaplan-Meier; Table 15.1). All implant failures occurred during the first year of follow-up and were counted as early failures. No failures of the prostheses occurred, rendering a 100% survival rate. The estimated patient-related cumulative survival rates (CSRs) after 5 years of follow-up were 94.5% for G1 and 96.4% for G2 (Kaplan-Meier; Table 15.2 and Fig 15.4). Survival curves did not differ significantly between the two groups ($p = 0.645$, log-rank test). At 5 years of follow-up, 94 of the 110 patients had readable radiographs (86%). The bone level was on average −1.56 mm (SD = 0.89 mm) overall; −1.45 mm (SD = 0.77 mm) for G1 (maxilla: −1.44 mm [SD = 0.88 mm], mandible: 1.42 mm [SD = 0.82 mm]) and −1.67 mm (SD = 0.99 mm) for G2 (Table 15.3; maxilla: 1.72 mm [SD = 1.03 mm], mandible: 1.63 mm [SD = 1.01 mm]). The difference in marginal bone level between the two groups was nonsignificant ($p = 0.414$).

The incidence rate of mechanical complications (considering both interim and definitive prostheses) over the 5 years of follow-up was significant between the two groups with 0.16 [(45/55)/5] for G1 and 0.13 [(35/55)/5] for G2 ($p = 0.032$). For G1, the type of mechanical complications were fracture of the prosthesis (41 patients), abutment screw loosening (21 patients), and prosthetic screw loosening (6 patients), with 21 patients presenting more than one complication. While for G2 there were fractures of the prosthesis in 31 patients (23 patients with natural teeth as opposing dentition and 8 patients with removable prosthesis as opposing dentition), abutment screw loosening in 12 patients (11 patients with natural teeth as opposing dentition and 1 patient with removable prosthesis as opposing dentition) and prosthetic screw loosening in 2 patients (both with natural teeth as opposing dentition), with 9 patients presenting more than one complication (all with natural teeth as opposing dentition). For G1, the majority of complications occurred in the interim prosthesis ($n = 29$ patients; fractured prostheses = 28 patients) compared to the definitive prosthesis ($n = 16$ patients; fractured prostheses = 13 patients), and 15 patients with complications in both prostheses; while for G2, the majority of complications occurred in the definitive prosthesis ($n = 19$ patients; fractured prostheses = 15 patients) compared to the interim prosthesis ($n = 16$ patients; fractured prostheses = 16 patients), and 2 patients with complications in both prostheses. Thirty patients (37.5%) suspected of being heavy bruxers experienced mechanical complications (18 patients in G1, 12 patients in G2). The prosthetic planning for patients who presented mechanical complications was adjusted in an attempt to resolve the complications. The loosening of prosthetic components was addressed by re-tightening the prosthetic components; the prosthesis fracture was addressed by mending the prosthesis (acrylic resin) or repairing the ceramic (metal ceramic prosthesis). The common strategy addressing both complications (prosthetic components loosening and fractures) was the adjustment of the occlusion and manufacture of a night-guard.

TABLE 15.2   Implant Survival of the Completely Edentulous Rehabilitations Using the Rehabilitation as Unit of Analysis (Kaplan-Meier Product Limit Estimator); Survival Distribution Between the 2 Study Groups

Time (Months)	Status (0 = Nonfailure; 1 = Failure[a])	Cumulative Proportion Surviving at the Time		No. of Cumulative Events	No. of Patients at Risk
		Estimate	Std. Error		
Group 1 (Double Full-Arch Rehabilitations)					
0	0	–	–	0	55
3	1	0.982	0.018	1	54
6	1	0.964	0.025	2	53
7	1	0.945	0.031	3	52
12	0	–	–	3	52
24	0	–	–	3	52
36	0	–	–	3	52
48	0	–	–	3	52
60	0	–	–	3	52
Group 2 (Single Full-Arch Rehabilitations)					
0	0	–	–	0	55
3	1	0.982	0.018	1	54
10	1	0.964	0.025	2	53
12	0	–	–	2	53
24	0	–	–	2	53
36	0	–	–	2	53
48	0	–	–	2	53
60	0	–	–	2	53

Difference between groups in survival was not significant ($p = 0.645$, log-rank test).

[a]Failure was defined as the first implant to fail in one patient.

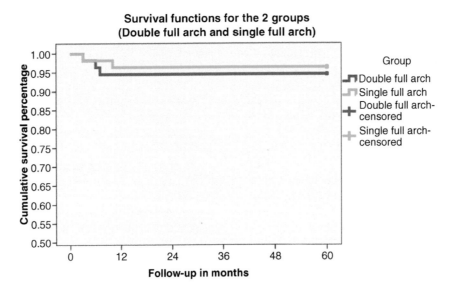

FIGURE 15.4   Survival estimation for both groups using the patient as unit of analysis and calculated through the Kaplan-Meier product limit estimator. No significant difference was registered between the two survival curves ($p = 0.645$, log-rank test).

TABLE 15.3   Marginal Bone Level, Situated Apically to the Implant Platform, After 5 Years of Follow-up with the Patient as Unit of Analysis in Groups 1 and 2

	Group 1: All-on-4 Double Full-Arch		Group 2: All-on-4 Single Full-Arch	
Average (mm)[a]	1.45[b]		1.67[b]	
Standard deviation (mm)	0.77		0.99	
Number	46		48	
Frequencies	*N*	*%*	*N*	*%*
0 mm	0	0.0%	1	2.1%
0.1–1.0 mm	15	32.6%	15	31.3%
1.1–2.0 mm	24	52.2%	17	35.4%
2.1–3.0 mm	4	8.7%	9	18.8%
>3.0 mm	3	6.5%	6	12.5%

[a]Overall marginal bone level was 1.56 mm (0.89 mm).
[b]Difference between groups in marginal bone level was not significant ($p = 0.414$).

The patient-related incidence rate of biological complications over the 5 years of follow-up for the two groups was 0.06 [(16/55)/5] for G1 and 0.05 [(14/55)/5] for G2, with no significant differences between the groups ($p = 0.669$). For G1, there were 15 incidences of peri-implant pathology and one fistulae formation ($n = 16$ implants, 7.2%); while for G2 there were 12 incidences of peri-implant pathology, one of suppuration and one abscess formation ($n = 14$ implants, 6.4%). Thirteen of the patients (G1: 7 patients; G2: 6 patients) with biological complications were smokers. Eighty-one percent of the patients (13/16) in G1 and 86% (12/14) of the patients in G2 presenting biological complications also presented mechanical complications.

DISCUSSION

The difference in survival rate between the two groups (G1: 94.5%; G2: 96.4%) was not significant; however, a significant difference was registered between both groups concerning mechanical complications. Therefore, the null hypothesis stating that there is no difference in the experimental and control group survival curves could be partially rejected. The overall 95.5% (patient-related) CSRs at 5 years for the immediate loading protocol in double full-arch rehabilitations and the overall marginal bone level of 1.56 mm apical to the implant platform after 5 years (group 1: 1.45 mm; group 2: 1.67 mm) was within the limits of previous reports on the rehabilitation of edentulous jaws using the same protocol in single full-arch rehabilitations.[13,19,30] In a longitudinal study on the survival of implants in the rehabilitation of the edentulous mandible using the All-on-4 treatment concept, a CSR of 94.8% at 5 years using the patient as unit of analysis was reported.[30] Another study evaluating the 5-year outcome of the same concept in the maxilla reported a 93% CSR using the patient as unit of analysis together with −1.95 mm of

marginal bone level.[13] An additional study evaluating the 5-year outcome of immediate function implants in completely edentulous maxillary rehabilitations with different degrees of bone resorption (low-to-high bone resorption) reported an 88.6% CSR using the patient as unit of analysis.[19] There were also no significant differences in marginal bone level or the incidence of biological complications between the two groups.

There was a significantly higher incidence of mechanical complications in double full-arch rehabilitations (occluding with implant-supported fixed prostheses) compared to single full-arch rehabilitations (occluding with natural teeth and removable dentures). A previous study reporting the long-term outcome of up to 10 years of a retrievable metal ceramic implant-supported fixed prostheses with milled titanium frameworks and all-ceramic crowns registered a twofold increase in the probability of crown fracture in the presence of a metal ceramic implant-supported fixed prosthesis opposing dentition.[31] A retrospective analysis of porcelain failures of implant-supported metal ceramic crowns and fixed partial dentures (FPDs) investigating patient- and implant-specific predictors of ceramic failure reported that metal ceramic prostheses (single crown or FPDs) had approximately 7 times higher odds of porcelain fracture and 13 times greater odds of a fracture requiring either repair or replacement when in occlusion with another implant-supported restoration, as compared to opposing a natural tooth.[32] Nevertheless, the explanation for this result cannot rule out other variables including not only a lack of proprioception by the patient and/or the lack of shock-absorbing capacity by the prosthesis, but also relating to technical failure in the manufacturing process, occlusion failure in controlling the occlusion following predetermined guidelines, or parafunctional movements by the patient, all these variables acting independently or in association.[31–33] In our study, 84% of the patients with mechanical complications were either suspect of being heavy bruxers or presented an implant-supported fixed prosthesis as opposing dentition. This implies that these patients may benefit from a prosthetic protocol including periodic clinical maintenance appointments in short intervals for occlusion evaluation and the use of a night-guard prescribed from the initial stage of implant rehabilitation to decrease the probability of mechanical complications. Nevertheless, these mechanical complications did not affect the long-term survival of the prostheses or the implants, demonstrating that those procedures are safe and effective.

The biological complication incidence rate, mainly peri-implant pathology, affected patients at a similar rate in both groups. These biological complications seemed to cluster in a determined number of patients, as 13 of the 16 patients in G1 (81%) and 12 of the 14 patients in G2 (86%) also presented mechanical complications, suggesting a synergetic effect between mechanical and biological complications, a situation that has been previously described in a systematic review investigating the effect of occlusal overload on peri-implant tissue health in the animal model.[34] Furthermore, biological complications occurred in 44% (7/16 patients) and 43% (6/14 patients) from G1 and G2, respectively, who were smokers. These results find parallels in the literature, where a recent systematic review reported smoking, together with history of periodontitis and poor oral hygiene as risk indicators for peri-implant pathology.[35]

The limitations of this study include: the retrospective design; being performed in a single center, which implies further validation in different social and cultural backgrounds; the different subgroups in G2 (single full-arch patients occluding with removable prostheses or natural teeth) as the amount of forces that can be generated by denture patients versus dentate patients is different; and the possible differences on the occlusal concept followed for the different subgroups, as these were chosen according to the specific conditions and treatment plan performed for the patient and not according to a specific inclusion criteria as a prospective study would imply. The strengths of this study include the long-term follow-up of 5 years and the use of a control group in the study design. Randomized controlled trials should be performed to confirm these results and investigate the effectiveness of using a controlled prosthetic protocol on the long-term outcome of double full-arch rehabilitated patients.

CONCLUSIONS

Rehabilitating double full-arch or single full-arch patients did not yield significant differences on implant survival and marginal bone level in the long-term follow-up; however, the incidence of mechanical complications registered was significantly higher for double full-arch patients than for single full-arch patients.

ACKNOWLEDGMENT

The authors thank Miss Andreia de Araújo and Mr. Sandro Catarino for all the help in data management.

REFERENCES

1. Cooper LF: The current and future treatment of edentulism. *J Prosthodont* 2009;18:116–122.
2. Brunello DL, Mandikos MN: Construction faults, age, gender, and relative medical health: factors associated with complaints in complete denture patients. *J Prosthet Dent* 1998;79:545–554.
3. MacEntee MI, Nolan A, Thomason JM: Oral mucosal and osseous disorders in frail elders. *Gerodontology* 2004;21:78–84.
4. Douglass CW, Shih A, Ostry L: Will there be a need for complete dentures in the United States in 2020? *J Prosthet Dent* 2002;87:5–8.
5. Zarb GA, Schmitt A: Implant therapy alternatives for geriatric edentulous patients. *Gerodontology* 1993;10:28–32.
6. Randow K, Ericsson I, Nilner K, et al: Immediate functional loading of Brånemark dental implants: an 18-month clinical follow-up study. *Clin Oral Implants Res* 1999;10:8–15.
7. Tarnow DP, Emtiaz S, Classi A: Immediate loading of threaded implants at stage 1 surgery in edentulous arches: ten consecutive case reports with 1- to 5-year data. *Int J Oral Maxillofac Implants* 1997;12:319–324.
8. Schnitman PA, Wohrle PS, Rubenstein JE, et al: Ten-year results for Brånemark implants immediately loaded with fixed prostheses at implant placement. *Int J Oral Maxillofac Implants* 1997;12:495–503.
9. Maló P, Rangert B, Nobre M: "All-on-Four" immediate-function concept with Brånemark System implants for completely edentulous mandibles: a retrospective clinical study. *Clin Implant Dent Relat Res* 2003;5:S2–S9.
10. Fazi G, Tellini S, Vangi D, et al: Three-dimensional finite element analysis of different implant configurations for a mandibular fixed prosthesis. *Int J Oral Maxillofac Implants* 2011;26:752–759.
11. Fermergard R, Astrand P: Osteotome sinus floor elevation and simultaneous placement of implants—a 1-year retrospective study with Astra Tech implants. *Clin Implant Dent Relat Res* 2008;10:62–69.
12. Agliardi EL, Pozzi A, Stappert CF, et al: Immediate fixed rehabilitation of the edentulous maxilla: a prospective clinical and radiological study after 3 years of loading. *Clin Implant Dent Relat Res* 2014;16:292–302.
13. Maló P, de Araújo Nobre M, Lopes A, et al: "All-on-4" immediate-function concept for completely edentulous maxillae: a clinical report on the medium (3 years) and long-term (5 years) outcomes. *Clin Implant Dent Relat Res* 2012;14 Suppl 1:e139–e150.
14. Hsu Y, Fu J, Hezaimi K, et al: Biomechanical implant treatment complications: a systematic review of clinical studies of implants with at least 1 year of functional loading. *Int J Oral Maxillofac Implants* 2012;27:894–904.

15. Wood MR, Vermilyea SG: A review of selected dental literature on evidence-based treatment planning for dental implants: report of the Committee on Research in Fixed Prosthodontics of the Academy of Fixed Prosthodontics. *J Prosthet Dent* 2004;92:447–462.

16. Gross MD: Occlusion in implant dentistry: a review of the literature of prosthetic determinants and current concepts. *Aust Dent J* 2008;53:S60–S68.

17. Maló P, de Araújo Nobre M, Lopes A, et al: Preliminary report on the outcome of tilted implants with longer lengths (20–25 mm) in low-density bone: one-year follow-up of a prospective cohort study. *Clin Implant Dent Relat Res* 2013; [Epub ahead of print] doi: 10.1111/cid.12144

18. Maló P, Rangert B, Nobre M: All-on-4 immediate-function concept with Brånemark System implants for completely edentulous maxillae: a 1-year retrospective clinical study. *Clin Implant Dent Relat Res* 2005;7:S88–S94.

19. Maló P, Nobre MD, Lopes A: The rehabilitation of completely edentulous maxillae with different degrees of resorption with four or more immediately loaded implants: a 5-year retrospective study and a new classification. *Eur J Oral Implantol* 2011;4:227–243.

20. Friberg B, Jemt T: Rehabilitation of edentulous mandibles by means of five TiUnite implants after one-stage surgery: a 1-year retrospective study of 90 patients. *Clin Implant Dent Relat Res* 2008;10:47–54.

21. Kim KS, Kim YL, Bae JM, et al: Biomechanical comparison of axial and tilted implants for mandibular full-arch fixed prostheses. *Int J Oral Maxillofac Implants* 2011;26:976–984.

22. Bevilacqua M, Tealdo T, Pera F, et al: Three-dimensional finite element analysis of load transmission using different implant inclinations and cantilever lengths. *Int J Prosthodont* 2008; 21:539–542.

23. Francetti L, Romeo D, Corbella S, et al: Bone level changes around axial and tilted implants in full-arch fixed immediate restorations: interim results of a prospective study. *Clin Implant Dent Relat Res* 2012;14:646–654.

24. Ogawa T, Dhaliwai S, Naert I, et al: Impact of implant number, distribution and prosthesis material on loading on implants supporting fixed prostheses. *J Oral Rehabil* 2010;37:525–531.

25. Gross MD: Occlusion in implant dentistry: a review of the literature of prosthetic determinants and current concepts. *Aust Dent J* 2008;53:S60–S68.

26. Papaspyridakos P, Chen C, Chuang S, et al: A systematic review of biologic and technical complications with fixed implant rehabilitations for edentulous patients. *Int J Oral Maxillofac Implants* 2012;27:102–110.

27. Balshi TJ, Wolfinger GJ: Immediate loading of Brånemark implants in edentulous mandibles: a preliminary report. *Implant Dent* 1997;6:83–88.

28. Esposito M, Grusovin MG, Achille H, et al: Interventions for replacing missing teeth: different times for loading dental implants. *Cochrane Database Syst Rev* 2009;21(1): CD003878.

29. von Elm E, Altman DG, Egger M, et al: STROBE Initiative. The Strengthening the Reporting of Observational Studies in Epidemiology (STROBE) statement: guidelines for reporting observational studies. *J Clin Epidemiol* 2008;61:344–349.

30. Maló P, de Araújo Nobre M, Lopes A, et al: A longitudinal study of the survival of All-on-4 implants in the mandible with up to 10 years of follow-up. *J Am Dent Assoc* 2011; 142:310–320.

31. Maló P, de Araújo Nobre M, et al: Retrievable metal ceramic implant-supported fixed prostheses with milled titanium frameworks and all-ceramic crowns: retrospective clinical study with up to 10 years of follow-up. *J Prosthodont* 2012;21:256–264.

32. Kinsel RP, Lin D: Retrospective analysis of porcelain failures of metal ceramic crowns and fixed partial dentures supported by 729 implants in 152 patients: patient-specific and implant-specific predictors of ceramic failure. *J Prosthet Dent* 2009;101:388–394.

33. Kim Y, Oh TJ, Misch CE, et al: Occlusal considerations in implant therapy: clinical guidelines with biomechanical rationale. *Clin Oral Implants Res* 2005;16:26–35.

34. Chambrone L, Chambrone LA, Lima LA: Effects of occlusal overload on peri-implant tissue health: a systematic review of animal-model studies. *J Periodontol* 2010;81:1367–1378.

35. Heitz-Mayfield LJ: Peri-implant diseases: diagnosis and risk indicators. *J Clin Periodontol* 2008;35:S292–S304.

16

THE INFLUENCE OF REHABILITATION CHARACTERISTICS IN THE INCIDENCE OF PERI-IMPLANT PATHOLOGY: A CASE-CONTROL STUDY

Miguel Alexandre De Araújo Nobre, RDH, MSC EPI,[1,2] and Paulo Maló, DDS, PHD[2]

[1]Preventive Medicine Unit, Faculty of Medicine, University of Lisbon, Portugal
[2]Maló Clinic, Lisbon, Portugal

Keywords
Peri-implant pathology; dental implants; rehabilitation characteristics.

Correspondence
Miguel de Araújo Nobre, Maló Clinic, Avenida dos Combatentes, 43, Andar 4 A, 1600-042 Lisboa, Portugal. E-mail: miguelnobre@fm.ul.pt; mnobre@maloclinics.com

Disclosure: This study was funded by a grant from Nobel Biocare Services AG (grant no. 2012-1126). Professor Maló is currently a consultant for Nobel Biocare.

Accepted October 5, 2013

Published in *Journal of Prosthodontics* January 2014; Vol. 23, Issue 1

doi: 10.1111/jopr.12114

ABSTRACT

Purpose: To investigate the influence of rehabilitation characteristics in the incidence of peri-implant pathology (P-iP).

Materials and Methods: A total of 1350 patients (270 with P-iP matched for age, gender, and time of follow-up with 1080 controls without P-iP) rehabilitated with dental implants were included. The effect of the independent variables [Implant length in millimeters (IL); implant diameter in millimeters; implant surface (IS); presence of cantilevers; implant:crown ratio (ICR), type of abutment (TA); abutment height; fracture of prosthetic components (FPCs); type of prosthetic reconstruction (TPR); type of material used in the prosthesis (TMUP); loosening of prosthetic components (LPCs); and passive misfit (PM) diagnosed within the previous year] was evaluated through bivariate analysis (chi-square), with level of significance of 5%. Crude odds ratios (OR) with 95% confidence intervals and the attributable fraction (AF) were calculated for the independent variables individually identified as factors associated with the incidence of peri-implant pathology.

Results: The following variables were identified as risk factors: machined IS ($p = 0.015$; OR = 1.46), 17° TA ($p = 0.000$; OR = 3.06), completely edentulous TPR ($p = 0.000$; OR = 2.49), TMUP ($p = 0.000$; metal-acrylic OR

$= 2.29$; acrylic $OR = 4.90$; metal-ceramic $OR = 8.43$), 1:1 ICR ($p = 0.002$; $OR = 1.54$), FPC ($p = 0.000$; $OR = 3.01$), LPC ($p = 0.000$; $OR = 4.15$), and PM ($p = 0.002$; $OR = 20.36$). The attributable fraction rendered the following theoretical potential reductions in the cases if the exposure to the variables was removed: IS (31.5%), TA (67.3%), TMUP (5.4% to 73.3%), ICR (35%), FPC (66.8%), LPC (73.8%), and PM (95.1%).

Conclusions: Within the limitations of this study, machined implant surfaces, 17° abutments, completely edentulous reconstructions, the type of metal used in the prosthesis, 1:1 implant:crown ratio, fracture of prosthetic components, loosening of prosthetic components, and passive misfit emerged as risk factors for the incidence of P-iP. Eliminating the exposure to these variables would, in theory, result in a significant reduction in the incidence of P-iP.

Peri-implant pathology is defined as "the term for inflammatory reactions with loss of supporting bone tissue surrounding the implant in function."[1] In a recent review, the prevalence of this pathology was reported with a wide range (12% to 43% of implant sites),[2] placing a question mark on the sensitivity of the epidemiological reports of this pathology.

The pathogenesis of peri-implant pathology can be described by two types:

1. classical (soft tissue apical to the bone) with dental plaque causing mucositis (reversible condition), which when left untreated, can lead to progressive destruction of the peri-implant tissue (peri-implant pathology) with resulting bone loss, and ultimately to implant loss,[3,4]

2. retrograde (bone to soft tissues), with bone loss occurring at the bone crest due to microfractures of the bone caused by overloading, loading too early, or occlusal lateral forces.[5]

Another problem is the low number of clinical studies found in the literature addressing the issue of risk factors for peri-implant pathology,[6-16] with the large majority focusing on implant outcome success/failure. The follow-up time represents a variable with influence in the incidence of peri-implant pathology. Tonetti[17] suggested the density function for implant loss decreases over time, while emerging data indicated an increase in the incidence of peri-implant pathology with follow-up time. Kourtis et al[18] pointed to peri-implant pathology as the main cause for late implant loss, and Maximo et al[7] registered a positive correlation between implant time of loading and incidence of peri-implant pathology.

An implant, as the functional unit of a rehabilitation, possesses different characteristics in the design that vary across different implant systems. Using Brånemark system implants (Nobel Biocare, Zurich, Switzerland) as reference, its length may vary between 7 and 18 mm in a standard implant, its diameter between 3.3 and 6 mm, and the surface between machined and porous (anodically oxidized).[19]

In generic terms, the longer the implant length, the longer the surface area for osseointegration and prosthetic support. Several studies reported lower survival rates for shorter implants.[20-22] This observation may be interpreted in two ways. First, shorter implants have a shorter bone-implant area, placing the implant more at risk for occlusal overload. Second, an infection in the coronal-apical direction may need less time to cause marginal bone resorption in a critical portion of the implant with established osseointegration, leading to an implant failure.

With regard to the implant surface, according to a meta-analysis by Esposito et al[23] in Brånemark implants with 3 years of follow-up, there were more cases of peri-implant disease in rough surface implants than with machined surface implants. The same finding was reported by Rosenberg et al[15] for implants with hydroxyapatite surface enhanced by patients' conditions (periodontally compromised). This may be due to ease of microbial adhesion to rough compared to the machined surface. Teughels et al[24] conducted a systematic review of the literature on the effect of material characteristics and/or surface topography of the implant in the development of the biofilm (plaque), concluding that implant surfaces with a higher degree of roughness ($R = 0.2$ μm) facilitate biofilm formation. In a retrospective evaluation of predisposing conditions for the occurrence of retrograde peri-implant pathology in Brånemark system implants, Quirynen et al[12] observed a higher incidence of retrograde peri-implant pathology in TiUnite (rough) (Nobel Biocare) implants.

The components of an implant-prosthetic rehabilitation (abutment, abutment screw, and crown/prosthesis) may relate to the occurrence of peri-implant pathology, to the extent that they are part of the equation when the disease occurs by occlusal overload.[25] Regarding the abutments, there is no evidence that the different surface topography influences the accumulation of plaque either in the animal model[26] or in a human model as evidenced by Van Assche et al[27] through a randomized clinical trial comparing the accumulation of plaque on different surfaces.

Regarding the type of prosthetic reconstruction, a higher incidence of implant failures and prosthetic complications have been observed in partially edentulous patients rehabilitated with a fixed partial prosthesis supported by two implants compared to a prosthesis supported by three or more implants.[28–30] This may occur due to a biomechanically unfavorable situation with respect to the number of implants supporting the structure.[31]

The type of restorative material used in the prosthesis ranges from acrylic, metal-acrylic, metal-ceramic, and to ceramic. The academic hypothesis of using acrylic as a means of reducing the concentration of occlusal stress on the bone/implant interface[32] acting as a shock absorbing agent has been postulated; this assumption is supported by finite element analysis studies and mathematical models.[33,34] However, there were no significant differences in marginal bone loss between implants restored with ceramic or acrylic in clinical studies.[35]

The presence of cantilevers in a fixed prosthesis has been considered a risk factor due to the considerable increase of occlusal load on the implants, especially the most distal implant.[32] These results have been supported by in vitro studies,[36–38] suggesting a maximum limit of a 15-mm-long cantilever in the mandible.[38] A recent meta-analysis from retrospective cohort studies concluded that there were no differences in bone loss in implants supporting a cantilever because of this factor per se.[39] However, Bragger et al[40] noted an increased incidence of prosthetic complications with a fixed implant-supported prosthesis supporting a cantilever.

The implant:crown ratio (ICR) has been theoretically considered a risk factor for the occurrence of prosthetic complications in implants. When the height of the pillar-crown complex is substantially increased, the leverage on the implant head increases, which in the presence of an increase of lateral forces may cause loosening of the prosthetic screws or fractured components.[41] However, this theory was not supported, and no evidence was found in clinical trials,[42] cohort studies,[43–45] or meta-analyses.[46]

Nevertheless, a recent prospective cohort study revealed a significant correlation between a less favorable ICR and marginal bone resorption.[47]

Mechanical complications include fracture of prosthetic components, loosening of prosthetic components, or lack of passive fit. The causes for fractures of prosthetic components can be varied: from clinical cases with functional and anatomical peculiarities, to parafunctional habits, to improper design of the prosthesis, or factors related to the characteristics of the materials.[48] For parafunctional habits, there is little clinical evidence that bruxism, in particular, has a causal relationship with the increase of implant failures.[49,50] However, there seems to be a broad consensus that excessive or improper occlusal stress can cause bone loss, if secondarily associated with bone characteristics.[51]

Implant-supported prostheses may be screwed or cemented. The advantages of a screwed prosthesis relate to the possibility of easily removing the prosthesis; however, problems with the screws are one of the most common mechanical complications. One retrospective study reported a 38% incidence of prosthetic screw loosening,[52] further supported by several clinical studies.[31,53–55] The screw is the weakest link in any implant system. In a theoretical analysis of metal fatigue in gold screws, the authors pointed out the importance of manufacturing a prosthesis with precision using sufficient implants to minimize fatigue.[56–58] However, Kallus and Bessing[59] reported that screw loosening is due to lack of passive fit of the prosthesis, the responsibility of the operator.

The significance of loosening has been discussed in the literature, in view of the possible bacterial colonization of those spaces as a possible role in the etiology of peri-implantitis.[60] This theory has evolved from observations in vitro[60] and in vivo.[61,62] It may cause leakage of bacteria into the peri-implant sulcus, inducing cellular infiltration localized at the implant/abutment interface, as shown in animals[63] and possibly in humans.[64,65] However, no epidemiological findings substantiate this hypothesis.

The aim of this study was to determine the influence of rehabilitation characteristics as possible factors associated with increased risk for the incidence of peri-implant pathology and consequent failure of the implant.

MATERIALS AND METHODS

This article was written following the STROBE (Strengthening the Reporting of Observational Studies in Epidemiology) guidelines.[66] This study was approved by the National Commission of Data Protection (Portugal) and the Faculty of Medicine-University of Lisbon Ethical Board.

The study population consisted of patients over 18 years, of both genders, rehabilitated with dental implants at the Center for Implantology and Fixed Oral Rehabilitation-Lisbon, Portugal. *Cases* were defined as the patients rehabilitated with dental implants at the Center for Implantology and Fixed Oral Rehabilitation-Lisbon diagnosed with peri-implant pathology. *Controls* were defined as patients rehabilitated with dental implants at the same center without diagnosis of peri-implant pathology.

Peri-implant pathology was diagnosed through: peri-implant pockets ≥5 mm diagnosed through probing of the peri-implant sulcus/pocket using a probe calibrated to 0.25 N (Click-Probe; Kerrhawe S.A., Bioggio Svizzera, Switzerland);[67] bleeding on probing;[67] bone loss visible to x-ray;[68] and attachment loss equal to or greater than 2 mm.[69] Inclusion criteria were: patients who underwent surgery to insert dental implants and followed at the clinical center; patients rehabilitated with implant-supported prostheses with a minimum follow-up of 1 year after surgery; patients who gave their informed consent to have their charts reviewed in this retrospective study. Exclusion criteria were: patients who had undergone surgery for placement of dental implants less than 1 year prior; patients who refused or were unable to give informed consent; prevalent cases of peri-implant pathology; patients whose medical records were incomplete or missing; patients who underwent immunosuppressive therapy; patients under 18 years of age.

This study was conducted between January and July 2009. The matching between cases and controls was carried for the demographic variables: age (2 years ≤ case age ≤ 2 years) and gender, due to high probability of association of these variables with implant failure: more prevalent in men,[14] and ages over 40 years[70] and follow-up time of implantation (2 months ≤ case follow-up ≤ 2 months), due to a possible correlation between the increase in follow-up time (exposure time) and the occurrence of peri-implant pathology.[17] A 1:4 relation between cases and controls was settled to optimize the number of cases needed.

The sample was obtained from a list of patients submitted to implant surgery. There were initially 1763 eligible patients (346 cases; 1417 controls); from these, 383 patients (66 cases and 317 controls) were excluded from the study; 181 patients had incomplete diagnosis (12 cases and 169 controls); 202 patients refused to participate (54 cases and 148 controls). From the 1380 patients (280 cases and 1100 controls), 30 patients (10 cases and 20 controls) were randomly selected to be included in the pilot study and consequently excluded from the study, reaching the final 1350 patients (270 cases and 1080 controls).

The sample consisted of 1350 individuals of both genders, divided by two groups: cases and controls. The average age of our sample was 55.8 years (standard deviation = 10.2 years), with a minimum of 28 years and a maximum of 88 years. The majority of participants were female (62.7%). The implants were inserted between February 1998 and November 2006. Peri-implant pathology was diagnosed, on average, 3 years after implant insertion.

Data collection consisted of indirect documentation, filling in the data on a digital form, and through consulting the patient's clinical file (record sheets, radiographs, medical questionnaire, and clinical diary). The independent variables were: implant length in millimeters (IL) (7 mm, 8.5 mm, 10 mm, 11.5 mm, 13 mm, 15 mm, 18 mm); implant diameter in millimeters (3 to 3.5 mm, 3.75 to 4.3 mm, 5 to 6 mm); implant surface (IS) (machined, oxidized); presence of cantilevers (0, ≥1); ICR (2:1, 1:1), type of abutment (TA) (straight: 0°; 17° angulated, 30° angulated); abutment height (1 mm, 2 mm, 3 mm, 4 mm, 5 mm); fracture of prosthetic components (FPCs) (absent, present); type of prosthetic reconstruction (TPR) (single teeth, partial rehabilitation, complete rehabilitation); type of material used in the prosthesis (TMUP) (ceramic, metal-ceramic, acrylic); loosening of prosthetic components (LPCs) (absent, present); passive misfit (PM) diagnosed within the previous year (absent, present).

Statistical Analysis

Univariate analysis for characterization of cases and controls in relation to the independent variables was performed. Bivariate analysis was conducted to evaluate the difference between the groups of cases and controls in relation to the independent variables. In nominal independent variables, the comparison between cases and controls was performed using the Chi-square test (upon presence of applicability conditions, otherwise the Fisher exact test was applied, with supplemental measures of Cramer's V or the contingency coefficient). Crude odds ratios (OR) with 95% confidence intervals were calculated for the variables significantly different in the bivariate analysis. Estimation of attributable fraction (AF) of peri-implant pathology for the cases exposed to the risk factors identified in the bivariate analysis was calculated through an equation[71] according to the odds ratio of exposure.

$$AF = \frac{A1+}{M1+} \frac{OR-1}{OR}$$

where AF = attributable fraction; A1+ = prevalence of the disease in the exposed; M1+ = prevalence of the disease; and OR = odds ratio.

RESULTS

The univariate analysis is described in Tables 16.1 to 16.5. Considering the implants, the sample revealed a majority of implants with 15 mm or more in length, 3.75 to 4.3 mm in diameter, and an oxidized surface. A majority of reconstructions were single teeth, without cantilevers, with metal-ceramic material used in the prosthesis, with a 1:1 ICR, and using straight abutments of 2 mm. Forty-three patients fractured a prosthetic component, 25 patients had loosening of prosthetic components, and 6 patients had passive misfit diagnosed within the previous year of the reference date.

The bivariate analysis resulted in significant differences between cases and controls for the variables IL, IS, TA, TPR, TMUP, ICR, FPC, LPC, and PM (Table 16.6) (abbreviations listed in Table 16.6). Crude OR with 95% CI are described in Table 16.7. Patients with biomechanical complications had a higher probability for incidence of peri-implant pathology, with PM, LPC, and FPC revealing a 20-fold, 4-fold, and 3-fold increase, respectively. Patients with complete edentulous rehabilitations (OR = 2.5), with TMUP of metal-ceramic, metal-acrylic, or acrylic, using 17° angulated abutments (OR = 3.1), with an ICR of 1:1 or more, or with machined surface implants also were more at risk for the incidence of the disease. The attributable risk fraction determined that the patients' suppression exposure to PM, LCP, FCP, metal-ceramic or acrylic TMUP, 17° abutments,

TABLE 16.1 Frequencies and Percentages of the Variables Related to the Characteristics of the Reconstruction

| | | Follow-up Time (Months) | | | | | Implant Length | | | | | | | |
		[1 to 3]	[3 to 5]	[5 to 10]	+10	Total	7 mm	8.5 mm	10 mm	11.5 mm	13 mm	15 mm	18 mm	Total
Cases	Number	164	71	34	1	270	4	18	20	16	43	153	16	270
	% w/group	60.7%	26.3%	12.6%	0.4%	100.0%	1.5%	6.7%	7.4%	5.9%	15.9%	56.7%	5.9%	100.0%
	% w/variable	19.6%	20.5%	20.6%	25.0%	20.0%	30.8%	25.7%	13.2%	15.2%	16.9%	22.9%	18.4%	20.0%
	% w/total	12.1%	5.3%	2.5%	0.1%	20.0%	0.3%	1.3%	1.5%	1.2%	3.2%	11.3%	1.2%	20.0%
Controls	Number	671	275	131	3	1080	9	52	132	89	211	516	71	1080
	% w/group	62.1%	25.5%	12.1%	0.3%	100.0%	0.8%	4.8%	12.2%	8.2%	19.5%	47.8%	6.6%	100.0%
	% w/variable	80.4%	79.5%	79.4%	75.0%	80.0%	69.2%	74.3%	86.8%	84.8%	83.1%	77.1%	81.6%	80.0%
	% w/total	49.7%	20.4%	9.7%	0.2%	80.0%	0.7%	3.9%	9.8%	6.6%	15.6%	38.2%	5.3%	80.0%
Total	Number	835	346	165	4	1350	13	70	152	105	254	669	87	1350
	% w/group	61.9%	25.6%	12.2%	0.3%	100.0%	1.0%	5.2%	11.3%	7.8%	18.8%	49.6%	6.4%	100.0%
	% w/variable	100.0%	100.0%	100.0%	100.0%	100.0%	100.0%	100.0%	100.0%	100.0%	100.0%	100.0%	100.0%	100.0%
	% w/total	61.9%	25.6%	12.2%	0.3%	100.0%	1.0%	5.2%	11.3%	7.8%	18.8%	49.6%	6.4%	100.0%

TABLE 16.2 Frequencies and Percentages of the Variables Related to the Characteristics of the Reconstruction

| | | Implant Diameter (mm) | | | | | Implant Surface | | | Presence of Cantilevers | | | Implant:Crown Ratio | | |
		[3 to 3.5]	[3.75 to 4.3]	[5 to 6]	0	Total	Machined	Oxidized	Total	0	≥1	Total	2:1	1:1	Total
Cases	Number	16	254	0	0	270	74	196	270	231	39	270	109	161	270
	% w/group	5.9%	94.1%	0%	0%	100.0%	27.4%	72.6%	100.0%	85.6%	14.4%	100.0%	40.4%	59.6%	100.0%
	% w/variable	15.0%	20.5%	0%	0%	20.0%	25.0%	18.6%	20.0%	19.5%	23.4%	20.0%	24.8%	17.7%	20.0%
	% w/total	1.2%	18.8%	0%	0%	20.0%	5.5%	14.5%	20.0%	17.1%	2.9%	20.0%	8.1%	11.9%	20.0%
Controls	Number	91	987	2	0	1080	222	858	1080	952	128	1080	330	750	1080
	% w/group	8.4%	91.4%	0.2%	0%	100.0%	20.6%	79.4%	100.0%	88.1%	11.9%	100.0%	30.6%	69.4%	100.0%
	% w/variable	85.0%	79.5%	100.0%	0%	80.0%	75.0%	81.4%	80.0%	80.5%	76.6%	80.0%	75.2%	82.3%	80.0%
	% w/total	6.7%	73.1%	0.1%	0%	80.0%	16.4%	63.6%	80.0%	70.5%	9.5%	80.0%	24.4%	55.6%	80.0%
Total	Number	107	1241	2	0	1350	296	1054	1350	1183	167	1350	439	911	1350
	% w/group	7.9%	91.9%	0.1%	0%	100.0%	21.9%	78.1%	100.0%	87.6%	12.4%	100.0%	32.5%	67.5%	100.0%
	% w/variable	100.0%	100.0%	100.0%	0%	100.0%	100.0%	100.0%	100.0%	100.0%	100.0%	100.0%	100.0%	100.0%	100.0%
	% w/total	7.9%	91.9%	0.1%	0%	100.0%	21.9%	78.1%	100.0%	87.6%	12.4%	100.0%	32.5%	67.5%	100.0%

TABLE 16.3 Frequencies and Percentages of the Variables Related to the Characteristics of the Reconstruction

Type of Abutment

		Straight (0°)	17° Angle	30° Angle	Total
Cases	Number	195	32	43	270
	% w/group	72.2%	11.9%	15.9%	100.0%
	% w/variable	18.2%	40.5%	21.4%	20.0%
	% w/total	14.4%	2.4%	3.2%	20.0%
Controls	Number	875	47	158	1080
	% w/group	81.0%	4.4%	14.6%	100.0%
	% w/variable	81.8%	59.5%	78.6%	80.0%
	% w/total	64.8%	3.5%	11.7%	80.0%
Total	Number	1070	79	201	1350
	% w/group	79.3%	5.9%	14.9%	100.0%
	% w/variable	100.0%	100.0%	100.0%	100.0%
	% w/total	79.3%	5.9%	14.9%	100.0%

Abutment Height

		1 mm	2 mm	3 mm	4 mm	5 mm	Total
Cases	Number	104	125	27	13	1	270
	% w/group	38.5%	46.3%	10.0%	4.8%	0.4%	100.0%
	% w/variable	20.1%	22.0%	16.7%	13.0%	25.0%	20.0%
	% w/total	7.7%	9.3%	2.0%	1.0%	0.1%	20.0%
Controls	Number	413	442	135	87	3	1080
	% w/group	38.2%	40.9%	12.5%	8.1%	0.3%	100.0%
	% w/variable	79.9%	78.0%	83.3%	87.0%	75.0%	80.0%
	% w/total	30.6%	32.7%	10.0%	6.4%	0.2%	80.0%
Total	Number	517	567	162	100	4	1350
	% w/group	38.3%	42.0%	12.0%	7.4%	0.3%	100.0%
	% w/variable	100.0%	100.0%	100.0%	100.0%	100.0%	100.0%
	% w/total	38.3%	42.0%	12.0%	7.4%	0.3%	100.0%

Fracture of Prosthetic Components (Previous Year)

		No	Yes	Total
Cases	Number	252	18	270
	% w/group	93.3%	6.7%	100.0%
	% w/variable	19.3%	41.9%	20.0%
	% w/total	18.7%	1.3%	20.0%
Controls	Number	1055	25	1080
	% w/group	97.7%	2.3%	100.0%
	% w/variable	80.7%	58.1%	80.0%
	% w/total	78.1%	1.9%	80.0%
Total	Number	1307	43	1350
	% w/group	96.8%	3.2%	100.0%
	% w/variable	100.0%	100.0%	100.0%
	% w/total	96.8%	3.2%	100.0%

TABLE 16.4 Frequencies and Percentages of the Variables Related to the Characteristics of the Reconstruction

Type of Prosthetic Reconstruction

		Single Teeth	Partial	Complete	Total
Cases	Number	91	32	147	270
	% w/group	33.7%	11.9%	54.4%	100.0%
	% w/variable	14.0%	16.5%	28.9%	20.0%
	% w/total	6.7%	2.4%	10.9%	20.0%
Controls	Number	557	162	361	1080
	% w/group	51.6%	15.0%	33.4%	100.0%
	% w/variable	86.0%	83.5%	71.1%	80.0%
	% w/total	41.3%	12.0%	26.7%	80.0%
Total	Number	648	194	508	1350
	% w/group	48.0%	14.4%	37.6%	100.0%
	% w/variable	100.0%	100.0%	100.0%	100.0%
	% w/total	7.9%	91.9%	0.1%	100.0%

Type of Material Used in the Prosthesis

		Ceramic	Metal-Ceramic	Metal-Acrylic	Acrylic	Total
Cases	Number	81	87	17	85	270
	% w/group	30.0%	32.2%	6.3%	31.5%	100.0%
	% w/variable	12.8%	35.4%	13.4%	24.9%	20.0%
	% w/total	6.0%	6.4%	1.3%	6.3%	20.0%
Controls	Number	554	159	110	257	1080
	% w/group	51.3%	14.7%	10.2%	23.8%	100.0%
	% w/variable	87.2%	64.6%	86.6%	75.1%	80.0%
	% w/total	41.0%	11.8%	8.1%	19.0%	80.0%
Total	Number	635	246	127	342	1350
	% w/group	47.0%	18.2%	9.4%	25.3%	100.0%
	% w/variable	100.0%	100.0%	100.0%	100.0%	100.0%
	% w/total	47.0%	18.2%	9.4%	25.3%	100.0%

Loosening of Prosthetic Components

		No	Yes	Total
Cases	Number	258	12	270
	% w/group	95.6%	4.4%	100.0%
	% w/variable	19.5%	48.0%	20.0%
	% w/total	19.1%	0.9%	20.0%
Controls	Number	1067	13	1080
	% w/group	98.8%	1.2%	100.0%
	% w/variable	80.5%	52.0%	80.0%
	% w/total	79.0%	1.0%	80.0%
Total	Number	1325	25	1350
	% w/group	98.1%	1.9%	100.0%
	% w/variable	100.0%	100.0%	100.0%
	% w/total	98.1%	1.9%	100.0%

TABLE 16.5 Frequencies and Percentages of the Variables Related to the Characteristics of the Reconstruction

| | | Passive Misfit Diagnosed Within Previous Year | | |
		No	Yes	Total
Cases	Number	265	5	270
	% w/group	98.1%	1.9%	100.0%
	% w/variable	19.7%	83.3%	20.0%
	% w/total	19.6%	0.4%	20.0%
Controls	Number	1079	1	1080
	% w/group	99.9%	0.1%	100.0%
	% w/variable	80.3%	16.7%	80.0%
	% w/total	79.9%	0.1%	80.0%
Total	Number	1344	6	1350
	% w/group	99.6%	0.4%	100.0%
	% w/variable	100.0%	100.0%	100.0%
	% w/total	99.6%	0.4%	100.0%

ICR of 1:1, or machined surface implants would have resulted in a drastic decrease in the incidence of peri-implant pathology (Table 16.7).

DISCUSSION

In this study, the presence of mechanical complications (fracture of prosthetic components, loosening of prosthetic components, or passive misfit) and some characteristics related to the reconstruction (implant length, implant surface, type of abutment, type of prosthetic reconstruction, type of material used in the prosthesis, and implant:crown ratio) led to a higher risk for the incidence of peri-implant pathology. In the presence of mechanical complications, although few studies in the literature focus on this topic, the importance of biomechanical problems is noted. These problems include passive misfit, which may be related to both mechanisms of developing disease, the retrograde (by increasing the burden shifted to the bone and possible bone loss), and the classical (by establishing the conditions for colonization of microflora between the remaining spaces of prosthetic components).[72] On the one hand, fracture of prosthetic components and loosening of prosthetic components can be regarded as "proxy" variables for the assessment of excessive or improper occlusal stress, factors that can cause bone loss around implants, if secondarily associated with bone characteristics.[51] On the other hand, loosening of prosthetic components may also play a facilitating role for the incidence of peri-implant pathology by allowing bacteria to colonize the space between the prosthetic components.[60–62,64,73] The loosening of prosthetic components, however, may be improved with the current TorqTite (Nobel Biocare AB) screws. In a study measuring the critical bending moment

(CBM) of abutments, Lee et al[74] reported that TorqTite screws result in higher CBM when tested, decreasing the probability of screw loosening.

Machined surfaces constituted a risk factor when compared to oxidized surfaces. This may be due to the osseoconductive properties of the oxidized surfaces,[75–77] resulting in an increased area of contact between bone and implant,[78,79] allowing a higher capacity of support and better resistance to occlusal loads, acting as a protective factor in the biomechanical component of the disease.

Regarding the type of abutment, our results are supported in the literature, as angulated abutments are associated with a greater amount of stress on prostheses and surrounding bone than that associated with straight abutments.[80] In the case of the type of prosthetic reconstruction, the majority of studies either did not differentiate between different types of rehabilitations or performed the study on only one type of rehabilitation. There is therefore the probability that the association of the type of prosthetic reconstruction with peri-implant pathology occurs in association with other variables. In a study with 15 years of follow-up in edentulous patients, Carlsson et al[81] found that in completely edentulous patients, although bone loss was limited, it was found to be associated with several factors, including tobacco use and oral hygiene habits as most important.

The type of material used in the prosthesis influenced the risk status of a patient developing peri-implant pathology, with metal-ceramic, metal-acrylic, and acrylic materials as risk factors when using ceramic material as reference. This potential effect of biological risk may be explained by the fact that the ceramic material can offer a lower retention on the accumulation of dental plaque due to its lower surface roughness compared with acrylic,[82] a basic condition for the development of classical peri-implant pathology. In a literature review, Bollen et al[82] designated a threshold roughness of dental materials of 0.2 μm, above which there is a simultaneous increase in the accumulation of dental plaque. In this context, Chan and Weber,[83] in a comparative study on the retention of plaque in various materials, observed that full ceramic crowns had a retention of soft matter by 32%, while the metal-ceramic and acrylic resin materials had a retention 90% and 152%, respectively.

An implant:crown ratio of 1:1 was a risk factor for the incidence of peri-implant pathology. A possible explanation is that the increased height of the abutment-crown complex could represent an increase of leverage over the head of the implant, which in the presence of lateral forces in the occlusion may, in turn, lead to loosening or fracture of prosthetic components.[84] In a recent prospective cohort study, Malchiodi et al[47] studied the influence of implant:crown ratio on implant success rates and crestal bone levels, reporting a statistically significant correlation between implant success rate and implant:crown ratio, and between

TABLE 16.6 Results from Bivariate Analysis for the Variables in the Group Implant with Significant Differences Between Cases and Controls. Relative Frequencies for Cases and Controls and Absolute Frequencies with 95% CI and _p_ Value Relative to the Statistical Test

	Cases Relative Frequency (CI 95% Proportion)	Controls Relative Frequency (CI 95% Proportion)	Absolute Frequency (CI 95% Proportion)	_p_
Implant length (mm) (IL)				
7	4/270 = 0.01 (0.00; 0.03)	9/1080 = 0.01 (0.00; 0.01)	13/1350 = 0.01 (0.00; 0.01)	0.037
8.5	18/270 = 0.07 (0.04; 0.10)	52/1080 = 0.05 (0.04; 0.06)	70/1350 = 0.05 (0.04; 0.06)	
10	20/270 = 0.07 (0.04; 0.11)	132/1080 = 0.12 (0.10; 0.14)	152/1350 = 0.11 (0.10; 0.13)	
11.5	16/270 = 0.06 (0.03; 0.09)	89/1080 = 0.08 (0.07; 0.10)	105/1350 = 0.08 (0.06; 0.09)	
13	43/270 = 0.16 (0.12; 0.20)	211/1080 = 0.20 (0.17; 0.22)	254/1350 = 0.19 (0.17; 0.21)	
15	153/270 = 0.57 (0.51; 0.63)	516/1080 = 0.48 (0.45; 0.51)	669/1350 = 0.50 (0.47; 0.52)	
18	16/270 = 0.06 (0.03; 0.09)	71/1080 = 0.07 (0.05; 0.08)	87/1350 = 0.06 (0.05; 0.08)	
Implant surface (IS)				
Mac	74/270 = 0.27 (0.22; 0.33)	222/1080 = 0.21 (0.18; 0.23)	296/1350 = 0.22 (0.20; 0.24)	0.015
Oxi	196/270 = 0.73 (0.67; 0.78)	858/1080 = 0.79 (0.77; 0.82)	1054/1350 = 0.78 (0.76; 0.80)	
Type of abutment (TA)				
0°	195/270 = 0.72 (0.67; 0.78)	875/1080 = 0.81 (0.79; 0.83)	1070/1350 = 0.79 (0.77; 0.81)	0.000
17°	32/270 = 0.12 (0.08; 0.16)	47/1080 = 0.04 (0.03; 0.06)	79/1350 = 0.06 (0.05; 0.07)	
30°	43/270 = 0.16 (0.12; 0.20)	158/1080 = 0.15 (0.13; 0.17)	201/1350 = 0.15 (0.13; 0.17)	
Type of prosthetic reconstruction (TPR)				
Sing	91/270 = 0.34 (0.28; 0.39)	557/1080 = 0.52 (0.49; 0.55)	648/1350 = 0.48 (0.45; 0.51)	0.000
Par	32/270 = 0.12 (0.08; 0.16)	162/1080 = 0.15 (0.13; 0.17)	194/1350 = 0.14 (0.12; 0.16)	
Tot	147/270 = 0.54 (0.49; 0.60)	361/1080 = 0.33 (0.31; 0.36)	508/1350 = 0.38 (0.35; 0.40)	
Type of material used in the prosthesis (TMUP)				
Cer	81/270 = 0.30 (0.25; 0.35)	554/1080 = 0.51 (0.48; 0.54)	635/1350 = 0.47 (0.44; 0.50)	0.000
M-C	87/270 = 0.32 (0.27; 0.38)	159/1080 = 0.15 (0.13; 0.17)	246/1350 = 0.18 (0.16; 0.20)	
M-A	17/270 = 0.06 (0.03; 0.09)	110/1080 = 0.10 (0.08; 0.12)	127/1350 = 0.09 (0.08; 0.11)	
Acr	85/270 = 0.31 (0.26; 0.37)	257/1080 = 0.24 (0.21; 0.26)	342/1350 = 0.25 (0.23; 0.28)	
Implant:crown ratio (ICR)				
2:1	109/270 = 0.40 (0.35; 0.46)	330/1080 = 0.31 (0.28; 0.33)	439/1350 = 0.33 (0.30; 0.35)	0.002
1:1	161/270 = 0.60 (0.54; 0.65)	750/1080 = 0.69 (0.67; 0.72)	911/1350 = 0.67 (0.65; 0.70)	
Fractures of prosthetic components within previous year (FPC)				
Yes	18/270 = 0.07 (0.04; 0.10)	25/1080 = 0.02 (0.01; 0.03)	43/1350 = 0.03 (0.02; 0.04)	0.000
No	252/270 = 0.93 (0.90; 0.96)	1055/1080 = 0.98 (0.97; 0.99)	1307/1350 = 0.97 (0.96; 0.98)	
Loosening or decementations of prosthetic components within the previous year (LPC)				
Yes	12/270 = 0.04 (0.02; 0.07)	13/1080 = 0.01 (0.01; 0.02)	25/1350 = 0.02 (0.01; 0.03)	0.000
No	258/270 = 0.96 (0.93; 0.98)	1067/1080 = 0.99 (0.98; 0.99)	1325/1350 = 0.98 (0.97; 0.99)	
Passive misfit diagnosed within the previous year (PM)				
Yes	5/270 = 0.02 (0.00; 0.03)	1/1080 = 0.00 (0.00; 0.00)	6/1350 = 0.00 (0.00; 0.01)	0.002
No	265/270 = 0.98 (0.97; 1.00)	1079/1080 = 1.00 (1.00; 1.00)	1344/1350 = 1.00 (0.99; 1.00)	

Mac: Machined; Oxi: Oxidized; Sing: Single; Par: Partial; Tot: Total; Cer: Ceramic; M-C: Metal-ceramic; M-A: Metal-acrylic; Acr: Acrylic.

bone loss and implant:crown ratio, concluding that from the biomechanical point of view, implant:crown ratio would appear to be the main parameter capable of influencing implant success and crestal bone loss.

The importance of controlling risk factors for the incidence of peri-implant pathology was illustrated through the estimation of the AF for peri-implant pathology of the cases exposed. In this exercise, the suppression of exposure to the majority of variables would produce a drastic reduction in the percentage of cases. Taking passive misfit as reference, the suppression of exposure to this risk factor could result in a reduction of 95% of the cases exposed. In these situations, this would mean a consequent reduction in the population at risk, another assumption of the common interpretation of AF in public health (as potentially reducing the number of cases).[71]

TABLE 16.7 **Crude Odds Ratio (OR) with Corresponding 95% Confidence Intervals (CI) and Attributable Risk Fraction Calculations for the Variables Significantly Associated with the Incidence of Peri-implant Pathology**

	Odds Ratio (OR)	95% CI of the OR Upper and Lower Bounds	Attributable Risk Fraction AF = $\frac{A1+}{M1+} \frac{OR-1}{OR}$
Implant length			
18 mm	1.0		
15 mm	1.97	[0.54; 7.21]	
13 mm	1.54	[0.72; 3.29]	
11.5 mm	0.67	[0.33; 1.38]	
10 mm	0.80	[0.37; 1.71]	
8.5 mm	0.90	[0.48; 1.70]	
7 mm	1.32	[0.74; 2.33]	
Implant surface			
Oxidized	1.0		
Machined	1.46	[1.08; 1.98]	31.47
Straight (0°)	1.00		
Type of abutment			
17° angulated	3.06	[1.90; 4.91]	67.27
30° angulated	1.22	[0.84; 1.77]	
Type of prosthetic reconstruction			
Single teeth	1.0		
Partial	1.21	[0.78; 1.88]	
Complete	2.49	[1.86; 3.34]	57.88
Type of material used in the prosthesis			
Ceramic	1.0		
Metal-ceramic	8.43	[5.56; 12.77]	73.28
Metal-acrylic	2.29	[1.23; 4.27]	5.39
Acrylic	4.90	[3.17; 7.56]	55.80
Implant:crown ratio			
2:1	1.0		
1:1	1.54	[1.17; 2.03]	35.01
Fractures of prosthetic components within/previous year			
No	1.0		
Yes	3.01	[1.62; 5.61]	66.83
Loosening/decementations of prosthetic components within/ previous year			
No	1.0		
Yes	4.15	[1.90; 9.06]	73.81
Passive misfit diagnosed within/previous year			
No	1.0		
Yes	20.36	[2.37; 174.99]	95.09

While framing the significance of controlling risk factors in the general background of implant rehabilitation success, it is important to point out that despite all variables identified in this study as risk factors, the patient's healing and response may also play an important role in success, reflected in the recently proposed notions of osseosufficiency ("the state where host and implant interface reflects the combined capacity to promote and perpetuate successful osseointegration") and osseoseparation ("depleted marginal bone levels that occur with or without an accompanying gingivitis").[85] The limitations of this study are the retrospective design and the lack of control for the possible confounders. The effect of these variables should be tested using prospective study designs, controlling for the presence of other variables of interest in the etiopathogenesis of the peri-implant pathology through multivariable analysis.

CONCLUSIONS

Passive misfit of the prosthesis, loosening of prosthetic components, fracture of components, with complete edentulous rehabilitations, with metal-ceramic, metal-acrylic, or acrylic resin prostheses, using 17° angulated abutments, with an implant:crown ratio of 1:1 or more, or implants with a machined surface were significantly associated with an increased risk in the incidence of peri-implant pathology. The hypothetical removal of exposure of the majority of these variables could result in a drastic decrease in disease incidence. More studies with stronger designs should be performed to attest the causal relationship between these variables with peri-implant pathology.

REFERENCES

1. Albrektsson T: Consensus report of session IV. In Lang NP (ed): *Proceedings of the First European Workshop on Periodontology*. London, Quintessence, 1994, pp. 365–369.
2. Zitzmann NU, Berglundh T: Definition and prevalence of peri-implant diseases. *J Clin Periodontol* 2008;35:S286–S291.
3. Pontoriero R, Tonelli MP, Carnevale G, et al: Experimentally induced peri-implant mucositis. A clinical study in humans. *Clin Oral Implants Res* 1994;5:254–259.
4. Mombelli A: In vitro models of biological responses to implant microbiological models. *Adv Dental Res* 1999;13:67–72.
5. Meffert RM: Research in implantology at Louisiana State University School of Dentistry. *Int J Oral Implantol* 1990;6:15–21.
6. Ferreira SD, Silva GL, Cortelli JR, et al: Prevalence and risk variables for peri-implant disease in Brazilian subjects. *J Clin Periodontol* 2006;33:929–935.
7. Maximo MB, de Mendonca AC, Alves JF, et al: Peri-implant diseases may be associated with increased time loading and

generalized periodontal bone loss: preliminary results. *J Oral Implantol* 2008;34:268–273.

8. Rutar A, Lang NP, Buser D, et al: Retrospective assessment of clinical and microbiological factors affecting periimplant tissue conditions. *Clin Oral Implants Res* 2001;12:189–195.

9. Zhou W, Han C, Li D, et al: Endodontic treatment of teeth induces retrograde peri-implantitis. *Clin Oral Implant Res* 2009;20:1326–1332.

10. Karoussis IK, Muller S, Salvi GE, et al: Association between periodontal and peri-implant conditions: a 10-year prospective study. *Clin Oral Implants Res* 2004;15:1–7.

11. Roos-Jansaker AM, Renvert H, Lindahl C, et al: Nine- to fourteen-year follow-up of implant treatment. Part III: factors associated with peri-implant lesions. *J Clin Periodont* 2006;33:296–301.

12. Quirynen M, Vogels R, Alsaadi G, et al: Predisposing conditions for retrograde peri-implantitis, and treatment suggestions. *Clin Oral Implants Res* 2005;16:599–608.

13. Serino G, Strom C: Peri-implantitis in partially edentulous patients: association with inadequate plaque control. *Clin Oral Implants Res* 2009;20:169–174.

14. Aloufi F, Bissada N, Ficara A, et al: Clinical assessment of peri-implant tissues in patients with varying severity of chronic periodontitis. *Clin Implant Dent Relat Res* 2009;11: 37–40.

15. Rosenberg ES, Cho SC, Elian N, et al: A comparison of characteristics of implant failure and survival in periodontally compromised and periodontally healthy patients: a clinical report. *Int J Oral Maxillofac Implants* 2004;19:873–879.

16. Haas R, Haimbock W, Mailath G, et al: The relationship of smoking on peri-implant tissue: a retrospective study. *J Prosthet Dent* 1996;76:592–596.

17. Tonetti MS: Determination of the success and failure of root-form osseointegrated dental implants. *Adv Dent Res* 1999;13:173–180.

18. Kourtis SG, Sotiriadou S, Voliotis S, et al: Private practice results of dental implants. Part I: survival and evaluation of risk factors. Part II: surgical and prosthetic complications. *Implant Dent* 2004;13:373–385.

19. Nobel Biocare AB: Parallel-walled implants. Branemark System. Nobel Biocare, 2009.

20. Friberg B, Jemt T, Lekholm U: Early failures in 4,641 consecutively placed Branemark dental implants: a study from stage 1 surgery to the connection of completed prostheses. *Int J Oral Maxillofac Implants* 1991;6:142–146.

21. Bahat O: Treatment planning and placement of implants in the posterior maxillae: report of 732 consecutive Nobelpharma implants. *Int J Oral Maxillofac Implants* 1993;8:151–161.

22. Buser D, Mericske-Stern R, Bernard JP, et al: Long-term evaluation of non-submerged ITI implants. Part 1: 8-year life table analysis of a prospective multi-center study with 2359 implants. *Clin Oral Implants Res* 1997;8:161–172.

23. Esposito M, Coulthard P, Thomsen P, et al: Interventions for replacing missing teeth: different types of dental implants. *Cochrane Database Syst Rev* 2005;25:CD003815.

24. Teughels W, Van Assche N, Sliepen I, et al: Effect of material characteristics and/or surface topography on biofilm development. *Clin Oral Implants Res* 2006;17(Suppl 2): 68–81.

25. Uribe R, Penarrocha M, Sanchis JM, et al: Marginal peri-implantitis due to occlusal overload. A case report. *Med Oral* 2004;9:160–162, 159–160.

26. Zitzmann NU, Abrahamsson I, Berglundh T, et al: Soft tissue reactions to plaque formation at implant abutments with different surface topography. An experimental study in dogs. *J Clin Periodontol* 2002;29:456–461.

27. Van Assche N, Coucke W, Teughels W, et al: RCT comparing minimally with moderately rough implants. Part 1: clinical observations. *Clin Oral Implants Res* 2012;23:617–624.

28. Lekholm U, van Steenberghe D, Herrmann I, et al: Osseointegrated implants in the treatment of partially edentulous jaws: a prospective 5-year multicenter study. *Int J Oral Maxillofac Implants* 1994;9:627–635.

29. Parein AM, Eckert SE, Wollan PC, et al: Implant reconstruction in the posterior mandible: a long-term retrospective study. *J Prosthet Dent* 1997;78:34–42.

30. Gunne J, Jemt T, Linden B: Implant treatment in partially edentulous patients: a report on prostheses after 3 years. *Int J Prosthodont* 1994;7:143–148.

31. Rangert B, Jemt T, Jorneus L: Forces and moments on Branemark implants. *Int J Oral Maxillofac Implants* 1989;4:241–247.

32. Skalak R: Biomechanical considerations in osseointegrated prostheses. *J Prosthet Dent* 1983;49:843–848.

33. Davis DM, Rimrott R, Zarb GA: Studies on frameworks for osseointegrated prostheses. Part 2. The effect of adding acrylic resin or porcelain to form the occlusal superstructure. *Int J Oral Maxillofac Implants* 1988;3:275–280.

34. Gracis SE, Nicholls JI, Chalupnik JD, et al: Shock-absorbing behavior of five restorative materials used on implants. *Int J Prosthodont* 1991;4:282–291.

35. Naert I, Quirynen M, van Steenberghe D, et al: A six-year prosthodontic study of 509 consecutively inserted implants for the treatment of partial edentulism. *J Prosthet Dent* 1992;67:236–245.

36. Awadalla HA, Azarbal M, Ismail YH, et al: Three-dimensional finite element stress analysis of a cantilever fixed partial denture. *J Prosthet Dent* 1992;68:243–248.

37. White SN, Caputo AA, Anderkvist T: Effect of cantilever length on stress transfer by implant-supported prostheses. *J Prosthet Dent* 1994;71:493–499.

38. van Zyl PP, Grundling NL, Jooste CH, et al: Three-dimensional finite element model of a human mandible incorporating six osseointegrated implants for stress analysis of mandibular cantilever prostheses. *Int J Oral Maxillofac Implants* 1995;10:51–57.

39. Aglietta M, Siciliano VI, Zwahlen M, et al: A systematic review of the survival and complication rates of implant supported fixed dental prostheses with cantilever extensions after an observation period of at least 5 years. *Clin Oral Implants Res* 2009;20:441–451.

40. Bragger U, Aeschlimann S, Burgin W, et al: Biological and technical complications and failures with fixed partial dentures

(FPD) on implants and teeth after four to five years of function. *Clin Oral Implants Res* 2001;12:26–34.

41. Renouard F, Rangert B: *Risk Factors in Implant Dentistry: Simplified Clinical Analysis for Predictable Treatment.* Chicago, Quintessence, 1999.

42. Blanes RJ, Bernard JP, Blanes ZM, et al: A 10-year prospective study of ITI dental implants placed in the posterior region. II: influence of the crown-to-implant ratio and different prosthetic treatment modalities on crestal bone loss. *Clin Oral Implants Res* 2007;18:707–714.

43. Schulte J, Flores AM, Weed M: Crown-to-implant ratios of single tooth implant-supported restorations. *J Prosthet Dent* 2007;98:1–5.

44. Tawil G, Aboujaoude N, Younan R: Influence of prosthetic parameters on the survival and complication rates of short implants. *Int J Oral Maxillofac Implants* 2006;21:275–282.

45. Rokni S, Todescan R, Watson P, et al: An assessment of crown-to-root ratios with short sintered porous-surfaced implants supporting prostheses in partially edentulous patients. *Int J Oral Maxillofac Implants* 2005;20:69–76.

46. Blanes RJ: To what extent does the crown-implant ratio affect the survival and complications of implant-supported reconstructions? A systematic review. *Clin Oral Implants Res* 2009;20(Suppl 4): 67–72.

47. Malchiodi L, Cucchi A, Ghensi P, et al: Influence of crown-implant ratio on implant success rates and crestal bone levels: a 36-month follow-up prospective study. *Clin Oral Implants Res* 2013, Feb 12. doi: 10.1111/clr.12105 [Epub ahead of print].

48. Preoteasa E, Murariu CM, Ionescu E, et al: Acrylic resin reinforcement with metallic and nonmetallic inserts. *Revista medico-chirurgicala a Societatii de Medici si Naturalisti din Iasi* 2007;111:487–493.

49. Balshi TJ, Ekfeldt A, Stenberg T, et al: Three-year evaluation of Branemark implants connected to angulated abutments. *Int J Oral Maxillofac Implants* 1997;12:52–58.

50. Balshi TJ, Wolfinger GJ: Immediate loading of Branemark implants in edentulous mandibles: a preliminary report. *Implant Dent* 1997;6:83–88.

51. Proceedings of the 1996 World Workshop in Periodontics. *Ann Periodontol* 1996;1:816–820.

52. Becker W, Becker BE: Replacement of maxillary and mandibular molars with single endosseous implant restorations: a retrospective study. *J Prosthet Dent* 1995;74:51–55.

53. Zarb GA, Schmitt A: The longitudinal clinical effectiveness of osseointegrated dental implants: the Toronto study. Part III: problems and complications encountered. *J Prosthet Dent* 1990;64:185–194.

54. Jemt T: Failures and complications in 391 consecutively inserted fixed prostheses supported by Branemark implants in edentulous jaws: a study of treatment from the time of prosthesis placement to the first annual checkup. *Int J Oral Maxillofac Implants* 1991;6:270–276.

55. Jemt T, Linden B, Lekholm U: Failures and complications in 127 consecutively placed fixed partial prostheses supported by Branemark implants: from prosthetic treatment to first annual checkup. *Int J Oral Maxillofac Implants* 1992;7:40–44.

56. Patterson EA, Johns RB: Theoretical analysis of the fatigue life of fixture screws in osseointegrated dental implants. *Int J Oral Maxillofac Implants* 1992;7:26–33.

57. Morgan MJ, James DF, Pilliar RM: Fractures of the fixture component of an osseointegrated implant. *Int J Oral Maxillofac Implants* 1993;8:409–414.

58. Sakaguchi RL, Borgersen SE: Nonlinear finite element contact analysis of dental implant components. *Int J Oral Maxillofac Implants* 1993;8:655–661.

59. Kallus T, Bessing C: Loose gold screws frequently occur in full-arch fixed prostheses supported by osseointegrated implants after 5 years. *Int J Oral Maxillofac Implants* 1994;9:169–178.

60. Quirynen M, Bollen CM, Eyssen H, et al: Microbial penetration along the implant components of the Branemark system. An in vitro study. *Clin Oral Implants Res* 1994;5:239–244.

61. Quirynen M, van Steenberghe D: Bacterial colonization of the internal part of two-stage implants. An in vivo study. *Clin Oral Implants Res* 1993;4:158–161.

62. Persson LG, Lekholm U, Leonhardt A, et al: Bacterial colonization on internal surfaces of Branemark system implant components. *Clin Oral Implants Res* 1996;7:90–95.

63. Ericsson I, Persson LG, Berglundh T, et al: Different types of inflammatory reactions in peri-implant soft tissues. *J Clin Periodontol* 1995;22:255–261.

64. Lekholm U, Adell R, Lindhe J, et al: Marginal tissue reactions at osseointegrated titanium fixtures. II. A cross-sectional retrospective study. *Int J Oral Maxillofac Surg* 1986;15:53–61.

65. Adell R, Lekholm U, Rockler B, et al: Marginal tissue reactions at osseointegrated titanium fixtures. I. A 3-year longitudinal prospective study. *Int J Oral Maxillofac Surg* 1986;15:39–52.

66. von Elm E, Altman DG, Egger M, et al: The Strengthening the Reporting of Observational Studies in Epidemiology (STROBE) statement: guidelines for reporting observational studies. *Epidemiology* 2007;18:800–804.

67. De Araujo Nobre M, Capelas C, Alves A, et al: Non-surgical treatment of peri-implant pathology. *Int J Dent Hyg* 2006;4:84–90.

68. Esposito M, Hirsch JM, Lekholm U, et al: Biological factors contributing to failures of osseointegrated oral implants. I. Success criteria and epidemiology. *Eur J Oral Sci* 1998;106:527–551.

69. Fiorellini JP, Weber HP: Clinical trials on the prognosis of dental implants. *Periodontol* 2000;4:98–108.

70. Moy PK, Medina D, Shetty V, et al: Dental implant failure rates and associated risk factors. *Int J Oral Maxillofac Implants* 2005;20:569–577.

71. Rothman KJ, Greenland S: *Modern Epidemiology.* Philadelphia, Lippincott-Raven, 1998.

72. Sahin S, Cehreli MC: The significance of passive framework fit in implant prosthodontics: current status. *Implant Dent* 2001;10:85–92.

73. Adell R, Lekholm U, Rockler B, et al: Marginal tissue reactions at osseointegrated titanium fixtures. I. A 3-year longitudinal prospective study. *Int J Oral Maxillofac Surg* 1986;15:39–52.

74. Lee FK, Tan KB, Nicholls JI: Critical bending moment of four implant-abutment interface designs. *Int J Oral Maxillofac Implants* 2010;25:744–751.

75. Ivanoff CJ, Widmark G, Johansson C, et al: Histologic evaluation of bone response to oxidized and turned titanium microimplants in human jawbone. *Int J Oral Maxillofac Implants* 2003;18:341–348.

76. Huang YH, Xiropaidis AV, Sorensen RG, et al: Bone formation at titanium porous oxide (TiUnite) oral implants in type IV bone. *Clin Oral Implants Res* 2005;16:105–111.

77. Xiropaidis AV, Qahash M, Lim WH, et al: Bone-implant contact at calcium phosphate-coated and porous titanium oxide (TiUnite)-modified oral implants. *Clin Oral Implants Res* 2005;16:532–539.

78. Albrektsson TJC, Lundgren AK, Sul Y, et al: Experimental studies on oxidized implants. A histomorphometrical and biomechanical analysis. *Appl Osseointegration Res* 2000;1:15–17.

79. Zechner W, Tangl S, Furst G, et al: Osseous healing characteristics of three different implant types. *Clin Oral Implants Res* 2003;14:150–157.

80. Cavallaro J, Jr., Greenstein G: Angled implant abutments: a practical application of available knowledge. *J Am Dent Assoc* 2011;142:150–158.

81. Carlsson GE, Lindquist LW, Jemt T: Long-term marginal periimplant bone loss in edentulous patients. *Int J Prosthodont* 2000;13:295–302.

82. Bollen CM, Lambrechts P, Quirynen M: Comparison of surface roughness of oral hard materials to the threshold surface roughness for bacterial plaque retention: a review of the literature. *Dent Mater* 1997;13:258–269.

83. Chan C, Weber H: Plaque retention on teeth restored with full-ceramic crowns: a comparative study. *J Prosthet Dent* 1986; 56:666–671.

84. Renouard F, Rangert B: *Risk Factors in Implant Dentistry: Simplified Clinical Analysis for Predictable Treatment.* Chicago, Quintessence, 1999.

85. Zarb G, Koka S, Albrektsson T: Editorial: hyperbole, clinical dissonance, and scratching the surface: complication or disease? *Int J Prosthodont* 2013, 26:311.

17

CONCEPTS FOR DESIGNING AND FABRICATING METAL IMPLANT FRAMEWORKS FOR HYBRID IMPLANT PROSTHESES

Carl Drago, dds, ms,[1] and Kent Howell, dmd, ms[2]

[1]Clinical Director, Eon Clinics, Waukesha, WI, formerly, Associate Professor, Department of Restorative and Prosthetic Dentistry, The Ohio State University College of Dentistry, Columbus, OH

[2]Prosthodontist, Southwest Dental Group, Scottsdale, AZ, formerly, Advanced Prosthodontics, The Ohio State University, Columbus, OH

The article is associated with the American College of Prosthodontists' journal-based continuing education program. It is accompanied by an online continuing education activity worth 1 credit. Please visit www.wileyonlinelearning.com/jopr to complete the activity and earn credit.

Keywords
Implant framework design; cantilever extensions; CAD/CAM milling; implant hybrid prostheses.

Correspondence
Carl Drago, Eon Clinics, 20700 Swenson Dr., Pewaukee, WI 53072. E-mail: carl.drago@gmail.com

Supported in part by The Ohio State University College of Dentistry.

Dr. Drago is a consultant for Biomet 3i.

Accepted September 9, 2011

Published in Journal of Prosthodontics July 2012; Vol. 21, Issue 5

doi: 10.1111/j.1532-849X.2012.00835.x

ABSTRACT

Edentulous patients have reported difficulties in managing complete dentures; they have also reported functional concerns and higher expectations regarding complete dentures than the dentists who have treated them. Some of the objectives of definitive fixed implant prosthodontic care include predictable, long-term prostheses, improved function, and maintenance of alveolar bone. One of the keys to long-term clinical success is the design and fabrication of metal frameworks that support implant prostheses. Multiple, diverse methods have been reported regarding framework design in implant prosthodontics. Original designs were developed empirically, without the benefit of laboratory testing. Prosthetic complications reported after occlusal loading included screw loosening, screw fracture, prosthesis fracture, crestal bone loss around implants, and implant loss. Numerous authors promoted accurately fitting frameworks; however, it has been noted that metal frameworks do not fit accurately. Passively fitting metal implant frameworks and implants have not been realized. Biologic consequences of ill-fitting frameworks were not well understood. Basic engineering principles were then incorporated into implant framework designs; however, laboratory testing was lacking. It has been reported that I- and L-beam designs were the best clinical option. With the advent of CAD/CAM protocols, milled titanium frameworks became quite popular in implant prosthodontics. The purpose of this article is to discuss current and past literature regarding implant-retained frameworks for full-arch, hybrid restorations. Benefits, limitations, and complications associated with this type of prosthesis will be reviewed. This discussion will include the relative inaccuracy of casting/implant fit and improved accuracy noted with CAD/CAM framework/implant fit; cantilever extensions relative to the A/P implant spread; and mechanical properties associated with implant frameworks including I- and L-beam designs. Guidelines will be proposed for use by clinicians and laboratory technicians in designing implant-retained frameworks.

Edentulous patients have reported difficulties in managing complete dentures. Marachlioglou et al reported that patients had higher expectations regarding their complete dentures than did the dentists who treated them. Dentists reported that dentures would bring fewer benefits to patients than did the patients.[1] Patients with complete dentures have also reported decreased masticatory function in that they avoided certain food types because they were simply unable to chew them.[2] Lin et al reported the results of a clinical study investigating the relationship between chewing ability and diet among elderly edentulous patients. Approximately 58% of the subjects reported dissatisfaction with their dentures; 51% reported discomfort on chewing. Patient satisfaction or dissatisfaction with their dentures during mastication significantly impacted the diet of these elderly edentulous patients.[3]

Clinical denture issues may be related to loss of alveolar bone after tooth extraction. Dental implants, in addition to providing increased retention and support for prostheses, also have been reported to maintain alveolar bone volume.[4] Endosseous implants are thought to maintain bone width and height as long as implants remain anchored in bone with healthy, biologic attachments.[5]

HISTORICAL PERSPECTIVE

Two of the objectives regarding definitive implant prosthodontic treatments were the design and fabrication of accurately fitting, strong metal frameworks to splint multiple implants. Frameworks also served as the foundation for retaining fixed-implant prostheses on a long-term basis. Over the years, multiple, diverse methods have been used for implant framework design and fabrication; different materials have also been used, including, but not limited to, noble/base metal alloys and various ceramic materials (Figs 17.1–17.3).

Original Framework Designs for Fixed Hybrid Prostheses

Zarb and Jansson[6] stated that frameworks (fixed prostheses) could be designed in one of the two ways: (1) where metal

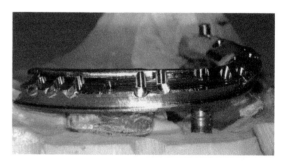

FIGURE 17.1 Clinical image of a mandibular fixed hybrid prosthesis approximately 13 years post insertion. Note the extreme wear/abrasion of the artificial teeth; the implant framework on the patient's right side was exposed secondary to occlusal abrasion.

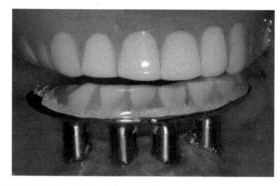

FIGURE 17.2 Clinical image of a mandibular implant CAD/CAM framework for a fixed hybrid implant prosthesis. This framework was made using an L-beam design. Facial and lingual finish lines were machined for finishing the processed acrylic resin.

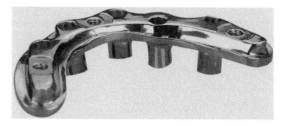

FIGURE 17.3 CAD image of a mandibular implant-retained framework designed as an I-bar. The facial and lingual finish lines were machined similar to the L-beam design in Figure 17.2.

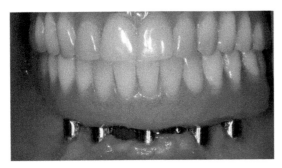

FIGURE 17.4 Clinical image of an acrylic resin wraparound mandibular fixed implant hybrid prosthesis. The cast metal framework was completely enveloped within the hybrid prosthesis.

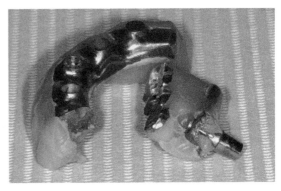

FIGURE 17.5 Laboratory image of a fractured fixed, implant-retained mandibular prosthesis. This prosthesis fractured through the distal cylinder on the patient's right side. The fracture also included the occlusal portion of the implant. The exact cause of this failure was unknown, although the vertical height of the framework appeared to be approximately 3+ mm.

frameworks comprised the bulk of the prostheses, and artificial teeth and minimal denture bases were the only non-metallic components. (2) Implant fixed prostheses consisting mostly of acrylic resin denture bases (wraparound design) and artificial teeth, with minimally sized metal frameworks (Fig 17.4).[6] Implant treatment was based on basic prosthodontic principles that included preliminary and definitive impressions, jaw relation records, wax try-in, metal framework try-in (with and without the artificial teeth), and insertion of definitive prostheses. Frameworks were fabricated according to the following criteria: bulk for strength, adequate access for oral hygiene procedures, minimal display of metal on the facial and occlusal surfaces, and strategic thinning of implant frameworks to allow for retention of acrylic resin denture teeth and denture bases. In removable partial denture (RPD) design, it was noted that retentive portions of RPD frameworks should allow for 1.5 mm thickness of resin. Thickness was also necessary to minimize the potential fracture of the acrylic resin base material surrounding metal frameworks.[7] These principles have been extrapolated to fixed implant framework design. It is interesting to note that in an early implant textbook, no mention was made of the lengths of the cantilevered segments.[6]

Numerous authors have reported on prosthetic maintenance issues with fixed implant prostheses. Zarb and Jansson noted that implant frameworks were vulnerable to fracture, especially at the junctions between distal abutments and cantilevered segments.[6] Zarb and Schmitt reported clinical problems that included: abutment screw fracture, gold alloy retaining screw fracture, and framework fractures (12/13 occurred in the cantilevered portions of the frameworks).[8] Relative to framework fracture, Zarb and Schmitt suggested design changes including cantilevered segments not exceeding 20 mm, increased cross-sectional surface areas, and using casting alloys with higher yield and tensile strengths compared to the alloys used in original osseointegrated prostheses. They also stated that prosthodontic treatment included a series of clinical steps that were mostly empirical, and that treatment invariably was accompanied by varying degrees of problems (Figs 17.5 and 17.6).

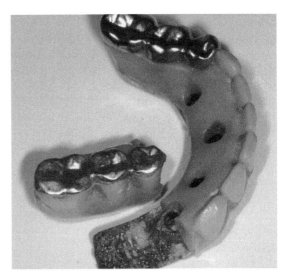

FIGURE 17.6 Laboratory image of a fixed, implant-retained mandibular prosthesis where a relatively long distal cantilevered prosthetic segment separated from the metal framework. The implants were placed in a relatively straight line, with minimal A/P spread. Note also the limited vertical thickness of the acrylic resin denture base; this indicated minimal interarch clearance.

Oral/facial symmetries and lip contours may be significantly influenced by appropriate/inappropriate maxillary tooth positions, vertical dimension, and/or the need for flanges of varying thicknesses for lip support.[9,10] Upper lip peri-oral activity may be far more revealing of maxillary gingival tissues than the corresponding activity of the lower lip.

Esthetic demands tend to be more dramatic with maxillary prostheses than mandibular prostheses. As per Zarb and Schmitt,[8] unlike mandibular implant prostheses where

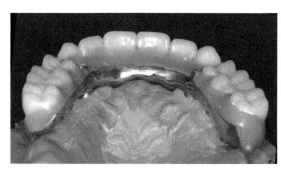

FIGURE 17.7 Laboratory palatal image of a maxillary fixed, implant-retained prosthesis. Note the junction between the prosthesis and the replica soft tissues in the anterior segment. This type of design is thought to facilitate phonetics.

hygienic type designs have proven to be functionally and esthetically acceptable, maxillary implant prostheses demand different sized and shaped labial/buccal flanges that may or may not compensate for optimal esthetics (including lip support), phonetics, and masticatory function (food impaction between intaglio surfaces and edentulous areas). If flanges are fabricated for upper lip support and phonetics, they may not be readily reduced for access for adequate peri-implant oral hygiene procedures (Fig 17.7). Maxillary prostheses impact speech significantly more than do mandibular prostheses. Patients have also identified speech as a major factor in perceived satisfaction of their prostheses.[11–15]

Maxillary functional issues are different from those encountered in edentulous mandibles. Maxillary complete dentures tend to predictably restore original soft tissue contours, tooth positions, and arch forms. Maxillary complete dentures, relative to tongue movements, are generally negligible; speech is not usually impaired. Functional demands for maxillary hybrid implant prostheses are complicated in that phonetics may be affected by hybrid designs and contours. Additionally, prosthetic gingival tissues are often required due to resorptive patterns of edentulous maxillae. Resorptive patterns in maxillae are dissimilar to mandibular resorption patterns: maxillae resorb superiorly, posteriorly, and medially; mandibles resorb inferiorly, anteriorly, and laterally.[16,17] Differences in maxillary and mandibular resorption patterns often lead to unfavorable implant and prosthetic relationships between opposing jaws.

Frameworks for the original fixed hybrid prostheses were waxed with gold alloy cylinders, cast with silver palladium alloys, and screwed into place with small retaining screws.[8] Fixed hybrid prostheses splinted implants together via a strong, rigid metallic unit that fulfilled the objectives of strength, support, non-tissue impingement, and non-interference to obtain the desired cosmetic results.[6] It is interesting to note that in chapter 15 of *Tissue Integrated Prostheses: Osseointegration in Clinical Dentistry* (Prosthodontic Complications), there was no mention of optimal framework design.[6,18–20]

In an early textbook, Glantz[21] stated that fixed implant prostheses were almost invariably extended distal to the most distal implants to create optimal functional balance between mandibular and maxillary prostheses. He stated that at the time (1985), there was no precise equation for describing functional deformation patterns of fixed prostheses with cantilevered pontics. He offered a complex equation where deformation of implant-retained, fixed prostheses was inversely related to the modulus of elasticity, width, and height (H) of frameworks and positively correlated with the amount of force and length (L) of frameworks. Therefore, for a given alloy with a known modulus of elasticity, taller (height) and thicker (width) frameworks resisted deformation better than thinner or more narrow frameworks. Therefore, the greater the force generated on a given framework, with increased framework lengths (cantilever), frameworks would be more likely to undergo deformation when compared to lesser forces and frameworks with decreased cantilever lengths.

Passively Fitting Implant Frameworks

Traditionally, implant frameworks were fabricated using the lost-wax technique and casting noble alloys. It has been well established that casting errors may be corrected using various soldering techniques.[22–24] It has been consistent from early reports regarding implant frameworks that passive, accurate fits should be obtained between implant frameworks and implant restorative components.[25] It has also been well established that implant frameworks cannot be made to fit passively.[26] Zarb and Jansson identified this in an early textbook by stating that if a clinical passive fit was not obtained, frameworks should be sectioned, an intraoral index made, and then the segments should be soldered.[27] Zervas et al reported in a laboratory study that soldering did not improve the casting misfit of three-unit fixed partial dentures (FPDs).[28] Rubenstein and Lowry reported in another laboratory study that assessed the accuracy of segmental indexing/soldering for full-arch frameworks, using two types of resin, that there were no significant differences noted between alloy/index combinations, except for angular changes around the Y-axis.[29]

Laser-welding of implant frameworks has also been studied. In a study undertaken to describe the effect of laser-welding conditions on material properties of welded frameworks, Uysal et al reported that, within the constraints of their finite element analysis, mechanical failure of welded joints should not be expected under simulated intraoral conditions.[30] Silva et al reported that implant frameworks may show a more precise adaptation between frameworks and implant restorative platforms when segments were sectioned and laser welded.[31] Hjalmarsson et al measured and compared the precision of fit of laser-welded (Cresco) and computer-numeric-controlled (CNC)-milled metal frameworks for implant-supported fixed complete prostheses.[26] Overall, the maximum 3D range of center point distortion was 279 µm. None of the frameworks presented a perfect, completely "passive" fit to any master cast; however, CNC frameworks had statistically significantly less vertical distortion than the Cresco groups. Other reports have resulted in similar findings.[32,33]

CAD/CAM frameworks have been found to fit more accurately than frameworks cast with gold alloys.[34,35] Implant framework fit and its effect on associated peri-implant bone levels has also been researched. Some authors have concluded that a perfect passive framework is impossible to achieve and arguably, unnecessary.[36-38] Although research regarding framework misfit as a cause of peri-implant bone loss is difficult to prove, others have described the value of excellent framework fit for optimal screw mechanics.[39,40]

Prosthetic Complications Associated with Fixed Implant Frameworks

Prosthetic complications have been defined as treatments, adjustments, or repairs of implant prostheses that became necessary secondary to unexpected events.[41,42] Zarb and Schmitt[5] identified three types of prosthetic complications: structural, cosmetic, and functional. Zarb and Schmitt[8] followed 46 patients treated with 274 implants (49 frameworks) for 4 to 9 years and reported a high incidence of prosthodontic complications associated with fixed implant prostheses: 9 abutment screw fractures (3.3%); 53 gold alloy screw fractures (19.3%); and 13 framework fractures (26.5%). It is important to note that Zarb and Schmitt's report included patients treated with early prosthetic protocols that included cast alloy frameworks, and minimal understanding of screw mechanics, torque, preload, and A/P spread. Contrast the above results with more recent reports. In a 5-year clinical study, Hjalmarsson et al reported on the clinical outcomes associated with screw-retained fixed implant prostheses made with laser welding versus frameworks made with milled commercially pure titanium. They noted significantly more complications in the laser-welded framework group than in the milled framework group.[43] Ortorp and Jemt reported the results of a 10-year clinical study, and noted the frequency of prosthetic complications was low, with similar clinical and radiographic results for CAD/CAM milled and cast gold alloy frameworks.[44] One prosthesis was lost in each group due to loss of implants; one prosthesis fractured in the CAD/CAM milled group. They noted more maintenance appointments were needed for maxillary prostheses.

Physical Properties of Metals Used in Fixed Implant Frameworks

Cast Noble Alloys Noble metals have been defined on the basis of their chemical and physical properties; noble alloys resist oxidation and corrosion by acids. Four noble metals are used in dental alloys: gold, palladium, silver, and platinum. These metals give noble metal alloys their inert intraoral properties. Alloys that contain more than 6% palladium are usually white/silver colored (Tables 17.1 and 17.2).[45]

There has been increased use of palladium/silver alloys in implant prosthodontics. These alloys provide mechanical properties similar to type III gold alloys, but at reduced cost. Increased amounts of silver increase ductility and lower hardness; silver also decreases tarnish resistance. Alloys with high palladium contents generally contain limited amounts of other noble metals.

Physical properties such as yield strength, Vickers Hardness, and ductility (% elongation) are properties clinicians and dental laboratory technicians consider when deciding which alloy should be used for dental frameworks.[45]

TABLE 17.1 Roles of Alloying Elements in Dental Noble Alloys

Property	Gold	Platinum	Palladium	Copper	Silver	Zinc	Iridium
Melting point °C (°F)	1063 (1945)	1769 (3224)	1552 (2829)	1083 (1981)	961 (1761)	420 (787)	2443 (4429)
Chemical activity	Inert	Inert	Mild	Very active	Active	Very active	Active
Approximate content (%)	50–95	0–20	0–12	0–17	0–20	0–2	0.005–0.1
Melting	Raises melting point mildly	Raises melting point rapidly	Raises melting point rapidly	Lowers melting point even below its own	Slight effect; may raise or sometimes lower mildly	Lowers melting point readily; in most solders	No effect
Tarnish resistance	Essential	Contributes	Increases tarnish resistance but less than Au and Pt	Contributes to tarnish in flame, or with sulfurous food	Tarnishes in presence of sulfur	Will tarnish, but in low percentages has little effect	Increased

TABLE 17.2   Composition and Properties of Dental Noble Alloys

Type	Composition				Vickers Hardness		Yield Strength, psi (MPa)		Ductility % Elongation
	Au	Pt	Pd	Ag	As Cast	Hardened	Quenched	Hardened	
III	74	0	4	12	130	157	38000 (262)	48000 (331)	39.4
IV	68.5	3	3.5	10.5	181	280	56400 (389)	101900 (703)	17
PFM	48.5	0	39.5	0	224	283	70500 (486)	87400 (603)	11

III Firmilay (Jelenko Co, New Rochelle, NY).
IV No.7 (Jelenko Co, New Rochelle, NY).
PFM Olympia (Jelenko Co, New Rochelle, NY).

Reproducible procedures resulting in consistent, accurate, strong castings with high yield strengths are critical for long-term successful metal frameworks. Stress resistance of alloys has an impact on the minimum dimensions in critical areas such as connector areas and cantilevers. Elastic modulus is also important because it determines the flexibility of metal frameworks. Flexibility is inversely proportionate to the elastic modulus—an alloy with a high elastic modulus will flex less under load than an alloy with a low elastic modulus. Casting accuracy is also important for fabrication of clinically acceptable frameworks.

Palladium/silver alloys usually contain about 50% to 60% palladium; most of the balance is silver. They generally exhibit satisfactory tarnish and corrosion resistance. The elastic modulus for this group of alloys is the most favorable of all the noble metal alloys and results in the least flexible castings.[45] One disadvantage with this group of alloys does not factor into frameworks for implant hybrid prostheses—the tendency to change to a green color with porcelain applications.

Cast Base Metal Alloys   Non-precious or base metal alloys are composed of non-noble metals, except for beryllium, a precious but non-noble metal. Most base metal alloys are based on combinations of nickel and chromium, although cobalt/chromium and iron-based alloys are also used. Corrosion resistance for base metal alloys depends on other chemical properties. After casting, a thin chromium oxide layer provides an impervious film that passivates the alloy surface. The layer is so thin that it does not dull the alloy surface. These alloys differ significantly from noble alloys, as they possess significant hardness, high yield strengths, and high elastic moduli. Elongation is equivalent to the gold alloys, but is countered by the high yield strength. Base metal alloys are significantly less expensive than noble alloys, but this may be negated by higher labor costs associated with finishing and polishing procedures. Allergies associated with nickel and nickel-containing alloys have been documented.[46] Inhaling dust from grinding nickel- and beryllium-containing alloys should be avoided.

Milled Titanium Frameworks   Ti and Ti alloys are well suited for use in clinical dentistry because they have excellent corrosion resistance, low specific gravity, and excellent biocompatibility, are inexpensive, and possess mechanical properties similar to cast gold alloys. Ti and its alloys are difficult to cast due to their high melting points, low density, and reactivity with elements in casting investments.[47]

Milled Zirconium Frameworks   Zirconia has been available for use in restorative dentistry as a dental ceramic replacement for metal frameworks in fixed and implant prosthodontics. The type of zirconia used in dentistry is yttria tetragonal zirconia polycrystal (Y-TZP). Y-TZP is a monophase ceramic material formed by directly sintering crystals together without any type of intervening matrix to form a dense, polycrystalline structure. Yttria is added to zirconia to stabilize and maintain the material's physical properties at lower temperatures than would otherwise occur without yttria.

The flexural strength of zirconia oxide materials has been reported to be 900 to 1100 MPa.[48] There are three main types of zirconia used in clinical dentistry: fully sintered or Hot Isostatic Pressing (HIP); partially sintered zirconia; and non-sintered or "green state" zirconia. The latter two types are softer than HIP zirconia and more cost efficient to mill. After milling, zirconia frameworks are sintered in furnaces at 1350 to 1500°C where the final shapes, strengths, and physical properties are achieved. Partially sintered zirconia frameworks are milled 20% to 25% larger than the actual frameworks to allow for shrinkage during the sintering process.[49]

Larsson and Vult von Steyern reported the results of a clinical study that compared clinical performances of 2- to 5-unit implant-supported, all-ceramic restorations fabricated with two zirconia systems.[50] They concluded that all-ceramic, implant-supported fixed dental prostheses of two to five units were reasonable treatment alternatives. One system in their study exhibited an unacceptable amount of porcelain veneer fractures and was not recommended for the type of treatment evaluated in their trial.

Guess et al performed a literature review for citations published from 1990 through 2010 regarding zirconia in clinical dentistry.[51] They reported high biocompatibility, low bacterial surface adhesion, and favorable chemical properties of zirconia ceramics. Zirconia, stabilized with yttrium oxide, exhibited high flexural strength and fracture toughness. Preliminary clinical data confirmed high stability of zirconia abutments and also as framework material for implant crowns and fixed dental prostheses. Zirconia abutment or framework damage was rarely reported; however, as also noted by Larsson and Vult von Steyern, porcelain veneer fractures were common technical complications in implant-supported zirconia restorations. Porcelain veneer failures were thought to be related to differences in coefficients of thermal expansion between core and veneering porcelains, and their respective processing techniques. Guess et al[51] concluded that since clinical long-term data were missing, clinicians should proceed with caution relative to designing extensive implant-borne zirconia frameworks.

Accuracy of framework/implant fit has long been a topic of discussion. Guichet et al, in a laboratory study, reported an average marginal opening of 46.7 μm for screw- and cement-retained fixed dental prostheses.[52] Upon screw tightening, marginal openings for the screw-retained group decreased an average of 65% to an average of 16.5 μm. The prostheses in both groups were made after master casts had been verified; however, it should be noted that there were no significant differences in marginal adaptation between the groups prior to screw tightening or cementation. Screw tightening did result in a statistically significant difference. Guichet et al noted that their results compared favorably with the results of other studies.[53,54] They further noted that the fit of one-piece castings continues to be controversial when passive fit is a criterion for clinical acceptability. The effects of soldering, as compared to one-piece castings, according to the authors, merits continued study.

One-piece casting procedures have produced stable and relatively homogeneous frameworks.[55] Cast metal frameworks are subject to expansion and contraction that may result in porosity and/or distortion of individual castings. Wichmann and Tschernitschek reported the results of a clinical study where almost one third of the evaluated castings exhibited casting defects.[56] Multiple studies have reported that CAD/CAM Ti frameworks achieve implant/framework fits superior to those obtained with cast metal frameworks.[57–60] In a laboratory study, Al-Fadda et al reported that CAD/CAM milled frameworks demonstrated significantly less error when compared to cast frameworks (33.7 μm vs. 49.2 μm) in the vertical axis; differences in the horizontal plane were 56 μm and 85 μm, respectively.[59]

In general, most clinical studies regarding implant prosthodontics have reported on implant and prosthesis cumulative survival rates (CSRs). Framework design has not been extensively discussed or reviewed. Interest in CAD/CAM technology for implant restorations has been increasing for multiple reasons, including that frameworks and abutments

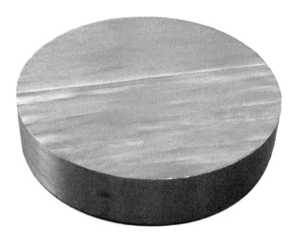

FIGURE 17.8 Titanium alloy blank prior to placement into milling machine for milling a CAD/CAM implant framework (Biomet 3i, Palm Beach Gardens, FL).

may be machined from solid blanks of material (Fig 17.8). Blanks are more homogeneous than conventional castings; physical properties are generally better. CAD/CAM technologies have eliminated conventional waxing, casting, and finishing procedures, along with the inaccuracies associated with these procedures. CAD/CAM frameworks produced commercially are generally less expensive for clinicians than cast metal frameworks, as they do not contain noble metals. CAD/CAM frameworks may be designed completely with computer software programs (Fig 17.9), or they may be waxed to certain specifications by dental technicians, scanned, and then milled in a procedure called "copy milling." The latter frameworks generally will not result in the decreased costs associated with CAD frameworks designed in CAD, as significant labor costs will be incurred in developing the wax/resin framework patterns (Figs 17.10 and 17.11).

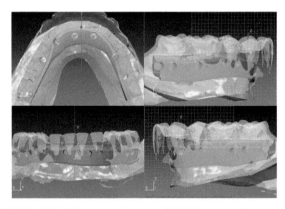

FIGURE 17.9 Representative set of JPEG images of a proposed design for a CAD/CAM mandibular implant framework/hybrid prosthesis. Note the "ghosted" images of the teeth. These types of images are sent to clinicians and laboratory technicians for input prior to milling.

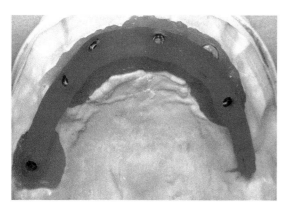

FIGURE 17.10 Laboratory occlusal image of a resin pattern, fabricated by a dental laboratory technician with specific contours, in preparation for a copy-milled CAD/CAM framework (North Shore Dental Laboratories, Lynn, MA).

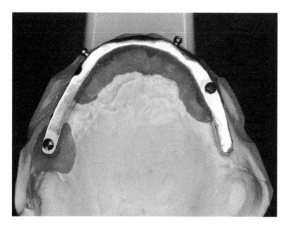

FIGURE 17.11 Laboratory occlusal image of the milled titanium alloy framework consistent with the resin pattern in Figure 17.10 (North Shore Dental Laboratories).

Based on the above studies, differences in accuracy of fit (CAD/CAM vs. cast frameworks) have been statistically significant; however, clinical significance has not been established. Some clinicians may not wish to use soldered frameworks as opposed to one-piece castings or milled frameworks. Specific clinical guidelines relative to framework fabrication have not been established. Among the factors clinicians may consider in fabricating fixed implant frameworks are: biocompatibility/type of alloy/type of ceramic, CAD/CAM (digital/copy mill), lost-wax technique, and expense. The authors of this article prefer to use CAD/CAM milled frameworks due to the accuracy of fit, biocompatibility/homogeneity of milled Ti alloy blanks, and decreased costs.

Design Considerations

Implant frameworks must be rigid to support fixed prostheses. Frameworks with cantilevered, freestanding segments

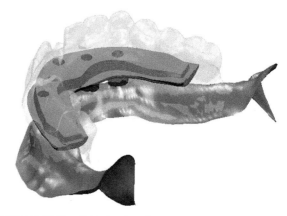

FIGURE 17.12 CAD implant framework with a modified I-bar design. The apical buccal and lingual portions of the framework were designed for use as finish lines for the denture base portion of the hybrid prosthesis.

have areas of high stress at or distal to the posterior abutments, and may compromise the structural integrity of inadequately designed frameworks.[5] Framework fracture may be avoided with optimal, mechanically designed frameworks. I-beam designs have been proposed to strengthen cantilevered portions of frameworks.[61] Taylor stated that cast alloy frameworks must have at least 3 mm of vertical bulk to provide sufficient rigidity to frameworks.[62] Rasmussen stated that I-beam-designed frameworks maximized resistance to occlusal loading and minimized permanent deformation under stress.[63] I-beams also provide rigidity and strength to frameworks with minimal increased bulk and weight (Fig 17.12). Rasmussen published his results in a clinical report where he incorporated I-beam framework designs into 35 prostheses, followed those patients for 3 years, and reported zero prosthetic failures.

Staab and Stewart evaluated two parameters regarding implant framework design (L, I, elliptical, and oval): beam deflection and maximum normal stress.[64] They noted that each of the tested designs could be viable clinically. They also reported that the I-beam design deflected less and experienced the smallest maximum normal stress of the tested designs. Elliptical designs deflected the most. The L design experienced the largest normal stress. Staab and Stewart noted the effectiveness of any framework design clinically could not be easily identified from a simple, static analysis; they also noted that the numerical differences they observed among the different designs were based on conditions that they decided upon for their experimental evaluation. Staab and Stewart[64] basically concurred with Cox and Zarb[61] and Rasmussen,[63] but did not propose that only I-beam configurations strengthened framework cantilevered segments.

Von Gonten et al stated that relative to framework design, consideration should be given to limit the amount of acrylic resin to retain artificial denture teeth.[65] Assuming rigid fixation to implants, areas of high stress concentrations in implant frameworks were focused at or just distal to the most posterior abutments in an arch, and would likely compromise the structural integrity of incorrectly designed frameworks.[63] Stress concentrations in these areas can be considerably greater than the mean applied force. Effective distribution of applied forces during mastication and clenching may be diminished by cantilevered segments deforming under stress. The worst-case scenario would be metal fatigue and fracture. Framework fractures may be minimized with proper design considerations.

Von Gonten et al described the fabrication of a mandibular fixed implant-supported framework with a more extensive cast alloy framework than was found in frameworks designed prior to 1995.[65] Their design consisted of an L-beam with extended vertical wall height lingually. The authors speculated that this provided increased resistance to cantilever stress and would resist fracture better than frameworks designed as I-beams (Fig 17.13). Von Gonten et al stated that this design was consistent with desirable physical properties, was readily maintainable by patients, and could be produced with available methods and materials. Von Gonten et al acknowledged that the L-beam design required significantly more alloy (12–14 pennyweights) and would be significantly more expensive than frameworks fabricated with I-beam designs. Unfortunately, the authors did not provide scientific evidence that the L-beam design resulted in more successful implant frameworks.

It is interesting to note that framework design characteristics have not been extensively reviewed or described. Sadowsky, in a 1997 comprehensive review article, described numerous characteristics of frameworks relative to adaptation to soft tissues, cleansibility, anterior/posterior (A/P) spread, and cantilever length, but was unable to cite definitive laboratory studies where variables were evaluated and conclusions drawn that would be helpful to clinicians designing implant frameworks.[66]

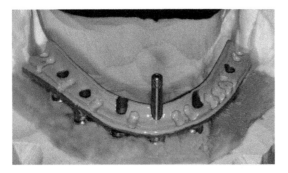

FIGURE 17.13   Example of a CAD/CAM milled framework with the L-beam design. Teeth are supported apically by the horizontal component of the L-beam design. The framework is designed to provide adequate support for the artificial teeth and denture base to minimize the risks of denture tooth/base fracture.

A/P spread has been discussed by several authors.[67,68] It was defined by English as the distance between the line connecting the two most distal implants and the center of the implant most distant to that line.[67] The A/P spread provides a macroscopic measure of the geometric distribution of the implants. Cantilever length and A/P spread are essential factors regarding distribution of occlusal loads. Some authors have suggested that cantilever lengths of 1.5 and A/P spreads of 2 be guides for maximum allowable cantilever lengths.[67,68] A cantilever length/A/P spread ratio of 2 was determined to be optimal by choosing implant forces equal to twice the applied loads as the failure criteria.[69] Cantilever lengths of 1.5 times the A/P spread were determined empirically for prostheses supported by five implants after considering clinical conditions that might biomechanically compromise the biologic and/or prosthetic outcomes of clinical cases.[69] Beumer et al recommended a minimum of six implants with an A/P spread of at least 20 mm and sufficient bone in the second premolar areas to support 10 mm implants.[70]

English recommended cantilever lengths be 1.5 times the A/P spread, but shorter in poor quality bone.[67] Due to bending moments, the presence of load-bearing cantilevers increase forces distributed to implants, possibly up to two or three times the applied loads on a single implant.[71] McAlarney and Stavropoulos observed that cantilever lengths seen clinically were often lower than those deemed optimal by clinicians for restoration of structure, function, and esthetics.[69]

The Rationale for Cantilever Length   McAlarney and Stavropoulos investigated possible relationships between calculated clinical cantilever length variables that included number and distribution of implants, arch placement, and clinically optimal cantilevers. For a set number of implants, the relationship between calculated cantilever length and A/P spread was linear.[70] The sum of the lengths on both sides versus prosthesis length between the most distal implants was linear, regardless of the number of implants. Predicted clinical success was defined as calculated length greater than the clinicians' optimal length. Satisfaction rates were 100%, 56%, 33%, 8%, and 0% for cases supported by 8 and 7, 6, 5, 4, and 3 implants (44% overall), respectively. Ninety-eight percent of cases with A/P spreads greater than 11.1 mm were satisfactory. McAlarney and Stavropoulos concluded that in 98% of all clinical cases studied with an A/P spread greater than 11.1 mm, the maximum cantilever length calculated through the mathematical model was greater than the cantilever length desired by the clinicians restoring the cases; the calculated maximum permissible cantilever lengths as calculated varied linearly with the A/P spread.

McAlarney and Stavropoulos also investigated the ratio that existed between cantilever length (CL) and the A/P spread, as this ratio is often used as an indication of CL in implant-supported prostheses.[69] They reported that although there was a trend of increasing CL with increasing AP spread, indiscriminate use of a single CL:AP ratio as an indication for cantilevers may not be prudent, because CL is also a function of the number of implants and the distribution of implants between the most anterior and posterior implants. Also, previously reported CL:AP ratios may be too high for different clinical situations. They reported that a CL:AP spread ratio of 2 was too great for all the cases studied, and that a ratio of 1.5 was too great for all cases except for six implant cases. It was interesting to note that the ratios varied by a factor greater than 3.

A/P Spread and the "All-on-Four" Protocol Implant treatment in edentulous maxillae may be quite challenging and more difficult compared to mandibular implant treatment as atrophic, edentulous maxillae generally consist of less-dense bone; several anatomic areas also preclude implant placement (nasal cavity, maxillary sinus).[72,73] Malo et al introduced a concept they termed "All on Four." This protocol called for placement of four maxillary implants: two vertical and two distally tilted implants, placed parallel to the anterior walls of the maxillary sinus (Fig 17.14).[74] One of the tenets of this treatment concept was that patients who were edentulous for many years usually warranted bone grafting in the maxillary sinus to compensate for minimal alveolar bone volumes posteriorly. For these patients to be treated with dental implants, sinus grafting would be warranted, and introduced additional surgical procedures, morbidity, and costs. Malo et al proposed reconstructing edentulous maxillary patients with a total of four implants: two anterior implants vertically placed and two posterior tilted implants where the tilted implants were placed anterior and parallel to the anterior sinus walls. The posterior implants required angled abutments for the prosthetic procedures (Fig 17.15). This specific implant arrangement provided for consistently large A/P spreads.

A recent (2010) publication detailing the "All-on-4" protocol reported the CSR for maxillary implants was 98.36%; mandibular implants was 99.73%.[75] Patients were

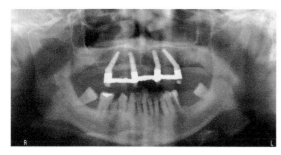

FIGURE 17.14 Panoramic radiograph of a patient treated with the "All-on-4" protocol. The two distal implants were placed parallel to the anterior wall of the maxillary sinus.

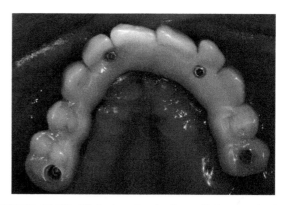

FIGURE 17.15 Clinical occlusal view of the prosthesis in Figure 17.14. The tilts of the distal implants were corrected with angled abutments. The A/P spread was significantly increased if compared to the A/P spread of four vertically placed implants.

followed for 4 to 59 months. Sixty-one maxillary prostheses and 93 mandibular prostheses were placed and followed; at the time the study results were published, the prosthetic CSR was 86%. The authors reported no differences in marginal bone loss between axial and tilted implants.

Guidelines for Implant-Retained Hybrid Frameworks

1. *Frameworks must be fabricated from materials and protocols that allow passive and accurate fit between frameworks and implants and/or abutments.* CAD/CAM fabricated frameworks generally provide better, more accurate fit than do cast frameworks.[57–60] Milled frameworks from solid blanks of Ti or Ti alloys are homogeneous; defects within CAD/CAM frameworks are minimal when compared to defects noted within cast frameworks.[57,58]

2. *Frameworks must be designed to resist tensile and compressive forces associated with mastication and parafunctional habits.* Frameworks need to be of adequate thickness buccally/lingually, and vertically. Thickness will depend on the type of metal and fabrication process used for each specific framework, the number and length of implants, the type of supporting bone, and the opposing occlusion. Carr and Stewart recommended cast bars be approximately 7 mm tall and 6 mm wide; one-piece castings were imprecise and inaccurate when evaluated for passive fit.[76] CAD/CAM milled frameworks may have slightly smaller dimensions. One manufacturer (Biomet 3i, Palm Beach Gardens, FL) only specifies that the minimum vertical height for milled bars is 2.5 mm. Two other manufacturers' websites (Nobel Biocare; Cagenix) did not contain any information relative to thickness for their bars. I-beam designs may be the best designs for implant-retained hybrid prostheses.[61,63,64]

3. *Framework design has evolved into a series of clinical and laboratory procedures that incorporate principles of fixed and removable prosthodontics; prostheses are more successful if frameworks are designed consistent with predetermined tooth positions.* Frameworks must be designed with adequate space (1.5 to 2 mm) for prosthetic materials: acrylic resin/composite resin/reinforced polymeric materials.[77] Retentive elements for denture base materials should be designed as integral parts of implant frameworks. Adequate thickness is necessary to minimize the potential for denture base fracture. Acrylic resin retention may be accomplished with nailhead retentive elements, retentive loops, or undercut areas randomly placed throughout frameworks. Retentive elements should be placed such that they will not interfere with tooth placement. Junctions of acrylic resin and metal finish lines should have retentive undercuts.[77] Resins are mechanically attached to metal frameworks; well-developed and distinct finish lines minimize stain and seepage of intraoral fluids into and around the resin/metal junction. Malodors may be caused by deposits at the resin/metal interface; separation between resin and metal may eventually lead to deterioration of denture bases.

There has been considerable research relative to acrylic resin retention in removable partial prosthodontics. In a laboratory study (80 chrome/cobalt frameworks), Lee et al concluded that significantly increased force was required to separate "primed" acrylic resin from RPD metal frameworks when compared to unprimed specimens.[78] Forces required to dislodge acrylic resin from RPD frameworks decreased in the following order: primed metal with beads (highest) > primed mesh > primed lattice > smooth metal plate (lowest). Primed latticework acrylic resin retention was significantly less retentive than the other three primed designs. In a similar study, Bulbul and Kesim reported that shear bond strengths (SBS) varied according to metal type, metal primer, and acrylic resin.[79] The SBS was highest between base metal and heat-polymerized resin with metal primer. SBS between noble metal and acrylic resin, for all control groups, was the lowest $(0.4 \pm 0.07\,\text{MPa})$ $(p < 0.001)$. For Ti, the highest SBS was observed for Meta Fast primed specimens; the lowest for the control group. For base metal, the highest SBS was for Metal Primer; the lowest for the control group. For the noble metal group, the highest SBS was for Alloy Primer; the lowest for the control group $(p < 0.001)$. Bulbul and Kesim concluded that metal primers were associated with increased adhesive bonding between acrylic resins and the metal alloys tested. Bonding values were higher for resin to base metal alloy RPDs when compared to noble and Ti alloys.

Clinicians must determine the appropriate location of the artificial teeth prior to designing frameworks. In edentulous patients, waxed denture prostheses must be constructed so that they may be imaged/scanned prior to proceeding with framework design. Matrices or facial cores are not needed for scanning CAD/CAM frameworks; however, they are helpful for technicians setting artificial teeth onto the frameworks prior to the framework/wax try-in.

4. *Cantilever extensions are dependent on: type of metal used in the frameworks, number and location of implants.* Base metal alloys flex less than noble alloy frameworks. Frameworks supported by three implants, with an A/P spread equivalent in millimeters to frameworks supported by six implants with the same A/P spread, should be designed with smaller cantilevers when compared to the six-implant-supported framework. Cantilever extensions may extend up to 1.5 of the A/P spread. Cantilevers may also be shortened depending on the above factors.

CONCLUSIONS

This article presented a review of current and past literature regarding implant-retained frameworks for full-arch, hybrid restorations. Benefits, limitations, and complications associated with fixed implant prostheses were discussed including the relative inaccuracy of casting/implant fit and improved accuracies noted with CAD/CAM framework/implant fit; cantilever extensions that were initially designed arbitrarily versus frameworks designed relative to the A/P implant spread; and the mechanical properties associated with implant frameworks including I- and L-beam designs. Guidelines were proposed for use by clinicians and laboratory technicians in designing implant-retained frameworks. Further clinical and laboratory research continues to be warranted to test the efficacy of the proposed guidelines.

REFERENCES

1. Marachlioglou CR, Dos Santos JF, Cunha VP, et al: Expectations and final evaluation of complete dentures by patients, dentist and dental technician. *J Oral Rehabil* 2010;3:518–524.
2. Gjengedal H, Berg E, Boe OE, et al: Self-reported oral health and denture satisfaction in partially and completely edentulous patients. *Int J Prosthodont* 2011;24:9–15.
3. Lin YC, Chen JH, Lee HE, et al: The association of chewing ability and diet in elderly complete denture patients. *Int J Prosthodont* 2010;23:127–128.
4. Jemt T: Single implants in the anterior maxilla after 15 years of follow-up: comparison with central implants in the edentulous maxilla. *Int J Prosthodont* 2008;21:400–408.

5. Zarb G, Schmitt A: Edentulous predicament. 1. A prospective study of the effectiveness of implant supported fixed prostheses. *J Am Dent Assoc* 1996;127:59–72.

6. Zarb G, Jansson T: Prosthodontic procedures. In Branemark PI, Zarb G, Albrektsson T (eds): *Tissue Integrated Prostheses: Osseointegration in Clinical Dentistry.* Chicago, Quintessence, 1985, pp. 250–251.

7. Carr AB, McGivney GP, Brown DT (eds): Denture base considerations. In *McCracken's Removable Partial Prosthodontics* (ed 11). St. Louis, Elsevier Mosby, 2005, p. 131.

8. Zarb GA, Schmitt A: The longitudinal clinical effectiveness of osseointegrated dental implants: the Toronto study. Part III: problems and complications encountered. *J Prosthet Dent* 1990;64:185–194.

9. Graser C, Myers M, Iranpour B: Resolving esthetic and phonetic problems associated with maxillary implant-supported prostheses. A clinical report. *J Prosthet Dent* 1989;62:376–378.

10. Henry P: Future therapeutic directions for management of the edentulous predicament. *J Prosthet Dent* 1998;79:100–106.

11. Marcus PA, Joshi J, Jones JA, et al: Complete edentulism and denture use for elders in New England. *J Prosthet Dent* 1996;76:260–266.

12. Jemt T, Book K, Lindén B, et al: Failures and complications in 92 consecutively inserted overdentures supported by Brånemark implants in severely resorbed edentulous maxillae: a study from prosthetic treatment to first annual check-up. *Int J Oral Maxillofac Implants* 1992;7:162–167.

13. Naert I, Quirynen M, van Steenberghe D, et al: A study of 589 consecutive implants supporting complete fixed prostheses. Part II: prosthetic aspects. *J Prosthet Dent* 1992;68:949–956.

14. Heydecke G, McFarland DH, Feine JS, et al: Speech with maxillary implant prostheses: ratings of articulation. *J Dent Res* 2004;83:236–240.

15. Springer NC, Chang C, Fields HW, et al: Smile esthetics from the layperson's perspective. *Am J Orthod Dentofacial Orthop* 2011;139:e91–e101.

16. Tallgren A: The continuing reduction of the residual alveolar ridges in complete denture wearers: a mixed-longitudinal study covering 25 years. 1972. *J Prosthet Dent* 2003;89:427–435.

17. Atwood D, Coy W: Clinical, cephalometric, and densitometric study of reduction of residual ridges. *J Prosthet Dent* 1971;26: 280–295.

18. Hulterstrom M, Nilsson U: Cobalt-chromium as a framework material in implant-supported fixed prostheses: a preliminary report. *Int J Oral Maxillofac Implants* 1991;6:475–480.

19. Goll GE: Production of accurately fitting full-arch implant frameworks. Part I: clinical procedures. *J Prosthet Dent* 1991;66:377–384.

20. Bergendal B, Palmqvist S: Laser welded titanium frameworks for fixed prostheses supported by osseointegrated implants: a 2-year multicenter study report. *Int J Oral Maxillofac Implants* 1995;10:199–206.

21. Glantz PO: Aspects of prosthodontic design. In Branemark PI, Zarb G, Albrektsson T (eds): *Tissue Integrated Prostheses:*

Osseointegration in Clinical Dentistry. Chicago, Quintessence, 1985, pp. 329–330.

22. Jemt T: Three-dimensional distortion of gold alloy castings and welded titanium frameworks. Measurements of the precision of fit between completed implant prostheses and the master casts in routine edentulous situations. *J Oral Rehabil* 1995;22: 557–564.

23. Moon PC, Eshleman JR, Douglas HB, et al: Comparison of accuracy of soldering indices for fixed prostheses. *J Prosthet Dent* 1978;40:35–38.

24. Sutherland JK, Hallam RF: Soldering technique for osseointegrated implant prostheses. *J Prosthet Dent* 1990;63:242–244.

25. Zarb GA, Jansson T: Laboratory procedures and protocol. In Branemark PI, Zarb G, Albrektsson T (eds): *Tissue Integrated Prostheses: Osseointegration in Clinical Dentistry.* Chicago, Quintessence, 1985, p. 303.

26. Hjalmarsson L, Ortorp A, Smedberg JI, et al: Precision of fit to implants: a comparison of Cresco™ and Procera® implant bridge frameworks. *Clin Implant Dent Relat Res* 2010;12: 271–280.

27. Zarb GA, Jansson T. Prosthodontic procedures. In Branemark PI, Zarb G, Albrektsson T (eds): *Tissue Integrated Prostheses: Osseointegration in Clinical Dentistry.* Chicago, Quintessence, 1985, p. 262.

28. Zervas PJ, Papazoglou E, Beck FM, et al: Distortion of three-unit implant frameworks during casting, soldering, and simulated porcelain firings. *J Prosthodont* 1999;8:171–179.

29. Rubenstein JE, Lowry MB: A comparison of two solder registration materials: a three-dimensional analysis. *J Prosthet Dent* 2006;95:379–391.

30. Uysal H, Kurtoglu C, Gurbuz R, et al: Structure and mechanical properties of Cresco-Ti laser-welded joints and stress analyses using finite element models of fixed distal extension and fixed partial prosthetic designs. *J Prosthet Dent* 2005;93:235–244.

31. Silva TB, De Arruda Nobilo MA, Pessanha Henriques GE, et al: Influence of laser-welding and electroerosion on passive fit of implant-supported prosthesis. *Stomatologija* 2008;10: 96–100.

32. Eliasson A, Wennerberg A, Johansson A, et al: The precision of fit of milled titanium implant frameworks (I-Bridge) in the edentulous jaw. *Clin Implant Dent Relat Res* 2010;12: 81–90.

33. Al-Fadda SA, Zarb GA, Finer Y: A comparison of the accuracy of fit of 2 methods for fabricating implant-prosthodontic frameworks. *Int J Prosthodont* 2007;20:125–131.

34. Drago C, Saldarriaga RL, Domagala D, et al: Volumetric determination of the amount of misfit in CAD/CAM and cast implant frameworks: a multicenter laboratory study. *Int J Oral Maxillofac Implants* 2010;25:920–929.

35. Takahashi T, Gunne J: Fit of implant frameworks: an in vitro comparison between two fabrication techniques. *J Prosthet Dent* 2003;89:256–260.

36. Hermann JS, Schoolfield JD, Schenk RK, et al: Influence of the size of the microgap on crestal bone changes around titanium implants. A histometric evaluation of unloaded non-submerged

implants in the canine mandible. *J Periodontol* 2001;72: 1372–1383.

37. King GN, Hermann JS, Schoolfield JD, et al: Influence of the size of the microgap on crestal bone levels in non-submerged dental implants: a radiographic study in the canine mandible. *J Periodontol* 2002;73:1111–1117.

38. Sahin S, Cehreli MC: The significance of passive framework fit in implant prosthodontics: current status. *Implant Dent* 2001;10:85–92.

39. Binon PP: The effect of implant/abutment hexagonal misfit on screw joint stability. *Int J Prosthodont* 1996;9:149–160.

40. McGlumphy EA, Mendel DA, Holloway JA: Implant screw mechanics. *Dent Clin North Am* 1998;42:71–89.

41. Taylor TD, Agar, JR: Twenty years of progress in implant prosthodontics. *J Prosthet Dent* 2002;88:89–95.

42. Taylor TD, Agar JR, Vogiatzi T: Implant prosthodontics: current perspective and future directions. *Int J Oral Maxillofac Implants* 2000;15:66–75.

43. Hjalmarsson L, Smedberg JI, Pettersson M, et al: Implant level prostheses in the edentulous maxillae: a comparison with conventional abutment level prostheses after 5 years of use. *Int J Prosthodont* 2011;24:158–167.

44. Ortorp A, Jemt T: CNC milled titanium frameworks supported by implants in the edentulous jaw: a 10 year comparative clinical study. *Clin Implant Dent Relat Res* 2009 Aug 17; epub ahead of print.

45. O'Brien WJ: *Dental Materials and Their Selection* (ed 4). Chicago, Quintessence, 2008, pp. 196–197.

46. Moffa JP: Biological effects of nickel-containing dental alloys. Council on Dental Materials, Instruments, and Equipment. *J Am Dent Assoc* 1982;104:501–505.

47. Pieralini AR, Benjamin CM, Ribeiro RF, et al: The effect of coating patterns with spinel-based investment on the castability and porosity of titanium cast into three phosphate-bonded investments. *J Prosthodont* 2010;19:517–522.

48. White S, Mildus V, McLaren E: Flexural strength of a layered zirconia and porcelain dental all-ceramic system. *J Prosthet Dent* 2005;94:125–131.

49. Keough B, Kay H, Sager R: A ten-unit all ceramic anterior fixed partial denture using YTZP zirconia. *Pract Proced Aesthet Dent* 2006;16:37–43.

50. Larsson C, Vult von Steyern P: Five-year follow-up of implant-supported Y-TZP and ZTA fixed dental prostheses. A randomized, prospective clinical trial comparing two different material systems. *Int J Prosthodont* 2010;23:555–561.

51. Guess P, Alt W, Strub J: Zirconia in fixed implant prosthodontics. *Clin Implant Dent Relat Res* 2010 Dec 22; epub ahead of print.

52. Guichet D, Caputo A, Choi H, et al: Passivity of fit and marginal opening in screw- or cement-retained implant fixed partial denture designs. *Int J Oral Maxillofac Implants* 2000;15: 239–246.

53. Sorensen J, Avera S, Tomas C: Comparison of interface fidelity of implant systems [abstract 2191]. *J Dent Res* 1991;70:540.

54. Keith S, Miller B, Woody R, et al: Marginal discrepancy of screw-retained and cemented metal-ceramic crowns on implant abutments. *Int J Oral Maxillofac Implants* 1999;14: 369–378.

55. Gunne J, Jemt T, Linden B: Implant treatment in partially edentulous patients: a report on prostheses after 3 years. *Int J Prosthodont* 1994;7:143–148.

56. Wichmann M, Tschernitschek H: Quality assurance by X-ray structure analysis. *Dtsch Zahnarztl Z* 1993;48:682–688.

57. Jemt T, Back T, Petersson A: Precision of CNC-milled titanium frameworks for implant treatment in the edentulous jaw. *Int J Prosthodont* 1999;12:209–215.

58. Ortorp A, Jemt T, Back T, et al: Comparisons of precision of fit between cast and CNC-milled titanium implant frameworks for the edentulous mandible. *Int J Prosthodont* 2003;16:194–200.

59. Al-Fadda SA, Zarb GA, Finer Y: A comparison of the accuracy of fit of 2 methods for fabricating implant-prosthodontic frameworks. *Int J Prosthodont* 2007;20:125–131.

60. Drago C, Saldarriaga R, Domagala D, et al: Volumetric determination of the degree of misfit in CAD/CAM and cast implant frameworks: a multicenter laboratory study. *Int J Maxillofac Implants* 2010;25:920–929.

61. Cox J, Zarb G: Alternative prosthodontic superstructure designs. *Swed Dent J Suppl* 1985;28:71–75.

62. Taylor TD: Prosthodontic complications associated with implant therapy. *Oral Maxillofac Surg Clin North Am* 1991;3:979–992.

63. Rasmussen EJ: Alternative prosthodontic technique for tissue integrated prostheses. *J Prosthet Dent* 1987;57:198–204.

64. Staab GH, Stewart RB: Theoretical assessment of cross sections for cantilevered implant supported prostheses. *J Prosthodont* 1994;3:23–30.

65. von Gonten AS, Teojilo M, Woohy G: Modifications in the design and fabrication of mandibular osseointegrated fixed prostheses frameworks. *J Prosthodont* 1995;4:82–89.

66. Sadowsky SJ: The implant-supported prosthesis for the edentulous arch: design considerations. *J Prosthet Dent* 1997;78: 28–33.

67. English C: Critical A-P spread. *Implant Soc* 1990;1:2–3.

68. McAlarney ME, Stavropoulos DN: Determination of cantilever length anterior-posterior spread assuming failure criteria to be the compromise of the prosthesis retaining screw-prosthesis joint. *Int J Oral Maxillofac Implants* 1996;11:331–319.

69. McAlarney ME, Stavropoulos DN: Theoretical cantilever lengths versus clinical variables in fifty-five clinical cases. *J Prosthet Dent* 2000;83:332–343.

70. Beumer J, Hamada M, Lewis S: A prosthodontics overview. *Int J Prosthodont* 1993;6:126–130.

71. Takayama T: Biomechanical considerations on osseointegrated implants. In Hobo S, Ichida E, Garcia L (eds): *Osseointegration and Occlusal Rehabilitation*. Chicago, Quintessence, 1989, pp. 265–280.

72. Tallgren A: The continuing reduction of the residual alveolar ridges in complete denture wearers: a mixed-longitudinal study covering 25 years. *J Prosthet Dent* 1972;27:120–132.

73. Atwood D, Coy W: Clinical, cephalometric, and densitometric study of reduction of residual ridges. *J Prosthet Dent* 1971;26: 280–295.

74. Malo P, Rangert B, Nobre M: All on 4 immediate-function concept with Branemark System implants for completely edentulous maxillae: a 1-year retrospective clinical study. *Clin Implant Dent Relat Res* 2005;7(Suppl 1):S88–S94.

75. Agliardi E, Panigatti S, Cleric M, et al: Immediate rehabilitation of the edentulous jaws with full fixed prostheses supported by four implants: interim results of a single cohort prospective study. *Clin Oral Implants Res* 2010;21: 459–465.

76. Carr AB, Stewart RB: Full-arch implant framework casting accuracy: preliminary in vitro observation for in vivo testing. *J Prosthodont* 1993;2:2–8.

77. Carr AB, Brown DT: Denture base considerations. In Carr AB, Brown DT (eds): *McCracken's Removable Partial Prosthodontics* (ed 12). St. Louis, Elsevier Mosby, 2011, p. 106.

78. Lee G, Engelmeier R, Gonzalez M, et al: Force needed to separate acrylic resin from primed and unprimed frameworks of different designs. *J Prosthodont* 2010;19:14–19.

79. Bulbul M, Kesim B: The effect of primers on shear bond strength of acrylic resins to different types of metals. *J Prosthet Dent* 2010;103:303–308.

18

COMPLICATIONS AND PATIENT-CENTERED OUTCOMES WITH AN IMPLANT-SUPPORTED MONOLITHIC ZIRCONIA FIXED DENTAL PROSTHESIS: 1 YEAR RESULTS

BRYAN LIMMER, DMD, MS,[1] ANNE E. SANDERS, MS, PHD,[2] GLENN RESIDE, DMD, MS,[3] AND LYNDON F. COOPER, DDS, PHD, FACP[1]

[1]Department of Prosthodontics, University of North Carolina School of Dentistry, Chapel Hill, NC
[2]Department of Dental Ecology, University of North Carolina School of Dentistry, Chapel Hill, NC
[3]Department of Oral and Maxillofacial Surgery, University of North Carolina School of Dentistry, Chapel Hill, NC

The article is associated with the American College of Prosthodontists' journal-based continuing education program. It is accompanied by an online continuing education activity worth 1 credit. Please visit www.wileyhealthlearning.com/jopr to complete the activity and earn credit.

Keywords
Dental implant; edentulism; mandible; zirconia; dental prosthesis; OHIP-49.

Correspondence
Bryan Limmer DMD, MS, 5161 E. Arapahoe Rd., Ste #255 Centennial, CO 80122. E-mail: drbryanlimmer@gmail.com

Research support from an American College of Prosthodontists Education Foundation (ACPEF) grant.

The authors deny any conflicts of interest.

Accepted July 10, 2013

Published in *Journal of Prosthodontics* June 2014; Vol. 23, Issue 4

doi: 10.1111/jopr.12110

ABSTRACT

Purpose: To characterize the number and type of complications that occur with a monolithic zirconia fixed dental prosthesis (MZ-FDP) supported by four endosseous implants in the edentulous mandible over time and to quantify the impact of treatment on oral health quality of life (OHQoL).

Methods: Seventeen edentulous participants were enrolled. New conventional dentures were fabricated for each participant. Four Astra Tech Osseospeed TX implants (Dentsply) were then placed in the parasymphyseal mandible, and after a period of healing, a full-arch monolithic zirconia prosthesis (Zirkonzahn) was inserted. Complication data were recorded and OHQoL was evaluated using the Oral Health Impact Profile (OHIP-49), administered on four occasions: enrollment; implant surgery; and 6- and 12-month recalls.

Results: Sixty-eight implants were placed in 17 edentulous individuals aged 30 to 78 (mean 57.9 years). Implant survival was 94% from the subject perspective and 99% from

---

the implant perspective. Prosthesis survival was 88%. Twelve complications occurred in ten participants, whereas seven participants remained complication free. Both OHIP-49 severity and extent scores decreased significantly between enrollment and 12-month recall ($p < 0.001$). The mean OHIP-49 severity score at baseline was 94.8 (95% confidence interval [CI]: 73.9, 115.8) and declined an average of 76.8 (95% CI: −91.3, −62.3) units per participant. The mean OHIP-49 extent score at baseline was 17.2 (95% CI: 10.8, 23.6) and declined 16.3 (95% CI: −20.2, −12.4) units per participant on average.

Conclusions: Implant survival was high, and few complications related to the MZ-FDP were observed. The most common prosthetic complication was tooth chipping in the opposing maxillary denture, which accounted for 50% of all complication events. Substantial and clinically important improvements in OHQoL were achieved with both conventional dentures and the implant-supported MZ-FDP. The data of this short-term study indicate that the implant-supported MZ-FDP is a therapeutic option with particular advantages in the edentulous mandible that warrants further long-term study.

The prevalence of edentulism in the United States is declining. Yet continued population growth, current dental practice trends, and an increased proportion of older individuals within the population generate a continued need for edentulous therapy.[1] Edentulism results in reduced oral and social function.[2,3] It is associated with poorer health status across a wide range of measures, including physical health, nutrition, disability, and self-esteem.[2] Conventional dentures address the problems associated with edentulism, but do so incompletely and introduce their own set of related problems.[3] The rapid rate of bone resorption observed in the edentulous mandible is of particular concern due to the accompanying instability of a mandibular denture, often the most troublesome complaint of denture patients.[4,5]

Dental implant therapy offers advantages over conventional denture therapy in the treatment of mandibular edentulism by providing significant improvements in prosthesis function and comfort, as well as by aiding alveolar bone preservation.[6–10] The current literature shows a high level of biologic success when using four to six implants with a fixed prosthesis in the edentulous parasymphyseal mandible.[11–17] However, the degree of prosthetic success and the magnitude of improvement in patient-centered outcomes for the wide variety of possible prosthesis designs are either debated or unknown.[18–22]

The most commonly used and most commonly studied implant-supported fixed dental prosthesis (FDP) is the metal-acrylic hybrid prosthesis, which comes with a particular set of technical problems.[21,22] Common complications for the metal-acrylic hybrid include fracture of the acrylic veneer, wear or debonding of the resin denture teeth, and screw/abutment loosening or fracture.[21,22] Different prosthesis designs and materials may have entirely different prosthetic outcomes, but little data are available. Zirconia-based materials have generated considerable interest for dental applications and have the potential to address some of the problems previously encountered in the metal-acrylic hybrid.[23] In addition to favorable physical and biologic properties, zirconia can be manipulated using computer aided design/computer aided manufacturing (CAD/CAM) technology.[23] The ability to precisely design a full-arch prosthesis in the virtual world, to store those design files indefinitely, and to predictably fabricate such a device in a highly automated fashion may fundamentally change access to care for the edentulous population. Zirconia is currently used in endodontic dowels, dental implants, dental implant abutments, single crowns, and multiunit FDPs with varying degrees of success.[24] The use of zirconia, specifically monolithic zirconia, has not been rigorously investigated in the fabrication of a full-arch fixed prosthesis. Aside from clinical reports, few longitudinal clinical studies on full-arch zirconia (layered or monolithic) exist.[25,26]

In addition to biologic and prosthetic outcomes, patient-centered outcomes are becoming more important in evaluating the overall success of a prosthetic therapy.[18,20,29,36] Oral health quality of life (OHQoL) is the most used measure of patient perception, and is considered a more complete valuation of oral disease and its treatment than general measures of "satisfaction."[27] Further, the Oral Health Impact Profile (OHIP) has emerged as one of the most powerful and widely accepted tools for the assessment of OHQoL.[20] The 49-item OHIP (OHIP-49)[28] was developed on the basis of the 1980 World Health Organization's International Classification of Impairments, Disabilities, and Handicaps (ICIDH). In accordance with the ICIDH, the OHIP-49 comprises seven subscales to evaluate impairment (functional limitation, physical pain, psychological discomfort), disability (physical, psychological, and social disability), and handicap resulting from dental conditions. Assessment of OHQoL in conjunction with biologic and prosthetic outcomes provides additional insights regarding the impact that possible complications have on the perception of dental therapy.

The purpose of this study was to investigate the biologic and technical complications of a full-arch monolithic zirconia

FDP (MZ-FDP) supported by four implants in the edentulous mandible over a period of 1 year and to quantify the change in OHQoL.

MATERIALS AND METHODS

This was an Institutional Review Board (IRB)-approved, prospective clinical study using a single-arm design. A consecutive sample of 17 participants was screened and enrolled according to the inclusion and exclusion criteria.

Inclusion and Exclusion Criteria

Patients aged 18 to 80 at time of enrollment, American Society of Anesthesiologists (ASA) Class I or II, and who were completely edentulous in both the maxilla and mandible or those possessing a terminal dentition requiring extraction were eligible for inclusion. Patients were excluded if they met any of the following criteria: history of radiotherapy in the head and neck region, uncontrolled diabetes, known alcohol and/or drug abuse, taking medication that might significantly interfere with coagulation and/or patients with bleeding disorders, smoking greater than ten cigarettes per day, vertical bone height less than 10 mm, unrealistic esthetic expectations, and/or psychological problems that prevent acceptance of a removable prosthesis. Pregnant women and ASA Class III or IV patients were also excluded.

Assessment and Conventional Denture Fabrication

A panoramic radiograph and diagnostic casts were used for initial diagnosis and planning. New conventional dentures were fabricated to establish functional and esthetic parameters. A traditional approach that included custom trays, a semi-adjustable articulator, a facebow transfer, and bilaterally balanced occlusion with shallow anterior guidance was employed. Phonares I denture teeth (Ivoclar Vivadent, Schaan, Liechtenstein) were used in the denture tooth setup, and a clinical remount was performed at the time of denture insertion. A radiographic guide was created by duplicating the mandibular denture in radiopaque acrylic. A cone beam computed tomography scan was acquired with the Galileos imaging system (Sirona Dental Company, Long Island City, NY), and the data used for evaluation of implant sites.

Surgical Procedures

Four Astra Tech Osseospeed TX implants (Dentsply, Molndal, Sweden) were surgically placed in the parasymphyseal mandible using a clear acrylic duplicate of the mandibular denture as a surgical guide.[32] The implants were tilted such that screw access holes exited anteriorly through the mandibular lateral incisors and posteriorly through the second

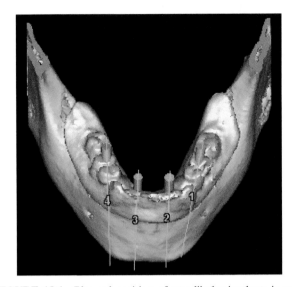

FIGURE 18.1 Planned position of mandibular implants in relation to mandibular prosthesis.

premolars (Fig 18.1). A resonance frequency analysis device (Osstell, Gothenburg, Sweden) was used to assess primary stability for immediate loading. Twenty degree UniAbutments were inserted, and an overdenture or a fixed interim prosthesis was provided following surgery. A postoperative panoramic radiograph was taken, and the participant was seen for follow-up.

Zirconia Prosthesis Fabrication

An abutment level impression was made, and a master cast produced (Fig 18.2). Maxillomandibular relationships were obtained, and the master cast was mounted against a cast of the upper denture. A polymethylmethacrylate mock-up of the future prosthesis was then fabricated and evaluated intraorally to confirm fit, esthetics, phonetics, and occlusion (Fig 18.3). The mock-up was then scanned, milled out of monolithic zirconia, stained, and sintered by a dental

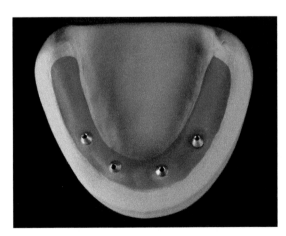

FIGURE 18.2 Master cast.

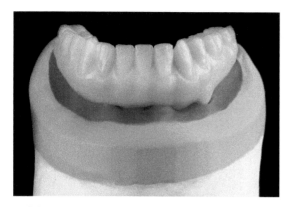

FIGURE 18.3   Mock-up of mandibular prosthesis.

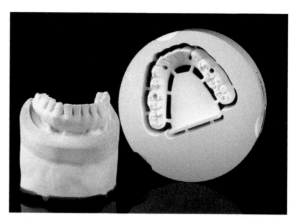

FIGURE 18.5   Milled green-state zirconia prosthesis.

laboratory (Zirkonzahn, Gais, Italy) (Figs 18.4–18.7). The definitive mandibular prosthesis was inserted approximately 16 weeks post-implant surgery. Participants were seen 6 and 12 months after prosthesis insertion for radiographic and clinical evaluation. They were educated on potential post-insertion complications of a biologic or technical nature and instructed to contact the clinic if any arose during the treatment or recall periods.

Biologic and Prosthetic Outcomes

Implant survival was defined as the implant being present and functional at the time of assessment. Prosthesis survival was defined as the prosthesis being present and functional at the

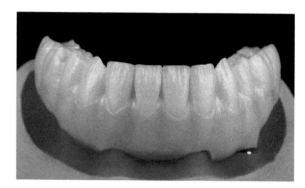

FIGURE 18.6   Stained, presintered zirconia prosthesis.

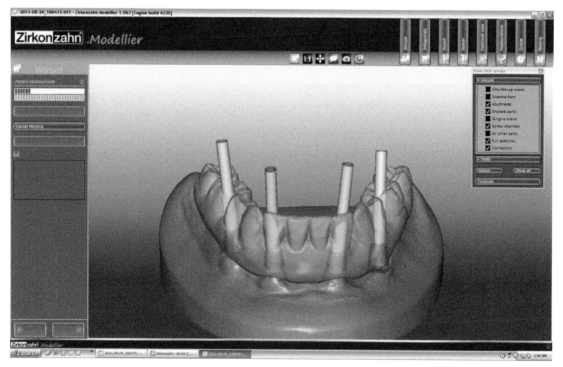

FIGURE 18.4   Scan and digital design of mandibular prosthesis.

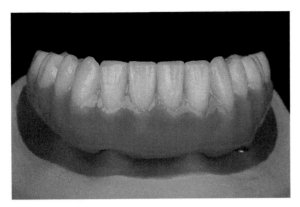

FIGURE 18.7 Sintered and polished definitive zirconia prosthesis.

time of assessment. Complications were broadly defined as any event that required additional treatment. The exact nature, frequency, and timing of each complication were recorded. Complications were classified as either biologic or technical.

OHIP

The OHIP-49 questionnaire was first administered at the time of enrollment to obtain baseline values. It was next administered immediately prior to implant surgery to assess the effect of conventional denture therapy, and at 6- and 12-month recall appointments to assess the effect of MZ-FDP therapy. Responses to each of the 49 OHIP items are made on a five-point ordinal scale.

Analytic Methods

Two OHIP-49 summary scores were computed as dependent variables. The *severity* score is the cumulative sum of ordinal responses across all items with a possible range of 0 to 196. For both scores, higher values denote worse OHQoL. The *extent* score is a count of the number of items a participant reports having experienced "very often" or "fairly often." In addition to these two summary scores, the seven OHIP-49 subscales were individually examined to identify factors associated with change in OHIP-49 scores. To account for multiple tests, Bonferroni correction reduced the critical significance threshold to $p < 0.0035$ ($p = 0.05/14$). These baseline associations were tested for statistical significance using one-way ANOVA. To correctly account for the hierarchical structure of the data set, serial measurements on the same individual at multiple time points, the statistical approach estimated covariance parameters using two-level fixed slope, random intercept variance components models. These were fitted using the *xtmixed* command in STATA version 12.0 SE statistical software (Stata Corporation, College Station, TX). The OHIP extent and severity scores were

the dependent variables, and time of OHIP-49 administration was the exposure of interest. Beta coefficients from the model are directly interpretable as within-subject change in mean OHIP-49 extent and severity scores.

RESULTS

Results are presented for 17 participants, 11 men and 6 women, who ranged in age from 30 to 78 years (mean 57.9 years) at enrollment. Eight were edentulous, and nine had a terminal dentition prior to enrollment.

Biologic and Prosthetic Outcomes

Sixty-eight implants were placed in 17 participants. One implant failed to integrate, resulting in patient-related and implant-related survival rates of 94% (16/17) and 99% (67/68), respectively. During the MZ-FDP observation period, 12 complications occurred in ten participants. In addition to the one implant failure, six participants chipped maxillary denture teeth, two broke one or more abutments, one had a loose abutment, one had a component of the MZ-FDP debond, and one fractured the distal extension of the MZ-FDP (Tables 18.1 and 18.2). Prosthesis survival was 88% (15/17); one prosthesis was lost due to fracture, and one was removed after implant failure. Over the MZ-FDP observation period, 41% (7/17) of the participants were complication-free.

TABLE 18.1 Complications by Participant During MZ-FDP Observation Period

Participant Number	Complication (Number of Occurrences)
1	Chipped denture tooth (1)
2	Chipped denture tooth (1)
	Fractured abutment (1)
3	Loose abutment (1)
4	
5	Fractured abutment (1)
6	Fractured MZ-FDP (1)
	Debonded component (1)
7	
8	Implant failure (1)
9	
10	Chipped denture tooth (1)
11	Chipped denture tooth (1)
12	
13	
14	Chipped denture tooth (1)
15	
16	Chipped denture tooth (1)
17	

TABLE 18.2 Complications by Type and Timing

	Post MZ-FDP Insertion (Number of Occurrences)
Biologic	Implant failure (1)
Technical	Chipped denture tooth (6)
	Fractured abutment (2)
	Loose abutment (1)
	Debonded component (1)
	Fractured MZ-FDP (1)

OHIP Scores

The mean OHIP-49 severity score at enrollment was 94.8 (95% confidence interval [CI]: 73.9, 115.8), and the lowest and highest severity scores were 45 and 168, respectively. Lowest and highest extent scores were 4 and 43, respectively, and the mean extent score was 17.2 (95% CI: 10.8, 23.6).

Differences in mean OHIP-49 severity and extent scores at baseline were not statistically significant on the basis of participant characteristics (Table 18.3). Over the entire observation period, mean OHIP-49 severity scores decreased significantly by an average of 76.8 (95% CI: −91.3, −62.3) units per participant from an enrollment high of 94.8 to 18.0 at 12 months after prosthesis insertion (Table 18.4, Fig 18.8A). A significant reduction in mean OHIP-49 severity score was observed at implant surgery, and a further significant reduction was noted at 6 months after prosthesis insertion; however, the small reduction seen at the 12-month recall was not statistically significant (Table 18.4, Fig 18.8A). Mean OHIP-49 extent scores decreased significantly by an average of 16.3 (95% CI: −20.2, −12.4) units per participant from enrollment to 12-month recall (Table 18.5, Fig 18.8B). The mean OHIP-49 extent score decreased significantly from enrollment to prior to implant surgery; however, the remaining changes were not statistically significant (Table 18.5, Fig 18.8B).

Significant ($p < 0.0035$) reductions from enrollment scores were observed across all seven dimensions between enrollment and immediately prior to surgery. Further significant reductions occurred in the 6 months post-insertion on dimensions of functional limitation, pain, psychological discomfort, and physical disability, but not on psychological disability, social disability, or handicap (Fig 18.9). No domain exhibited significant change between the 6- and 12-month recall visits.

DISCUSSION

We observed a high degree of implant survival in the edentulous mandible over the course of 1 year and found technical complications to be far more common than biologic. The most common technical complication noted was chipped denture teeth in the opposing removable prosthesis, which accounted for 50% (6/12) of all complication events during the observation period. The etiology of maxillary denture tooth chipping may reflect multiple aspects of this therapy, including potential limitations of tooth arrangement and the physical properties of the selected line of denture teeth. The manufacturer reports a higher inorganic filler content as compared to other available varieties. The higher

TABLE 18.3 Participant Characteristics and OHIP-49 Severity and Extent Scores at Enrollment [Mean (SD)] ($n = 17$)

	N (%)	Enrollment Mean (SD) OHIP Severity Score[a]	p-Value	Enrollment Mean (SD) OHIP Extent Score[b]	p-Value
All participants	17 (100.0)	94.8 (40.8)	. . .	17.2 (12.49)	. . . [c]
Sex					
Male	11 (64.7)	84.5 (33.1)	0.162	14.3 (10.4)	0.335
Female	6 (35.3)	113.8 (49.6)		22.5 (15.2)	
Age (years)					
<50	3 (17.7)	119.7 (34.9)	0.421	23.7 (9.1)	0.315
50 to 64	6 (35.3)	98.5 (53.2)		19.2 (17.1)	
≥65	8 (47.1)	82.8 (31.4)		13.3 (9.2)	
Mandible status, enrollment					
Edentulous	7 (41.2)	115.4 (42.6)	0.574	23.1 (15.0)	0.100
Terminal dentition	10 (58.8)	80.4 (34.4)		13.0 (8.9)	

[a]*Severity* is the sum of OHIP-49 responses (potential range 0 to 196); higher scores denote worse OHQoL.

[b]*Extent* is the number of "fairly often" or "very often" responses (potential range 0 to 49); higher scores denote worse OHQoL.

[c]". . ." in Tables 18.3–18.5 define how calculation of the OHIP extent score is different than the severity score. "Fairly often" and "very often" are specific options on the questionnaire that carry different weight in the calculation.

TABLE 18.4 **Mean OHIP-49 Severity[a] Scores at Enrollment and Changes in This Score During Treatment ($n = 17$)**

	Beta Coefficient	95% CI	p-Value
Enrollment (mean severity score)	94.8	73.9, 115.8	. . .
Prior to implant surgery (change since enrollment)	−47.2	−61.7, −32.7	<0.001
Six months post-implant surgery (change since enrollment)	−74.3	−88.8, −59.8	<0.001
Six months post-implant surgery (change since implant surgery)	−27.1	−41.6, −12.6	<0.001
12 months post-implant surgery (change since enrollment)	−76.8	−91.3, −62.3	<0.001
12 months post-implant surgery (change since implant surgery)	−29.6	−44.1, −15.1	<0.001
12 months post-implant surgery (change since 6 months postsurgery)	−2.5	−17.0, 12.0	0.773

[a]*Severity* is the sum of OHIP-49 responses (potential range 0 to 196); higher scores denote worse OHQoL.

TABLE 18.5 **Mean OHIP-49 Extent[a] Scores at Enrollment and Changes in This Score During Treatment ($n = 17$)**

	Beta Coefficient	95% CI	p-Value
Enrollment (mean extent score)	17.2	10.8, 23.6	. . .
Prior to implant surgery (change since enrollment)	−12.6	−16.6, −8.7	<0.001
Six months post-implant surgery (change since enrollment)	−15.9	−19.9, −12.0	<0.001
Six months post-implant surgery (change since implant surgery)	−3.3	−7.2, 0.6	0.100
12 months post-implant surgery (change since enrollment)	−16.3	−20.2, −12.4	<0.001
12 months post-implant surgery (change since implant surgery)	−3.6	−7.6, 0.3	0.068
12 months post-implant surgery (change since 6 months post-surgery)	−0.4	−4.3, 3.6	0.860

[a]*Extent* is the number of "fairly often" or "very often" responses (potential range 0 to 49); higher scores denote worse OHQoL.

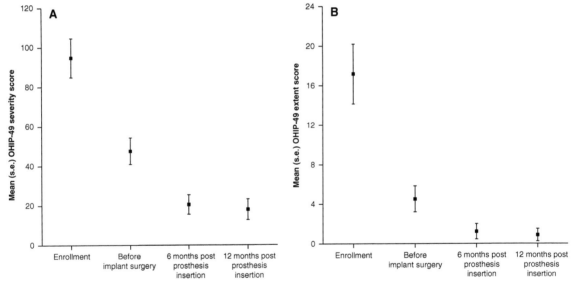

FIGURE 18.8 Mean (SE) OHIP-49 severity (A, left) and extent (B, right) scores at enrollment, immediately prior to implant surgery, 6 months post-insertion, and 12 months post-insertion. Scores prior to surgery and at 6 months postsurgery were significantly lower than at enrollment. The postsurgery score did not reduce significantly ($p = 0.685$) in the 6 months following surgery.

inorganic filler content adds wear resistance and superb esthetics, but may also increase the risk of chipping.[30] Interestingly, 67% (4/6) of participants who experienced minor chipping of maxillary incisors actually preferred to leave the defect unrepaired, as they felt it added uniqueness to their smile. Two recent systematic reviews on metal-acrylic prostheses report that denture tooth wear and denture tooth

fracture of either the implant-supported fixed prosthesis or the opposing complete denture are common issues with this therapy.[21,22] In this study, we only found chipping complications in the opposing complete denture, not with the zirconia prosthesis.

Few complications related specifically to the MZ-FDP were observed; however, one MZ-FDP did fracture 6 months

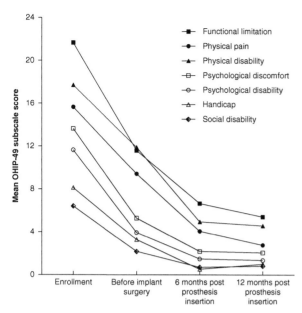

FIGURE 18.9 OHIP-49 subscale analysis. Significant ($p < 0.0035$) reductions from enrollment scores were observed across all seven dimensions between enrollment and immediately prior to surgery. Further significant reductions occurred in the 6 months post-insertion on dimensions of functional limitation, pain and discomfort, psychological discomfort, and physical disability, but not on psychological disability, social disability, or handicap. No domain exhibited significant change between the 6- and 12-month recall visits.

after insertion. The fracture occurred vertically through the entire body of the prosthesis, resulting in the loss of the distal cantilever segment on the affected side (Fig 18.10). Several factors may have contributed to this event: cantilever length, anterior-posterior (A-P) spread,[37] restorative dimension, and/or the material properties of zirconia.

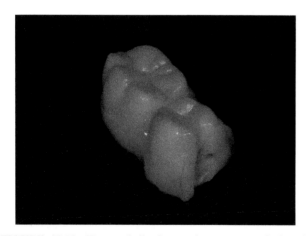

FIGURE 18.10 Fractured distal extension segment of zirconia prosthesis through screw access hole.

Each mandibular MZ-FDP possessed bilateral distal cantilevers, designed to restore first molar occlusion. Cantilever length and A-P spread varied with arch form, mental foramen position, and the accuracy of implant placement. The measured cantilever length of the fractured segment was approximately 17 mm, and the A-P spread was approximately 10 mm, yielding a ratio of 1.7 to 1. A ratio of approximately 1.5 to 1 is commonly recommended as the target value for distal extension cantilevers.[38–40] An increased ratio of cantilever length to A-P spread may have contributed to an unfavorable mechanical environment that led to the prosthesis fracture, as well as the two abutment fracture events. It is important to note that for this cohort, the mean cantilever length to A-P spread ratio was 2.0 (SD 0.82) to 1, with 77% (13/17) of the participants having a prosthesis with at least one side exceeding 1.5 to 1.

Vertical height of the prosthesis also varied with each participant in this study, depending on the amount of restorative space present after alveolectomy. A minimum restorative dimension, or distance from osseous crest to incisal edge, is thought necessary to allow adequate space for restorative materials, and thus adequate fracture resistance.[35] The vertical height of the distal segment in the fractured prosthesis was approximately 9 mm, which is notably smaller than the mean height of 13.2 mm (SD 3.2) for the other prostheses. Further, the fracture occurred at the distal screw access, where the prosthesis was smallest in cross-sectional area.

Finally, the MZ-FDP fracture could have been related to the material itself. Porosity in the original zirconia blank, post-sintering damage, and/or low temperature degradation of the zirconia may all contribute to an increased risk of material failure.[33,34]

One complication unique to the MZ-FDP was debonding of a single cementable unit observed in one participant (Fig 18.11). Fifteen of the 17 prostheses were made from a single block of zirconia; however, two participants required a prosthesis design variation where one or more single crowns or teeth could be cemented onto or into the main prosthesis to account for error in implant angulation. One limitation of this modification is that it either decreases retrievability or increases the risk of debonding, depending on which type of cement is selected. Another concern with this design modification is the potential reduction in cross-sectional area of the prosthesis.

The other primary aim of this study was to assess the within-subject change in OHIP-49 scores as the participant transitioned from baseline to conventional dentures and from conventional dentures to a mandibular MZ-FDP. Several important observations can be made from this OHIP-49 data. First, the construction of well-made, properly fitting dentures in participants with a terminal dentition or in participants with an ill-fitting prosthesis led to a significant change in OHQoL, indicated by the significant reduction of both OHIP-49 severity and extent scores between enrollment

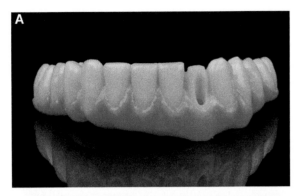

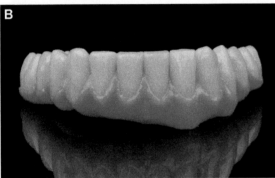

FIGURE 18.11 (A and B) Definitive zirconia prosthesis with cementable single unit missing and in place at lateral incisor site.

and implant surgery. This finding is consistent with that of several other studies evaluating the effect of complete dentures on OHQoL.[8,41,42] Second, participants with well-made, properly fitting conventional dentures achieved an additional significant improvement in OHQoL with a mandibular implant-supported MZ-FDP, illustrated by the significant decrease in OHIP-49 severity score from implant surgery to 6-month recall.

The lack of a statistically significant decrease in the OHIP-49 extent score for the interval between 6 and 12 months postinsertion does not undermine the significance of this treatment effect, but rather highlights several potential aspects of the study population, as well as the challenges of a questionnaire-based measure. The "very often" and "fairly often" responses within the population at baseline likely reflected social or esthetic variables more frequently, which were addressed reasonably well by a new set of conventional dentures, resulting in a large improvement in OHIP-49 extent scores at the second administration, and thus allowed little room for further improvement with the mandibular prosthesis at the third administration. The placebo effect may also be of clinical importance here by altering the extent responses after insertion of new conventional dentures, therefore masking further improvement at later evaluations.

Regardless of the nuances, the magnitude of reduction observed in both severity and extent scores is profound. A

study by John et al reported on the minimally important difference in OHIP-49 (severity) scores.[31] They found that a change of approximately six OHIP-49 units is required for patients to state that they feel at least "a little better," and that a change of about ten units is required for patients to state they feel "a lot better." Within the limitations of a questionnaire-based measure, the finding of our study, with a mean difference of 76.8 OHIP units, may indicate a profound change in QoL, vastly exceeding mere sense of improvement. Further, the degree of biologic and technical complications observed during the course of the study did not prevent these significant improvements in OHQoL.

CONCLUSIONS

A protocol for the treatment of mandibular edentulism using an implant-supported MZ-FDP was presented. Implant survival was high, and few complications related specifically to the MZ-FDP were observed. The most common technical complications were chipped teeth in the maxillary denture, possibly related to the particular type of denture teeth used. Substantial and clinically important improvements in OHQoL were achieved with the MZ-FDP. Specifically, well-made, properly fitting conventional dentures provide significant improvement in OHIP-49 scores among participants with a terminal dentition or an ill-fitting prosthesis, and the MZ-FDP significantly improved OHIP-49 scores for participants with well-made, properly fitting conventional dentures. The data of this short-term study indicate that the MZ-FDP is a viable therapeutic option with particular advantages in the edentulous mandible and warrants long-term study.

ACKNOWLEDGMENT

The authors wish to thank Dentsply (Molndal, Sweden), Zirkonzahn (Gais, Italy) for providing test materials.

REFERENCES

1. Douglass CW, Shih A, Ostry L: Will there be a need for complete dentures in the United States in 2020? *J Prosthet Dent* 2002;87:5–8.
2. Felton DA: Edentulism and comorbid factors. *J Prosthodont* 2009;18:88–96.
3. Cooper LF: The current and future treatment of edentulism. *J Prosthodont* 2009;18:116–122.
4. Tallgren A: The continuing reduction of the residual alveolar ridges in complete denture wearers: a mixed-longitudinal study covering 25 years. *J Prosthet Dent* 1972;27:120–132.

5. Allen PF, McMillian A, Walshaw D: A patient-based assessment of implant-stabilized and conventional complete dentures. *J Prosthet Dent* 2001;85:141–147.

6. Fueki K, Kimoto K, Ogawa T, et al: Effect of implant-supported or retained dentures on masticatory performance: a systematic review. *J Prosthet Dent* 2007;98:470–477.

7. Carlsson GE, Lindquist L: Ten-year longitudinal study of masticatory function in edentulous patients treated with fixed complete dentures on osseointegrated implants. *Int J Prosthodont* 1994;7:448–453.

8. Harris D, Hofer S, O'Boyle C, et al: A comparison of implant-retained mandibular overdentures and conventional dentures on quality of life in edentulous patients: a randomized, prospective, within-subject controlled clinical trial. *Clin Oral Implants Res* 2013;24:96–103.

9. Lindquist L, Rockler B, Carlsson G: Bone resorption around fixtures in edentulous patients treated with mandibular fixed tissue-integrated prostheses. *J Prosthet Dent* 1988;59:59–63.

10. Arvidson K, Bystedt H, Frykholm A, et al: Five year prospective follow up report of the AstraTech Dental Implant System in the treatment of edentulous mandibles. *Clin Oral Impl Res* 1998;9:225–234.

11. Adell R, Eriksson B, Lekholm U, et al: Long-term follow-up study of osseointegrated implants in the treatment of totally edentulous jaws. *Int J Oral Maxillofac Implants* 1990;5:347–359.

12. Brånemark PI, Svensson B, van Steenberghe D: Ten-year survival rates of fixed prostheses on four or six implants ad modum Brånemark in full edentulism. *Clin Oral Impl Res* 1995;6:227–231.

13. Eliasson A, Palmqvist S, Svensson B, et al: Five-year results with fixed complete-arch mandibular prostheses supported by 4 implants. *Int J Oral Maxillofac Implants* 2000;15:505–510.

14. Ekelund JA, Lindquist LW, Carlsson GE, et al: Implant treatment in the edentulous mandible: a prospective study on Brånemark System implants over more than 20 years. *Int J Prosthodont* 2003;16:602–608.

15. Attard NJ, Zarb GA: Long term treatment outcomes in edentulous patients with implant overdentures: the Toronto study. *Int J Prosthodont* 2004;17:417–424.

16. Bryant SR, MacDonald-Jankowski D, Kim K: Does the type of implant prosthesis affect outcomes for the completely edentulous arch? *Int J Oral Maxillofac Implants* 2007;22:117–139.

17. Malo P, Nombre M, Lopes A, et al: A longitudinal study of the survival of all-on-4 implants in the mandible with up to 10 years follow up. *J Am Dent Assoc* 2011;142:310–320.

18. Feine JS, Dufresne E, Boudrias P, et al: Outcome assessment of implant supported prostheses. *J Prosthet Dent* 1998;79:575–579.

19. Emami E, Heydecke G, Rompré PH, et al: Impact of implant support for mandibular dentures on satisfaction, oral and general health-related quality of life: a meta-analysis of randomized-controlled trials. *Clin Oral Implants Res* 2009;20:533–544.

20. Strassburger C, Kerschbaum T, Heydecke G: Influence of implant and conventional prostheses on satisfaction and quality of life: a literature review. Part II: qualitative analysis and evaluation of the studies. *Int J Prosthodont* 2006;19:339–348.

21. Brozini T, Petridis H, Tzanas K, et al: A meta-analysis of prosthodontic complication rates of implant supported fixed dental prostheses in edentulous patients after an observation period of at least 5 years. *Int J Oral Maxillofac Implant* 2011;26:304–331.

22. Papaspyridakos P, Chen C, Chuang S, et al: A systematic review of biologic and technical complications with fixed implant rehabilitations for edentulous patients. *Int J Oral Maxillofac Implants* 2012;27:102–110.

23. Manicone P, Iommetti PR, Raffaelli L: An overview of zirconia ceramics: basic properties and clinical applications. *J Dent* 2007;35:819–826.

24. Ozkurt Z, Kazazoglu E: Clinical success of zirconia in dental applications. *J Prosthodont* 2010;19:64–68.

25. Papaspyridakos P, Lal K: Complete arch implant rehabilitation using subtractive rapid prototyping and porcelain fused to zirconia prosthesis: a clinical report. *J Prosthet Dent* 2008;100:165–172.

26. Rojas-Viscaya F: Full zirconia fixed detachable implant-retained restorations manufactured from monolithic zirconia: clinical report after two years in service. *J Prosthodont* 2011;20:570–576.

27. Heydecke G: Implantologie: Wohlbefinden fur senioren. *Zahnarztl Mitt* 2000;90:52–57.

28. Slade GD, Spencer AJ: Development and evaluation of the oral health impact profile. *Comm Dent Health* 1994;11:3–11.

29. Brennan M, Houston F, O'Sullivan M, et al: Patient satisfaction and oral health related quality of life outcomes of implant overdentures and fixed complete dentures. *Int J Oral Maxillofac Implants* 2010;25:791–800.

30. Scientific Documentation SR Phonares. 2010. Ivoclar Vivadent. http://www.ivoclarvivadent.us/phonares/PDF/phonares-tech-doc.pdf. Accessed August 16, 2013.

31. John MT, Reissmann D, Szentpétery A, et al: An approach to define clinical significance in prosthodontics. *J Prosthodont* 2009;18:445–460.

32. Jensen O, Adams M, Cottam J, et al: The All-on-4 shelf: mandible. *J Oral Maxillofac Surg* 2011;69:175–181.

33. Denry I, Kelly JR: State of the art of zirconia for dental applications. *Dent Mater* 2008;24:299–307.

34. Lughi V, Sergo V: Low temperature degradation—aging—of zirconia: a critical review of the relevant aspects in dentistry. *Dent Mater* 2010;26:807–820.

35. Cooper L, Limmer B, Gates W: "Rules of 10"–guidelines for successful planning and treatment of mandibular edentulism using dental implants. *Compend Contin Educ Dent* 2012;33:328–334.

36. Thomason J, Heydecke G, Feine J, et al: How do patients perceive the benefits of reconstructive dentistry with regard to oral health quality of life and patient satisfaction? A systematic review. *Clin Oral Impl Res* 2007;18:168–188.

37. English C: The critical A-P spread. *Implant Soc* 1990;1:2–3.

38. Shackleton JL, Carr L, Slabbert JC, et al: Survival of fixed implant-supported prostheses related to cantilever lengths. *J Prosthet Dent* 1994;71:23–26.

39. Skalak R: Biomechanical considerations in osseointegrated prostheses. *J Prosthet Dent* 1983;49:843–848.

40. McAlarney M, Stavropoulos D: Theoretical cantilever lengths versus clinical variables in fifty-five clinical cases. *J Prosthet Dent* 2000;83:332–343.

41. Allen PF, Thomason JM, Jepson NJA, et al: A randomized controlled trial of implant retained mandibular overdentures. *J Dent Res* 2006;85:547–551.

42. Dierens M, Collaert B, Deschepper E, et al: Patient centered outcome of immediately loaded implants in the rehabilitation of fully edentulous jaws. *Clin Oral Impl Res* 2009;20: 1070–1077.

19

PROSTHETIC IMPROVEMENT OF PRONOUNCED BUCCALLY POSITIONED ZYGOMATIC IMPLANTS: A CLINICAL REPORT

Ataís Bacchi, DDS, MS, Mateus Bertolini Fernandes Dos Santos, DDS, MS, PHD, Marcele Jardim Pimentel, Mauro Antonio De Arruda Nóbilo, DDS, MS, PHD, and Rafael Leonardo Xediek Consani, DDS, MS, PHD

Department of Prosthodontics and Periodontics, Piracicaba Dental School, UNICAMP, Piracicaba, Brazil

Keywords
Zygomatic implants; prosthesis.

Correspondence
Ataís Bacchi, Piracicaba Dental School, UNICAMP—Prosthodontics and Periodontics, Av. Limeira, 901 Piracicaba SP 13414-903, Brazil. E-mail: atais_bacchi@yahoo.com.br

The authors deny any conflicts of interest.

Accepted September 24, 2013

Published in *Journal of Prosthodontics* August 2014; Vol. 23, Issue 6

doi: 10.1111/jopr.12148

ABSTRACT

This report presents a prosthetic technique for the improvement of surgically positioned, buccally placed zygomatic implants with the use of custom abutments for improved retention screw position and an esthetic implant reconstruction. The patient presented four zygomatic implants with pronounced buccal inclination. The anterior implants were inclined toward the location where the anterior artificial teeth should be placed during rehabilitation. As the manufacturer does not provide angulated abutments, we attempted the waxing and overcasting of a prosthetic abutment, repositioning the access holes of the prosthetic screws to a more palatal position. This clinical report demonstrates that abutment customization could be an interesting way to relocate the access holes of the prosthetic screws in cases of zygomatic implants with pronounced buccal inclination.

The oral rehabilitation of a patient with a severely resorbed edentulous maxilla represents a challenge for restorative dentistry. In many cases, these patients do not adapt to their conventional dentures and do not fit the inclusion criteria for receiving implants without a previous bone reconstruction. Techniques for the treatment of atrophic maxillae include composite grafts, Le Fort I osteotomy, iliac crest grafts, maxillary sinus grafts, and distraction osteogenesis.[1,2]

Journal of Prosthodontics on Dental Implants, First Edition. Edited by Avinash S. Bidra and Stephen M. Parel.
© 2015 American College of Prosthodontists. Published 2015 by John Wiley & Sons, Inc.

Although these reconstructive procedures present satisfactory results in increasing bone structure,[3,4] they cause discomfort to the patient, increase the risk of morbidity to donor and receptor sites, require a greater number of surgical procedures, and increase the length of treatment.[5,6] The zygomatic fixation technique is an alternative for the oral rehabilitation of these patients and differs from traditional treatment, where long implants are fixed in the zygomatic bone and in the alveolar process.[2] When compared to bone grafts, zygomatic implants can lead to a considerable reduction in the time of treatment period required (4 to 6 months) until the grafts can be loaded. Moreover, compared to grafting with autogenous bone, the placement of zygomatic implants avoids postoperative pain and reduces morbidity risk in the donor site.[7] The reduced number of zygomatic implants required for supporting fixed prostheses might also lead to less-expensive treatment.[7]

Indications for the zygomatic fixation technique are limited to cases of difficult resolution. Among the indications are treatment of atrophic maxillae[8–13] and treatment after tumor resection surgery in the maxillary bone.[14,15] This technique is also applicable for traumatic bone loss, congenital defects, unsuccessful bone graft augmentation, and patients who refuse bone graft augmentation.[16]

A modification in the original technique proposes the anchorage of two zygomatic implants in each hemi-arch, instead of the one zygomatic implant associated with conventional implants in the premaxillary region. The second zygomatic implant is placed mesially to the first, emerging in the canine or lateral incisor region, and these four implants are sufficient to rehabilitate the edentulous maxilla.[2,17] Other modifications, such as changes in the angulation of insertion, have been proposed to facilitate the surgical technique and improve predictability.[8]

The final positioning of implants orients the prosthetic treatment. The reduced option of abutments for zygomatic implants requires high precision in insertion, which can be achieved by auxiliary methods such as surgical guides and treatment planning with 3D software and prototypes.[1,18,19] The absence of reverse planning or reduced bone quantity may limit or complicate the positioning of the implants and, consequently, the prosthetic rehabilitation. This article provides a clinical report of the prosthetic management of four zygomatic implants with pronounced buccal inclination.

CLINICAL REPORT

A Caucasian female patient, 51 years old, sought prosthetic treatment in the Dental Clinics of Piracicaba Dental School. Upon initial examination, we observed a maxillary edentulous arch with a severely resorbed bone ridge and four zygomatic implants (External Hexagon, SIN; Sistemas de Implantes, São Paulo, Brazil). The opposite arch presented remaining teeth associated with a removable partial denture. The patient had panoramic presurgical radiography that showed frontal sinus pneumatization and a severe resorption of the posterior maxillary area. The pre- and postsurgical panoramic images are presented in Figure 19.1. Since the initial examination, a pronounced buccal inclination of the implants has been observed (Fig 19.2).

The impression copings (SIN) were adapted to the implants, and a functional impression was made with an open tray and poly(vinyl siloxane) impression material (Flextime; Heraeus Kulzer, São Paulo, Brazil). For the lower arch impression, we used a metallic tray and irreversible hydrocolloid material (Hydrogum; Zhermack, Badia Polesine, Italy). The casts were obtained with type IV dental stone (Herodent; Vigodent, Rio de Janeiro, Brazil). On the upper master cast, we created a record base with an occlusion rim, which was adjusted chairside. The casts were mounted in a semiadjustable articulator (Dentatus ARL; Dentatus, São Paulo, Brazil) by means of facebow (upper) and centric relation record (lower), and the teeth were waxed (Trilux; Vipi, Pirassununga, Brazil). Later, we performed a clinical evaluation of the occlusal relationship, lip support, and esthetics. A buccal index was made with the waxed prosthesis on the master cast to record the position of the artificial teeth using laboratory c-silicon material (Zetalabor;

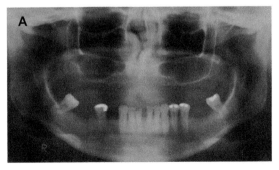 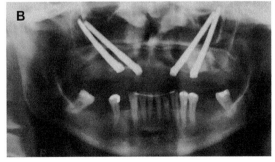

FIGURE 19.1   (A) Initial panoramic radiography showing the maxillary sinus pneumatization and (B) panoramic radiography after placement of the zygomatic implants.

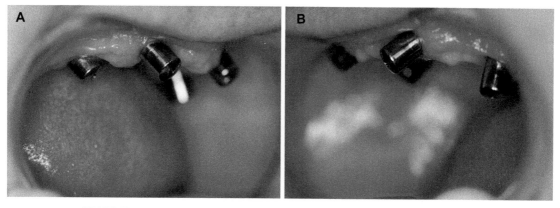

FIGURE 19.2 View of the implant inclinations in the (A) right and (B) left side.

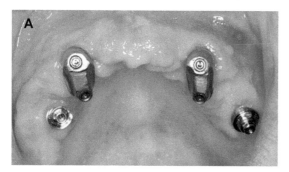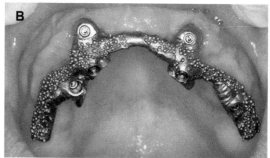

FIGURE 19.3 (A) Cast prosthetic abutments and (B) prosthetic framework.

Zhermack). This index was used to assist in the choice of the abutments and the construction of the framework.

Using the silicon index, we observed that the implants presented a pronounced buccal inclination in the direction of the anterior teeth; however, the implants' manufacturer did not offer angulated abutments for this type of implant. To overcome this limitation, we used straight mini-abutments on the implants. To correct the excessive inclination, we attempted the personalization of overcast prosthetic components with a palatine extension on the anterior mini-abutments, aiming to relocate the screws' access holes without affecting the esthetics. The prosthetic components were waxed and cast in cobalt-chromium alloy (Biosil F; DeguDent GmbH, Hanau, Germany) (Fig 19.3A). Then the prosthetic framework was also waxed and cast in Co-Cr alloy (Biosil F) (Fig 19.3B). During the course of treatment, the patient wore a provisional complete denture that injured the soft tissue in a localized region (Fig 19.3A). The complete denture was adjusted, and the lesion regressed normally.

The adaptation and passivity of the framework was examined in the mouth, followed by tooth waxing on the bar framework. After the esthetic and functional examination, the prosthesis was polymerized. On the day of installation, the anterior individualized components were screwed onto the mini-abutments with the prosthesis over them. The occlusal adjustments were realized, and the final aspect of the rehabilitation was recorded (Figs 19.4 and 19.5). The treatment has been followed for 18 months without any prosthetic complication.

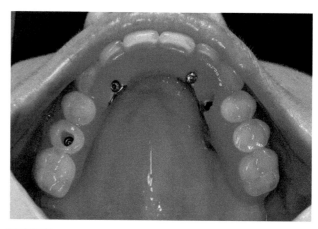

FIGURE 19.4 Occlusal view of the prosthesis showing the repositioning to the access holes of the prosthetic screws to a more palatal position.

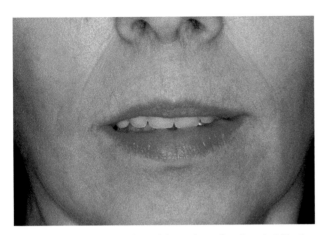

FIGURE 19.5 Frontal view of the patient after the rehabilitation.

DISCUSSION

Zygomatic fixation is only indicated in cases with difficult therapeutic resolutions, as in the treatment of an atrophic maxilla.[8–13] In this context, there are cases in which the posterior portion of the maxilla is extensively resorbed and/or has an accentuated pneumatization of the maxillary sinus, and cases of simultaneously anterior and posterior severe maxillary bone resorption.[9,10] In this report, the patient presented bone resorption and maxillary sinus pneumatization, common in cases of edentulous maxillae, that limited the insertion of conventional dental implants without bone reconstruction. Thus, fixation in distant sites was well indicated for reducing the presence of cantilevers.[17]

One modification of the initial zygomatic implant technique proposes the placement of four zygomatic implants with the anterior ones emerging in the canine or lateral incisor region.[2,17] In the patient presented here, the anterior implants emerged in the lateral incisor region, with a pronounced buccal inclination, which would compromise the esthetics of the prosthesis, since the screw access holes could be projected in the direction of the artificial teeth. The direction of the screw access holes was corrected by means of a customized, overcast component waxed with a palatine extension. Another possible way to correct this type of complication is to fabricate two metallic structures. The first (infrastructure) is screwed onto the implants to correct the problem of the implant inclination. The second (superstructure) is made to be screwed on to the infrastructure; however, this technique costs more and requires more occlusal space, which was not available in this case.

Cobalt-chromium alloy was used as the framework material for this patient. Initially, gold alloy was the material most

often used for framework fabrication, but, due to its high cost, alternative alloys were introduced in dentistry, among them Co-Cr, nickel-chromium, and titanium alloys.[20] Co-Cr alloys are harder and stronger among these materials, properties that have been shown to be important characteristics for an implant-supported framework.[20] Titanium alloys, as with Co-Cr alloys, present an adequate biocompatibility and resistance to corrosion; however, the cast procedures for Ti alloys have been considered to be more difficult and require more advanced technology.[21] Use of nickel-chromium alloys has been discouraged due to the possibility of allergic reaction and the carcinogenic potential of nickel.[21] Regarding the framework fabrication method, the overcastable components used for the present patient have shown to lead to a more passive framework than the entirely calcinable ones.[22] However, the most passive frameworks can be obtained from computer aided design/computer aided manufacturing (CAD/CAM) systems, which allow the fabrication of metallic and ceramic milled frameworks.[23] Despite these considerations, a CAD/CAM system was not used in this clinical report because they are still expensive for framework fabrication.

A high survival rate has been observed for zygomatic implants, ranging from 90.3 to 100%.[5,8,10,11,13,17,24] Moreover, patients with zygomatic implants present high levels of overall satisfaction, with minimal problems regarding hygiene and function.[5] Peñarrocha et al[25] obtained an overall average satisfaction rate of 90% in a study on satisfaction of patients rehabilitated with zygomatic implants (parameters evaluated were esthetics, function, ease of hygiene, comfort, and stability). Sartori et al[26] evaluated the satisfaction of patients rehabilitated with zygomatic fixtures and prostheses with regard to hygiene, esthetics, phonetics, and discomfort during chewing. The study concluded that treatment with zygomatic fixtures is predictable and reliable. The patients were satisfied with both implants and prostheses.[26] Thus, this type of rehabilitation has proved to be a viable treatment alternative for patients with severe maxillary resorption or maxillary sinus pneumatization,[8,27] increasing the predictability of outcomes, decreasing morbidity and treatment time, and avoiding bone grafts during treatment.[6]

Reverse planning is an important condition for implant placement, aiding in a correct final angulation. To avoid incorrect placement of the implants, we recommend the creation of surgical guides, which increase the predictability and safety of the technique and reduce surgical time.[28,29] Specialized professional training is also important for the success of treatment with zygomatic implants due to their greater technical complexity compared with conventional surgery for implant placement.[7,16,26] Moreover, the improper positioning of the implants is commonly observed and difficult to solve.

The use of an overcast component can relocate the position of the screw hole, relieving the esthetic region of the presence of the screw access.

CONCLUSION

The personalization of an overcast abutment was a viable solution for repositioning the screw access holes to a palatine region, solving the esthetic limitation caused by the accentuated buccal inclination of the malpositioned zygomatic implants.

REFERENCES

1. Stiévenart M, Malevez C: Rehabilitation of totally atrophied maxilla by means of four zygomatic implants and fixed prosthesis: a 6–40-month follow-up. *Int J Oral Maxillofac Surg* 2010;39:358–363.

2. Sharma A, Rahul GR: Zygomatic implants/fixture—a systematic review. *J Oral Implantol* 2013;39:215–224.

3. Clayman L: Implant reconstruction of the bone-grafted maxilla: review of the literature and presentation of 8 cases. *J Oral Maxillofac Surg* 2006;64:674–682.

4. Sjöström M, Sennerbey L, Nilson H, et al: Reconstruction of the atrophic edentulous maxilla with free iliac crest graft and implants: a 3-year report of a prospective clinical study. *Clin Implant Dent Relat Res* 2007;9:46–59.

5. Candel Martí E, Carrillo García C, Penarrocha Oltra D, et al: Rehabilitation of an atrophic posterior maxilla with zygoma implants: review. *J Oral Implantol* 2012;38:653–657.

6. Cordero EB, Benfatti CAM, Bianchini MA, et al: The use of zygomatic implants for the rehabilitation of atrophic maxillas with 2 different techniques: Stella and Extrasinus. *Oral Surg Oral Med Oral Pathol Oral Radiol Endod* 2011;112:e49–e53.

7. Chrcanovic BR, Abreu MH: Survival and complications of zygomatic implants: a systematic review. *Oral Maxillofac Surg* 2013;17:81–93.

8. Bedrossian ER, Stumpel LJ, Beckely M, et al: The zygomatic implant: preliminary data on treatment of severely resorbed maxillae. A clinical report. *Int J Oral Maxillofac Implants* 2002;17:861–865.

9. Ferrara ED, Stella JP: Restoration of the edentulous maxilla: the case for the zygomatic implants. *J Oral Maxillofac Surg* 2004;62:1418–1422.

10. Malavez C, Aberca M, Durdu F, et al: Clinical outcome of 103 consecutive zygomatic: a 6–48 months follow-up study. *Clin Oral Implant Res* 2004;15:18–22.

11. Aparicio C, Ouazzane W, Garcia R, et al: A prospective clinical study on titanium implants in the zygomatic arch for prosthetic rehabilitation of the atrophic edentulous maxilla with a follow-up of 6 months to 5 years. *Clin Implant Dent Relat Res* 2006;8:114–122.

12. Gálan-Gil S, Peñarrocha MD, Martínez JB, et al: Rehabilitation of severely resorbed maxillae with zygomatic implants: an update. *Med Oral Patol Oral Cir Bucal* 2007;12:e216–e220.

13. Kahnberg KE, Henry PJ, Hirsch JM, et al: Clinical evaluation of zygoma implant: 3-year follow-up at 16 clinics. *J Oral Maxillofac Surg* 2007;65:2033–2038.

14. Kreissl ME, Heydecke G, Metzger MC, et al: Zygoma implant-supported prosthetic rehabilitation after partial maxillectomy using surgical navigation: a clinical report. *J Prosthet Dent* 2007;97:121–128.

15. Boyes-Varley JG, Howes DG, Davidge-Pitts KD, et al: A protocol for maxillary reconstruction following oncology resection using zygomatic implants. *Int J Prosthodont* 2007;20:521–531.

16. Chrcanovic BR, Pedrosa AR, Custódio AL: Zygomatic implants: a critical review of the surgical techniques. *Oral Maxillofac Surg* 2013;17:1–9.

17. Parel SM, Brånemark MD, Ohrnell LO, et al: Remote implant anchorage for the rehabilitation of maxillary defects. *J Prosthet Dent* 2001;86:377–381.

18. Rosenfeld AL, Mandelaris GA, Tardieu PB: Prosthetically direct implant placement using computer software to ensure precise placement and predictable prosthetic outcomes. Part 2: rapid-prototype medical modeling and stereolithographic drilling guides requiring exposure. *Int J Periodontics Restorative Dent* 2006;26:347–353.

19. Bedrossian E: Laboratory and prosthetic considerations in computer-guided surgery and immediate loading. *J Oral Maxillofac Surg* 2007;65(7 Suppl 1):47–52.

20. Bacchi A, Consani RL, Mesquita MF, et al: Effect of framework material and vertical misfit on stress distribution in implant-supported partial prosthesis under load application: 3-D finite element analysis. *Acta Odontol Scand* 2013;71:1243–1249.

21. Barbosa GAS, Neves FD, Mattos MGC, et al: Implant/abutment vertical misfit of one-piece cast frameworks made with different materials. *Braz Dent J* 2010;21:515–519.

22. Bhering CL, Takahashi JM, Luthi LF, et al: Influence of the casting technique and dynamic loading on screw detorque and misfit of single unit implant-supported prostheses. *Acta Odontol Scand* 2013;71:404–409.

23. Paniz G, Stellini E, Meneghello R, et al: The precision of fit of cast and milled full-arch implant-supported restorations. *Int J Oral Maxillofac Implants* 2013;28:687–693.

24. Peñarrocha M, Gárcia B, Martín E, et al: Rehabilitation of severely atrophic maxillae with fixed implant-supported prostheses using zygomatic implants placed using the sinus slot technique: clinical report on a series of 21 patients. *Int J Oral Maxillofac Implants* 2007;22:645–650.

25. Peñãrrocha M, Carrillo C, Boronat A, et al: Level of satisfaction in patients with maxillary full-arch fixed prosthesis: zygomatic

versus conventional implants. *Int J Oral Maxillofac Implants* 2007;22:769–773.

26. Sartori EM, Padovan LEM, Sartori IAMS, et al: Evaluation of satisfaction of patients rehabilitated with zygomatic fixtures. *J Oral Maxillofac Surg* 2012;70:314–319.

27. Bedrossian ER, Stumpel LJ: Immediate stabilization at stage II of zygomatic implants: rationale and technique. *J Prosthet Dent* 2001;86:10–14.

28. Chow J, Hui E, Lee PK, et al: Zygomatic implants-protocol for immediate occlusal loading: a preliminary report. *J Oral Maxillofac Surg* 2006;64:804–811.

29. Koser LR, Campos PSF, Mendes CMC: Length determination of zygomatic implants using tridimensional computer tomography. *Braz Oral Res* 2006;20:331–336.

PART III

MANAGEMENT OF PATIENTS WITH MAXILLOFACIAL DEFECTS

20

IMPLANT-SUPPORTED FACIAL PROSTHESES PROVIDED BY A MAXILLOFACIAL UNIT IN A U.K. REGIONAL HOSPITAL: LONGEVITY AND PATIENT OPINIONS

S.M. Hooper, BDS, MSC,[1] T. Westcott, BDS,[2] P.L.L. Evans, MIMPT,[3] A.P. Bocca, MSC, FIMPT,[4] AND D.C. Jagger, BDS, MSC, PHD[5]

[1]Lecturer and Specialist in Restorative Dentistry, Department of Oral and Dental Science, Division of Restorative Dentistry, Bristol Dental School and Hospital, Bristol, U.K.

[2]Undergraduate Dental Student, Department of Oral and Dental Science, Division of Restorative Dentistry, Bristol Dental School and Hospital, Bristol, U.K.

[3]Maxillofacial Prosthodontist, Maxillofacial Prosthetic Unit, Morriston Hospital, Swansea, U.K.

[4]Laboratory Services Manager, Maxillofacial Prosthetic Unit, Morriston Hospital, Swansea, U.K.

[5]Professor of Restorative Dentistry, Department of Oral and Dental Science, Division of Restorative Dentistry, Bristol Dental School and Hospital, Bristol, U.K.

Keywords
Maxillofacial prostheses, implants.

Correspondence
Dr. D.C. Jagger, Department of Oral and Dental Science, Division of Restorative Dentistry, Bristol Dental School and Hospital, Lower Maudlin Street, Bristol BS1 2LY, U.K.
E-mail: D.C.Jagger@bris.ac.uk

Accepted June 30, 2004

Published in *Journal of Prosthodontics* March 2005; Vol. 14, Issue 1

doi: 10.1111/j.1532-849X.2005.00004.x

ABSTRACT

Purpose: The aim of this study was to acquire information on the types and longevity of implant-retained facial prostheses and the opinions of patients on several factors related to their prostheses.

Materials and Methods: A survey of 75 maxillofacial prosthetic patients currently under treatment and review at the Maxillofacial Unit, Morriston Regional Hospital was conducted through a 23-question postal questionnaire. These patients were selected as representative of a group of individuals receiving treatment or under review for the fabrication of maxillofacial prostheses.

Results: Of the prosthetic replacements, 83% were ear prostheses, 8% nose, 6% eye, and 2% combination prostheses. Of the 47 respondents, 8 (17%) reported that they were currently wearing their original prostheses. The remaining 39 (83%) respondents had all been provided with at least 1 replacement prosthesis. The mean lifetime of the prostheses was found to be 14 months (range: 4–36 months). The majority of replacement prostheses in this study were provided as a result of color fade or wear of the silicone material of the previous prosthesis. Individuals with no previous experience wearing a prosthesis had an unrealistic expectation of their prosthesis longevity, with a mean value of 17.8 months. In comparison, individuals with previous experience had reduced expectations, with a mean of 14.4 months. In terms of the patients' opinions of the overall quality of their prostheses, the results demonstrated that a large number of patients were satisfied. Thirty-five patients rated their prostheses as excellent and 9 as good. At 7–12 months, 4 patients rated their prostheses as excellent and 8 as good. At 13 months, 4 patients rated their prostheses as excellent and 5 as good.

Conclusions: It is important that advice be given to patients on the expected average longevity of their prostheses, together with information on factors affecting the longevity (i.e., environmental staining, cosmetics, and cleaning regimes). In this study, 26% of the replacement prostheses were provided due to color fading of the original prosthesis. This highlights the need for continuing research in the development of materials used for the construction of facial prostheses with improved properties, and in particular, improved color stability.

Maxillofacial prosthetics is concerned with the restoration and/or replacement of stomatognathic and associated facial structures by artificial substitutes that may or may not be removable.[1] It has been suggested that the area in and around the mouth is emotionally charged and strongly connected with self image. As an instrument of speech and eating, as well as a mirror of emotions, the mouth also has unique social and psychological implications and symbolic meaning. Disfigured individuals, lacking eyes, nose, ears, or facial tissues, may not be socially acceptable.[2] Loss of part of the face or having a congenitally missing ear, nose, or eye can have both a social and psychological impact on those affected.[3]

Maxillofacial prostheses aim to improve the esthetics of patients, and to restore, improve, and maintain the health of the hard and soft tissues. The effective accomplishment of these objectives should expedite patients' return to society.[4] Although many facial defects are rehabilitated for cosmetic and psychological reasons, oral defects also require rehabilitation for physiological reasons. There is often a need to restore separation between the oral/nasal structures that assist

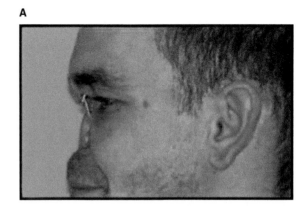

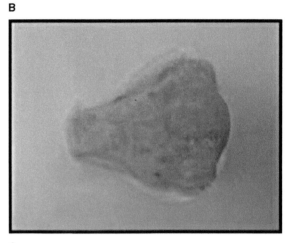

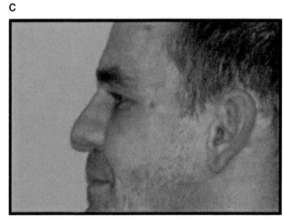

FIGURE 20.1   (A) Lateral view demonstrating a nasal defect and the position of dental implants for the retention of the nasal prosthesis. (B) Nasal prosthesis that will be attached to the implants shown in Figure 20.1A. (C) Implant-retained nasal prosthesis in situ.

the individual in speech and swallowing. Maxillofacial prostheses play an important part in rehabilitation following ablative surgery, congenital deformity, or trauma (Figs 20.1A–C and 20.2A–C). The psychological benefits and lifestyle improvement offered by maxillofacial prostheses have been well documented.[5,6] The physical and mental

A

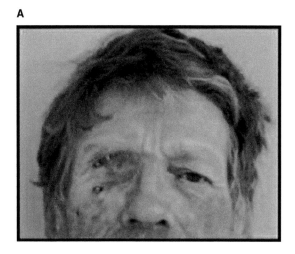

B

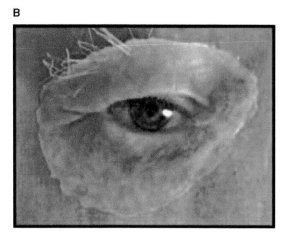

C

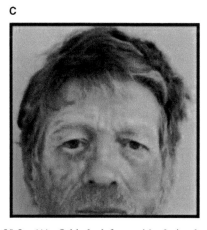

FIGURE 20.2 (A) Orbital defect with 3 implants in situ. (B) Orbital prosthesis that will be retained by the implants shown in Figure 20.2A. (C) Orbital prosthesis in situ.

well-being of these patients demand good organization and communication among the health professionals involved in their treatments. This is best achieved by multidisciplinary teams working in established centers. Maxillofacial prosthetic rehabilitation is a team effort involving restorative dentists, maxillofacial technicians, dieticians, speech and language therapists, physiotherapists, general medical practitioners, specialist nurses, and social workers.[4]

The clinical and laboratory production of a maxillofacial prosthesis is a time-consuming, labor-intensive, costly process. At Morriston Regional Hospital, Swansea, United Kingdom, the costs incurred for the provision of an orbital or auricular prosthesis have been calculated to be approximately £1,000–£1,500. This figure does not take into account additional costs incurred for repairs or remakes of prostheses. Replacement of prostheses may require patient appointment times of 4–5 hours. With the clinical, laboratory, and patient time expended in the construction of a prosthesis, it is essential that all factors are taken into account to maximize the longevity of the prosthesis. Prostheses with a short life span cannot only lead to patient disillusionment with the treatment, but also to excessive use of healthcare resources.

The longevity of a prosthesis is dependent on several factors, including the materials from which it is constructed and the behavioral factors of the wearer. The problems associated with the materials available for maxillofacial prostheses such as color fade, cracking, and splitting, together with the need for the development of improved materials, have been discussed by several authors.[7–11] Materials used for the fabrication of facial prostheses must ideally accept and retain intrinsic and extrinsic coloration. The appearance and mechanical strength must not be affected by sunlight or other environmental factors.[11] The ideal properties for materials used for the construction of prostheses should include compatibility with human tissue, flexibility, lightness, chemical and physical inertness, moldability, easy cleansing, durability, and ability to accept colorants.

Over the years, there have been several studies on the longevity of maxillofacial prostheses. Chen et al[12] reported an average prosthesis life of 10 months. Jani and Schaaf[13] reported that 69.6% of prostheses needed renewal within 1 year, with an additional 17.6% requiring renewal within an 18-month period. Jebreil,[14] however, reported renewal times of 6–9 months. Since publication of these studies, a number of advancements in the clinical techniques associated with the provision of maxillofacial prostheses and the materials from which they are constructed have been made. Significant advances in the field of material science has led to the production of new silicones with improved characteristics and improved methods of prosthesis coloration.[15]

A major change has been the increased use of extraoral endosseous implants, resulting in improved retention and stability of maxillofacial prostheses.[16] The use of dental implants for the retention and stability of facial prostheses has been shown to be effective and has eliminated the need for the use of adhesive tape. The use of implants has had a major impact on patients in that they are able to function in society, confident their defects may be less noticeable. The accumulation of the positive effects as a result of the use of implant-retained prostheses has undoubtedly improved the quality of life of patients.

The demand for maxillofacial prostheses is high, and there is a need to periodically evaluate the services provided. Many prostheses are rejected by patients due to patients' high expectations and lack of information provided regarding the prostheses.[15] It is through such investigations that factors related to success and failure of the prostheses may be identified, and the results used to produce prostheses with increased longevity and patient acceptability. The purpose of this study was to acquire information on the types and longevity of implant-retained facial prostheses and to assess the opinions of patients on several factors related to their prostheses from a group of patients currently under the care of the Maxillofacial Unit, Morriston Regional Hospital, Swansea.

MATERIALS AND METHODS

An initial pilot study was undertaken with questionnaires sent to 5 randomly selected maxillofacial patients currently under treatment and review at the Maxillofacial unit, Morriston Hospital. The survey was mailed to patients at their current addresses.

These patients were asked to complete the questionnaire, to comment on the design, and to identify any problems experienced in completing the questionnaires. An accompanying letter was written to explain the nature of this survey and inform the respondents that their replies would be anonymous and confidential. A stamped addressed envelope for reply was included. The results of the pilot study did not identify any problems with the questionnaire, the questionnaires were completed satisfactorily, and no changes were recommended. The remaining 70 questionnaires were posted, for a total of 75 surveys. The questionnaire was multiple choice, with structured tick-boxes. The number of free text responses was limited. The questionnaire was designed to obtain a patient history in terms of the maxillofacial prosthesis, i.e., prosthesis type, longevity of the prosthesis, possible reasons for prosthesis replacement, period of wear, and cleaning regimen.

TABLE 20.1   Study Population of Age Distribution

Age Grouping (Years)	Frequency	Percentage of Total
0–9	0	0
10–19	10	21.3
20–29	2	4.3
30–39	5	10.6
40–49	9	19.1
50–59	5	10.6
60–69	7	14.9
70–79	5	10.6
80–89	3	6.4
90–100	1	2.1

RESULTS

Of the 75 questionnaires sent, 47 were returned (32 males and 15 females), for a 63% response rate. The results were subjected to a statistical analysis using χ^2 and t-test. The results are presented in Tables 20.1–20.7.

The ages of respondents were grouped in 10-year groups from a 10–19 years group to a 90–100 years group. The age distribution of respondents is given in Table 20.1. In terms of employment status, 16 were recorded as employed, 19 retired, 10 in full-time education, and 2 as other.

The proportion of each type of prosthesis was ear 39 (83%), nose 4 (8.3%), orbit 3 (6.4%), and nose/orbit 1 (2.1%).

Of the 47 respondents, 8 (17%) reported they were currently wearing their original prostheses. The remaining 39 (83%) respondents had been provided with at least one replacement prosthesis. For the 39 patients who had been provided with replacement prostheses, the mean life span of their previous prostheses is given in Table 20.2. The mean lifetime of the prostheses was found to be 14 months (range: 4–36 months). Orbital prostheses had the longest life span (28 months), followed by ears (13 months), nose (12 months), and finally combination prostheses (4 months). Reasons for replacement prostheses included deterioration in color (12 (26%)), wear and tear (17 (36%)), poor fit (2 (4%)), prosthesis lost (2 (4%)), replacement at annual review (1 (2%)), and no response (13 (28%)). Respondents provided more than one answer to the question.

In terms of prosthesis daily wear, 4 (8%) of the respondents reported they wore the prostheses continuously, 30 (63%) during the day, 2 (4%) at school, 8 (17%) for social

TABLE 20.2   Longevity of Prosthesis

Prosthesis Type	All Prostheses	Nose	Ear	Orbit	Nose/Orbit
Mean lifetime	14 months	12 months	13 months	28 months	4 months
Min. lifetime recorded	4 months	12 months	4 months	12 months	4 months
Max. lifetime recorded	36 months	12 months	24 months	36 months	4 months

TABLE 20.3   Patients' Perception of Quality of Fit of the Prosthesis at the Edges

Quality of Edge	1 (Excellent)	2	3	4	5 (Poor)
New (*n* = 45)	31	12	2	0	0
0–6 months (*n* = 14)	4	6	3	1	0
7–12 months (*n* = 19)	5	5	4	4	1
13+ months (*n* = 12)	3	1	5	2	1

Applying the χ^2 test between results for: new and 0–6 months, $p = 0.014$; 0–6 months and 7–12 months, $p = 0.655$; 7–12 months and 13+ months, $p = 0.646$.

TABLE 20.4   Patients' Perception of the Degree of Comfort of Prosthesis

Comfort	1 (Excellent)	2	3	4	5 (Poor)
New (*n* = 45)	33	9	1	1	1
0–6 months (*n* = 14)	9	4	0	0	1
7–12 months (*n* = 19)	11	4	2	2	0
13+ months (*n* = 12)	8	1	3	0	0

Applying the χ^2 test between results for: new and 13+ months, $p = 0.08$.

TABLE 20.5   Patients' Perception of the Realism of Color Match

Color Match	1 (Excellent)	2	3	4	5 (Poor)
New (*n* = 45)	34	9	2	0	0
0–6 months (*n* = 14)	5	4	5	0	0
7–12 months (*n* = 19)	9	1	5	4	0
13+ months (*n* = 12)	3	1	3	4	1

Applying the χ^2 test between results for: new and 0–6 months, $p = 0.003$; 0–6 months and 7–12 months, $p = 0.097$; 7–12 months and 13+ months, $p = 0.545$.

TABLE 20.6   Patients' Perception of Realism of Prosthesis Shape and Reproduction of Fine Detail

	1 (Excellent)	2	3	4	5 (Poor)
Realism of shape (*n* = 45)	34	8	2	1	0
Realism of fine detail (*n* = 45)	34	9	2	0	0

TABLE 20.7   Patients' Overall Opinion of Prosthesis

Overall Opinion	Excellent	Good	Adequate	Poor
New (*n* = 45)	35	9	0	0
0–6 months (*n* = 14)	5	7	1	1
7–12 months (*n* = 19)	4	8	6	1
13+ months (*n* = 12)	4	5	2	1

Applying the χ^2 test between results for: new and 0–6 months, $p = 0.196$; 0–6 months and 7–12 months, $p = 0.288$; 7–12 months and 13+ months, $p = 0.178$.

outings, 2 (4%) on other occasions, and 1 (2%) did not provide a response. The number of hours per day that prostheses were worn was 0–3 (3 (6%)), 4–7 (4 (9%)), 8–11 (13 (28%)), 12–15 (19 (40%)), 16–19 (6 (13%)), 20–24 hours (1 (2%)), and no response (1 (2%)).

The results for difficulty associated with cleaning the implants were presented as a 5-point Likert Scale with a score of 1 for easy and 5 for difficult. Eighteen respondents reported a score of 1 (38%), 9 (19%) a score of 2, 12 (26%) a score of 3, 4 (9%) a score of 4, and 2 (4%) a score of 5. Two respondents did not provide a response.

The degree of difficulty experienced when inserting or removing the prosthesis was recorded using the Likert scale. Forty-one (87%) respondents reported no difficulty with a score of 1, 4 (9%) a score of 2, 1 (2%) a score of 4, and 1 (2%) a score of 5.

Patients' perceptions of the quality of fit of the prostheses at the edges are presented in Table 20.3. Patients' perceptions of degree of comfort are presented in Table 20.4. In terms of realism of color match of the prosthesis, the results are presented in Table 20.5. Patients' opinions of shape and fine detail of their prostheses when new are provided in Table 20.6. Patients were asked to give their prostheses overall scores for quality when new and at the present time. Scores were gathered as excellent, good, adequate, or poor. Each category was given a numerical value to enable a mean score to be calculated. The results are presented in Table 20.7.

DISCUSSION

In many instances our results were similar to previous studies, with a few exceptions. The distribution by patient gender (68% male, 32% female) demonstrated similar proportions of the sexes as reported in previous studies.[10,11] Previous studies reported a higher number of nose prostheses than the 8% here.[10,11]

The mean prosthesis life span in this survey, 14 months, was slightly longer than the values reported in previous studies.[12–14] A possible reason for this could be the introduction and use of improved materials for maxillofacial prostheses. Despite this improvement, the life spans of the prostheses were relatively short. The majority of replacement prostheses in this study were provided as a result of color fade or wear of the silicone material of the previous prostheses. No significant differences were attributed to sex or age of the respondents. One might expect an increase in longevity for ear prostheses provided for females with long hair, due to a possible reduction in environmental exposure as a result of protection by the hair. The limited longevity of facial prostheses can often be attributed to deterioration of the material from which they are constructed, and, in particular, due to color instability. Studies have reported that color fading is a common reason for patients disliking their prostheses. The discoloration of facial prostheses may be the result of intrinsic or extrinsic colorations secondary to environmental factors. It is a complex multifactorial phenomenon and may include several factors such as the intrinsic characteristics of the material, pigments, personal habits (cleaning regimes and use of cosmetics), and environmental staining (climate, fungal, and body oil accumulation).[10] It is important that research continues in this field.

Patient expectation of the longevity of their current prostheses did not significantly vary from the longevity of previous prostheses. Males had a mean prosthesis longevity of 11.4 months with an expectation of longevity of 14.3 months. Therefore, men tended to have an overestimated expectation of the longevity of their prostheses. Females had lower expectation of prosthesis longevity (15.8 months) than the life spans of previous prostheses worn (17.8 months).

A significant difference was observed in expected prosthesis life span among patients who had worn prostheses previously and those who were wearing their first prosthesis. The results demonstrated that those individuals with no previous experience had unrealistic expectations of prosthesis longevity, with a mean value of 17.8 months. In comparison, individuals with previous experience had reduced expectations with a mean of 14.4 months. This was an important finding, as unrealistic expectations of prosthesis longevity could be a potential cause of patient dissatisfaction with treatment. Average prosthesis longevity should be discussed during the formulation of the treatment plan for the achievement of realistic goals within the treatment provided.

Another problem identified by first-time wearers of prostheses was difficulty inserting and removing the prostheses. First-time wearers found this task significantly more difficult than patients with previous maxillofacial prostheses. This finding highlighted the importance of sufficient instruction in insertion and removal of the prosthesis.

In terms of quality of fit at the prosthesis edges, the results demonstrated that the patients' perceptions of the quality of fit was good upon insertion of the prosthesis and decreased with time. Regarding the degree of comfort (Table 20.4), the patient opinions demonstrated a high satisfaction with their new prostheses and decreased satisfaction as the prostheses aged. This is in agreement with a previous study.[17]

In terms of the patients' opinions of the overall quality of their prostheses, the results demonstrated that a large number of patients were satisfied, giving a score of excellent or good for their prosthesis.

CONCLUSIONS

Fabrication of maxillofacial prostheses is time-consuming, labor intensive, and costly. The results of this study demonstrated that for some patients the expected longevity of their prosthesis is higher than the actual longevity of the prosthesis. It is important, therefore, that advice is given to patients on the expected average longevity of their prosthesis, together with information on factors affecting the longevity at the first appointment. Many of the replacement prostheses were provided due to color fading of the original prostheses, highlighting the need for continuing research in the development of materials used for the construction of facial prostheses with improved properties—particularly improved color stability.

REFERENCES

1. Beumer J, Marunick M, Curtis T, et al: Acquired defects of the mandible: aetiology, treatment and rehabilitation. In Beumer J, Curtis TA, Marunick MT: *Maxillofacial Rehabilitation: Prosthodontic and Surgical Considerations*. St. Louis, Ishiyaku EuroAmerica, 1996.

2. Macgregor FC: Social and psychological implications of dentofacial disfigurement. *Angle Orthod* 1970;40:231–233.

3. Newton JT, Fiske J, Foote O, et al: Preliminary study of the impact of loss of part of the face and its prosthetic restoration. *J Prosthet Dent* 1999;82:585–590.

4. Ali A, Patton DW, Fardy MJ: Prosthodontic rehabilitation in the maxilla following treatment of oral cancer. *Dent Update* 1994;21:282–286.

5. Bailey LW, Edwards D: Psychological considerations in maxillofacial prosthetics. *J Prosthet Dent* 1975;34:533–538.

6. Sela M, Lowental U: Therapeutic effects of maxillofacial prostheses. *Oral Surg Oral Med Oral Pathol* 1980;50:13–16.

7. Lemon JC, Chambers MS, Jacobsen ML, et al: Colour stability of facial prostheses. *J Prosthet Dent* 1995;74:613–618.

8. Polyzois GL: Color stability of facial silicone prosthetic polymers after outdoor weathering. *J Prosthet Dent* 1999;82:447–450.

9. Gary JJ, Smith CT: Pigments and their application in maxillofacial elastomers: a literature review. *J Prosthet Dent* 1998;80:204–208.

10. Branemark PI, Tolman DE (eds): *Osseointegration in Craniofacial Reconstruction*. Chicago, Quintessence, 1998.

11. Polyzois GL, Tarantili PA, Frangou MJ, et al: Physical properties of a silicone prosthetic elastomer stored in simulated skin secretions. *J Prosthet Dent* 2000;83:572–577.

12. Chen MS, Udagama A, Drane JB: Evaluation of facial prostheses for head and neck cancer patients. *J Prosthet Dent* 1981;46:538–544.

13. Jani RM, Schaaf NG: An evaluation of facial prostheses. *J Prosthet Dent* 1978;39:546–550.

14. Jebreil K: Acceptability of orbital prostheses. *J Prosthet Dent* 1980;43:82–85.

15. Aziz T, Waters M, Jagger R: Surface modification of an experimental silicone rubber maxillofacial material to improve wettability. *J Dent* 2003;31:213–216.

16. Arcuri MR, Rubenstein JT: Facial implants. *Dent Clin North Am* 1998;42:161–175.

17. Markt JC, Lemon JC: Extraoral maxillofacial prosthetic rehabilitation at the M.D. Anderson Cancer Center: a survey of patient attitudes and opinions. *J Prosthet Dent* 2001;85:608–613.

21

IMMEDIATE OBTURATOR STABILIZATION USING MINI DENTAL IMPLANTS

GREGORY C. BOHLE, DDS,[1] WILLIAM W. MITCHERLING, DDS,[2] JOHN J. MITCHERLING, DDS,[3] ROBERT M. JOHNSON, DDS,[4] AND GEORGE C. BOHLE III, DDS, FACP[5]

[1]Resident, Department of Oral and Maxillofacial Surgery, Long Island Jewish Hospital, NY
[2]Chief, Department of Oral and Maxillofacial Surgery, St. Agnes Hospital, Baltimore, MD
[3]Chief, Department of Oral and Maxillofacial Surgery, The Good Samaritan Hospital, Baltimore, MD
[4]Department of Oral and Maxillofacial Surgery, Upper Chesapeake Medical Center, Baltimore, MD
[5]Director, Maxillofacial Prosthetics Program, Department of Surgery-Dental Service, Memorial Sloan-Kettering Cancer Center, New York, NY

Keywords
Maxillectomy; head and neck surgery; oral cancer; MTI; MDI; osseointegrated implants; endosseous implants.

Correspondence
George C. Bohle, III, Director, Maxillofacial Prosthetics Program, Department of Surgery-Dental Service, Memorial Sloan-Kettering Cancer Center, 1275 York Ave., New York, NY 10021. E-mail: bohleg@mskcc.org

Accepted April 18, 2007

Published in *Journal of Prosthodontics* August 2008; Vol. 17, Issue 6

doi: 10.1111/j.1532-849X.2008.00321.x

ABSTRACT

Edentulous patients with maxillary defects face a more challenging oral rehabilitation process than dentate patients. With the use of mini dental implants (MDIs), it is now possible to immediately increase obturator retention and stability. Implant patients can have a retentive obturator that enhances the overall efficacy of the prosthesis both in comfort and function.

Restoration of an edentulous patient with a maxillary defect poses a challenge to the treating prosthodontist. Without teeth to provide clasping, the prosthodontist has to rely on other means for retention and stabilization of the obturator. Brown advocates extensive use of the lateral walls of the defect to stabilize the prosthesis.[1] Several other authors have suggested resilient materials to engage key mucosal soft tissue undercuts to provide stabilization and retention,[2–6] and additional authors have advocated using conventional implants to retain and support the prosthesis.[7–14] This report

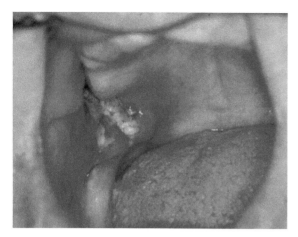

FIGURE 21.1   Preoperative photograph of maxillary tumor.

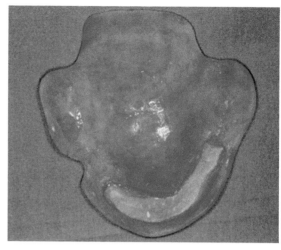

FIGURE 21.2   Surgical obturator with trough to fit over implants.

describes the use of mini dental implants (MDIs) placed coincident with a maxillectomy to aid in stabilization of the edentulous obturator.

CLINICAL REPORT

An 81-year-old, Caucasian male patient presented on referral from the Otolaryngology Head and Neck service with a diagnosis of a 3-cm, $T_2N_0M_0$, poorly differentiated squamous cell carcinoma of the right maxilla and sinus, approximating the bicuspid region and extending posteriorly to the hamular notch (Fig 21.1). Prior medical history was noncontributory; the patient was not taking any medications at the time of referral and had no known drug allergies. The patient was completely edentulous in the maxilla and had a partially edentulous mandible with right and left cuspids present. The patient wore a complete maxillary denture, which had been recently relined, and an acceptably fitting and retentive mandibular removable partial denture (RPD). A panoramic radiograph was obtained to evaluate the bone available for implant placement. The patient consented to placement of MDIs at the time of resection.

Two irreversible hydrocolloid impressions of the maxillary arch were made and poured in vacuum-mixed type III stone; the first for a permanent preoperative record and the second for a working cast. A surgical obturator was then fabricated using the working cast and the procedures demonstrated by Huryn and Piro[15] with the following modification to the aforementioned procedure: a wax rim, 6 mm high and 10 mm wide measured from the top of the ridge, was attached to the cast at the site of the proposed implants, and visible light-cured resin was used to fabricate the prosthesis. This wax rim forms a relieved trough to fit over the implants and allows for complete seating of the surgical obturator (Fig 21.2).

At the time of resection, four MDIs (MDI-MAX™, IMTEC Corp., Ardmore, OK), 2.4 × 13 mm, were placed

in the remaining maxilla. The implants were placed parallel to one another at a distance of 6 mm from the center of the adjacent implant. The number of implants will vary relative to the amount of remaining maxilla and in relationship to the maxillary sinus. Patients benefit from the placement of as many implants as possible. The implant sites were prepared using the 1.1-mm pilot drill to perforate the maxilla. The depth of the osteotomy sites is less than 3 mm, which provides maximum engagement of the implant to the bone. The finger driver was used for the initial seating, and once significant resistance was met, the winged thumb wrench was used until the implant would not advance any further. Finally, the ratchet wrench was used to complete the seating of the implant. All the threads were subgingival with only the collar of the implant and the retentive o-ball protruding. The implants were placed while waiting for the results of frozen sections, which did not extend the overall operative time. Once the implants were placed, the surgical obturator was fixed to the remaining maxillary ridge with 24-gauge stainless steel ligature wire (Fig 21.3).

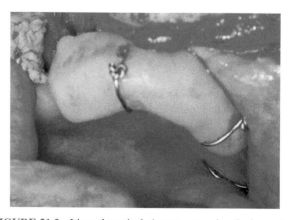

FIGURE 21.3   Ligated surgical obturator covering the immediate implants.

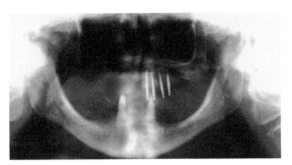

FIGURE 21.4 Postoperative Panorex demonstrating the mini implants in the remaining maxilla.

On postoperative day 5, the surgical obturator and packing was removed. The mouth was gently cleaned, and a postoperative panoramic radiograph and intraoral photographs were completed (Figs 21.4 and 21.5). At this point, the existing denture was modified and converted into the interim obturator prosthesis. Pressure-indicating paste was placed on the top of the o-ball, and the obturator was marked for the approximate implant location. The internal aspect of the denture was relieved to allow complete seating of the prosthesis intraorally with the retentive O-ring housings in place. The obturator portion was then formed with tissue conditioner (COE Comfort, Dentsply, York, PA) and trimmed to fit. Once the defect was sufficiently obturated, the retentive housings were incorporated into the prosthesis using autopolymerizing acrylic resin (Fig 21.6). The occlusion was adjusted using articulating paper and having the patient close. Over the ensuing weeks, the patient's range of motion improved, and the occlusion was further equilibrated with a clinical remount.

Upon successfully forming the obturator prosthesis and incorporating the retentive housings, the patient was instructed on the insertion, removal, and care of the prosthesis and implants. Removal should take place using both hands bilaterally and pulling straight down off the implants. Insertion takes some practice, but after a few days in front of the mirror the patient will be able to insert the prosthesis by feel. Using the dominant hand, have the patient use the

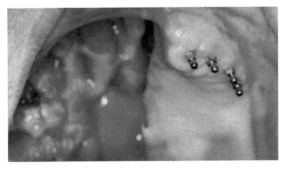

FIGURE 21.5 Postoperative intraoral photograph of the immediate implants.

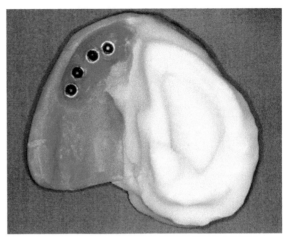

FIGURE 21.6 Completed interim obturator with resilient liner and incorporated O-ring housings.

prosthesis to move the cheek on the defect side laterally and direct the obturator portion first, the unaffected side can then be rotated into place. Once in the mouth, the patient will feel for the implants and press firmly in a superior direction using both hands until the prosthesis is fully seated. Discourage the patient from biting the prosthesis into place, as this could result in damage to the retentive O-rings, necessitating more frequent replacement.

Five weeks following surgery, the patient was treatment-planned for 33 fractions of external beam radiation therapy. Three months postradiation therapy, a primary impression of the maxilla and the surgical defect area was made with irreversible hydrocolloid for the fabrication of a definitive obturator. The impression was poured with type II stone, and the cast was used to construct a custom tray. The implant areas were marked with an indelible pen on the cast, which then transferred to the custom tray. Relief was provided in this area to ensure complete seating of the custom tray. The tray was then border molded, and a secondary impression was made with a 1:1 ratio of light and regular viscosity polysulfide. Once set, the impression material was removed from around the implants, and the metal retentive housings were placed on the implants. After roughing the custom tray with an acrylic bur, the retentive housings were attached using autopolymerizing acrylic resin as previously described. Implant analogues were placed into the incorporated housings, the impression was boxed, and type III stone was vacuum mixed and poured for the master cast (Fig 21.7). A base plate with O-ring housings was fabricated with a wax rim. Following wax rim modification, jaw relation records were made, and the casts were mounted. A wax trial denture was fabricated and tried in the patient's mouth to verify occlusal records, phonetics, and esthetics. Once the patient signed the consent for processing, the obturator was completed using heat-processed acrylic resin (Lucitone 199,

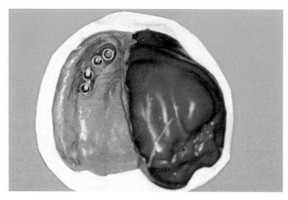

FIGURE 21.7 Secondary impression with laboratory analogs incorporated for the master cast.

Dentsply). The patient had experimented with a hollow and nonhollow designed obturator during the interim phase and was more comfortable with the nonhollow design. Using pressure-indicating paste, adjustments were made, and a remount was accomplished at the delivery appointment (Fig 21.8). The patient was then scheduled for recall appointments every 4 months, and after the 36-month follow-up period all the implants remain integrated without signs of mobility, radiolucency, or pain. The patient's oncologic and restorative prognosis is favorable and he will continue to be monitored for signs of recurrence or for implant failure.

DISCUSSION

The MDI described is a 2.4-mm diameter, self-advancing, single piece, threaded, roughened surface, titanium alloy (Ti-6Al-4V). This more open thread design allows for better penetration through cancellous bone compared to the smaller diameter, more-compact thread design used for denser bone.[16,17] This system differs from "transitional" or "modular" implants in that the surface treatment allows for osseointegration compared to transitional implant systems that have machine-polished titanium surfaces, which allow for counter

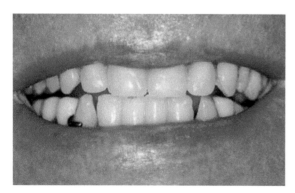

FIGURE 21.8 Completed treatment following surgery and radiation therapy.

torque removal once conventional implants have integrated.[18–28] Additionally, Kanie et al compared the mechanical properties of the mini transitional implant (MTI, Dentatus USA, New York, NY) and the MDI (IMTEC) and found that the MDI is stronger and more likely to integrate, making it suitable for long-term use.[29] Lastly, few reports are available describing the long-term success rate for MDIs.[30–32] These reports describe 32 2.4-mm × 13-mm—implants (Hi-Tec Implants, Herzlia, Israel) followed for 5 years; 27 total, 1.8-mm × 13-, 15-, and 17-mm, MDIs used as transitional implants followed for a median of 18 weeks; and a multi-institutional study of 1029 MDIs followed for 5 months to 8 years. The authors have an overall success rate of ≥92% but illustrate the disparity in reporting between short- and long-term survival and the need for further clinical research.

Once implanted, immediate use is of the utmost importance for patients needing oral rehabilitation of maxillectomy defects. Proper nutritional intake and the ability to communicate without nasality are necessary for physical and psychological healing. This immediate use is accomplished because the auto advancement thread pattern creates a stable, compacted bone interface rather than the bone healing toward the implant from a conventional osteotomy site. When conventional implants are placed in the maxilla, most practitioners will allow a minimum of 4 months healing time before second stage surgery is initiated, if the overall bone quality is favorable.[33] Some authors have suggested waiting 6 to 18 months following radiotherapy before placing conventional implants.[34] Although the exact timing of implant placement and restoration has not been established, using MDIs to enhance stabilization instantaneously improves the efficacy of the obturator.

Potential complications with this system are as with any implant system: bleeding, infection, discomfort, sinus perforation, nerve damage, lack of integration, mechanical overload, and soft tissue edema.

Note: The system described here now includes impression copings and brass analogs that accurately reproduce the implants and their positions for the master cast. At the time of this procedure, however, the impression copings were in development, so the choices were to register the implants in the impression material or in the housings.

CONCLUSION

Some practitioners find the use of mini implants controversial, as long-term survival data is sparse; however, immediate improvement in stabilization and retention of obturators can be accomplished with their aid. Placing these implants, preferably at the time of the ablative surgery, will shorten or hasten the recovery process of the edentulous patient as the obturator will be more efficacious. If planned in conjunction with the surgical team, the implants can be placed with little to no extension of the overall operative time. The patient can then begin adapting to the stable interim prosthesis quickly following packing removal and may be rehabilitated to a near presurgical level.[35]

REFERENCES

1. Brown K: Peripheral considerations in improving obturator retention. *J Prosthet Dent* 1968;20:176–181.

2. Payne AGL, Welton WG: An inflatable obturator for use following maxillectomy. *J Prosthet Dent* 1965;15:759–763.

3. Toremalm NG: A disposable obturator for maxillary defects. *J Prosthet Dent* 1973;29:94–96.

4. Schaaf NH: Obturators on complete dentures. *Dental Clin North Am* 1977;21:395–401.

5. Parr GR: A combination obturator. *J Prosthet Dent* 1979;41:329–330.

6. Taicher S, Rosen A, Arbree N, et al: A technique for fabrication of polydimethylsiloxane-acrylic resin obturators. *J Prosthet Dent* 1983;50:65–68.

7. Lorant JA, Roumanas E, Nishimura R, et al: Restoration of oral function after maxillectomy with osseous integrated implant retained maxillary obturators. *Am J Surg* 1994;168:412–414.

8. Roumanas ED, Nishimura RD, Davis BK, et al: Clinical evaluation of implants retaining edentulous maxillary obturator prostheses. *J Prosthet Dent* 1997;77:184–190.

9. Kabcenell J, Silken D, Kraut R: Restoration of a total maxillectomy patient using endosseous implants. *Int J Prosthodont* 1992;5:179–183.

10. Ihara K, Masaaki G, Miyahara A, et al: Multicenter experience with maxillary prostheses supported by Branemark implants: a clinical report. *Int J Oral Maxillofac Implants* 1998;13:531–538.

11. Mentag PJ, Kosinski TF: Increased retention of a maxillary obturator prosthesis using osteointegrated intramobile cylinder dental implants: a clinical report. *J Prosthet Dent* 1988;60:411–414.

12. Block MS, Guerra LR, Kent JN, et al: Hemimaxillectomy prosthesis stabilized with hydroxyapatite-coated implants: a case report. *Int J Oral Maxillofac Implants* 1987;2:111–113.

13. Niimi A, Ueda M, Kaneda T: Maxillary obturator supported by osseointegrated implants placed in irradiated bone: report of cases. *J Oral Maxillofac Surg* 1993;51:804–809.

14. Beumer J, III, Curtis TA, Marunick MT: *Maxillofacial Rehabilitation Prosthodontic and Surgical Considerations*. St. Louis, MO, Ishiyaku EuroAmerica, 1996, p. 258.

15. Huryn JM, Piro JD: The maxillary immediate surgical obturator prosthesis. *J Prosthet Dent* 1989;61:343–347.

16. English CE, Bohle III GC: Diagnostic, procedural, and clinical issues with the Sendax Mini Dental Implant™. *Compendium* 2003;24(Suppl. 1):3–25.

17. Shatkin TE, Shatkin S, Oppenheimer AJ: Mini dental implants for the general dentist. *Compendium* 2003;24(Suppl. 1): 26–35.

18. Sherine El Attar M, El Shazly D, et al: Study of the effect of using mini-transitional implants as temporary abutments in implant overdenture cases. *Implant Dent* 1999;8:152–158.

19. Simon H, Caputo AA: Removal torque of immediately loaded transitional endosseous implants in human subjects. *Int J Oral Maxillofac Implants* 2002;17:839–845.

20. Froum S, Emtiaz S, Bloom MJ, et al: The use of transitional implants for immediate fixed temporary prostheses in cases of implant restoration. *Pract Periodontics Aesthet Dent* 1998;10: 737–746.

21. Minsk L: Interim implants for immediate loading of temporary restoration. *Compend Contin Educ Dent* 2001;22:186–196.

22. Brown MS, Tarnow DP: Fixed provisionalization with transitional implants for partially edentulous patients: a case report. *Pract Periodontics Aesthet Dent* 2001;13:123–127.

23. Petrungaro PS: Fixed temporization and bone-augmented ridge stabilization with transitional implants. *Pract Periodontics Aesthet Dent* 1997;9:1071–1078.

24. Bichacho N, Landsberg CJ, Rohrer M, et al: Immediate fixed transitional restoration in implant therapy. *Pract Periodontics Aesthet Dent* 1999;11:45–51.

25. Petrungaro PS: Reconstruction of severely resorbed atrophic maxillae and management with transitional implants. *Implant Dent* 2000;9:271–277.

26. Nagat M, Nagaoka S, Mukunoki OL: The efficacy of modular transitional implant placed simultaneously with implant fixtures. *Compend Contin Educ Dent* 1999;20:39–42.

27. Zubery Y, Bichacho N, Moses O, et al: Immediate loading of modular transitional implants: a histologic and histomorphometric study in dogs. *Int J Periodontics Restorative Dent* 1999;19:343–353.

28. Bohsali K, Simon H, Kan JY, et al: Modular transitional implants to support the interim maxillary overdenture. *Compend Contin Educ Dent* 1999;20:975–978.

29. Kanie T, Nagat M, Ban S: Comparison of the mechanical properties of 2 prosthetic mini-implants. *Implant Dent* 2004;13:251–256.

30. Mazor Z, Steigmann M, Leshem R, et al: Mini-implants to reconstruct missing teeth in severe ridge deficiency and small interdental space: a 5-year case series. *Implant Dent* 2004;13: 336–341.

31. Ahn MR, An KM, Choi JH, et al: Immediate loading with mini dental implants in the fully edentulous mandible. *Implant Dent* 2004;13:367–372.

32. Bulard RA, Vance JB: Multi-clinic evaluation using mini-dental implants for long-term denture stabilization: a preliminary biometric evaluation. *Compend Contin Educ Dent* 2005;26:892–897.

33. Misch CE: *Contemporary Implant Dentistry* (ed 2). St. Louis, MO, Mosby, 1999, pp. 234, 598.

34. Marx RE, Johnson RP: Studies in the radiobiology of osteoradionecrosis and their clinical significance. *Oral Surg Oral Med Oral Pathol* 1987;64:379–390.

35. Bohle G 3rd, Rieger J, Huryn J, et al: Efficacy of speech aid prostheses for acquired defects of the soft palate and velopharyngeal inadequacy—clinical assessments and cephalometric analysis: a Memorial Sloan-Kettering study. *Head Neck* 2005;27:195–207.

22

PROSTHETIC RECONSTRUCTION OF A PATIENT WITH AN ACQUIRED NASAL DEFECT USING EXTRAORAL IMPLANTS AND A CAD/CAM COPY-MILLED BAR

CAROLINA VERA, DDS, MS,[1] CARLOS BARRERO, BDS, MS,[1] WILLIAM SHOCKLEY, MD,[2] SANDRA ROTHENBERGER,[1] GLENN MINSLEY, DMD,[1] AND CARL DRAGO, DDS, MS[3]

[1]Department of Prosthodontics, The University of North Carolina School of Dentistry, Chapel Hill, NC
[2]Department of Otolaryngology, The University of North Carolina School of Medicine, Chapel Hill, NC
[3]Eon Clinics, Waukesha, WI

The article is associated with the American College of Prosthodontists' journal-based continuing education program. It is accompanied by an online continuing education activity worth 1 credit. Please visit www.wileyhealthlearning .com/jopr to complete the activity and earn credit.

Keywords

Maxillofacial defects; maxillofacial prosthetics; extraoral implants; craniofacial implants; nasal prosthesis.

Correspondence

Carlos Barrero, BDS, MS, 343 Brauer Hall CB 7450, Prosthodontics Department, School of Dentistry University of North Carolina at Chapel Hill, Chapel Hill, NC 27599-7450. E-mail: carlos_barrero@dentistry.unc.edu

The authors deny any conflicts of interest.

Accepted October 22, 2013

Published in *Journal of Prosthodontics* October 2014; Vol. 23, Issue 7

doi: 10.1111/jopr.12165

ABSTRACT

Traditionally, patients with maxillofacial defects have been challenging to treat. A multitude of challenges associated with maxillofacial prosthetic treatment are not typically seen with patients who need conventional prosthodontic treatment. These types of patients generally require replacement of significant amounts of hard and soft tissues than do conventional prosthodontic patients. Most maxillofacial patients also warrant more emotional support than do conventional prosthodontic patients. Successful maxillofacial prosthetics still need to embrace the traditional goals of prosthodontic treatment: stability, support, retention, and esthetics. It is unlikely that a maxillofacial prosthesis will exactly duplicate the anatomy and function of missing or damaged structures. Although craniofacial implants (CFI's) have lower cumulative survival rates (CSR's) than intraoral endosseous implants, osseointegrated CFI's have proven to be significant adjuncts to improving retention of maxillofacial prostheses. However, CSR's of CFI's have been reported to be lower than CSR's for intraoral endosseous implants. Lately, computer-assisted design and computer-assisted machining (CAD/CAM) has been used in dentistry to facilitate fabrication of implant-supported frameworks. CAD/CAM protocols have numerous advantages over conventional casting techniques, including improved accuracy and biocompatibility, and decreased costs. The purpose of this paper is to review the literature on cumulative survival rates (CSR's) reported for CFI's and to illustrate the treatment of a maxillofacial patient using CFI's and a CAD/CAM copy-milled framework for retention and support of a nasal prosthesis.

Changes in midface and maxillofacial region anatomy due to acquired or congenital defects generally result in an array of physical changes and emotional patient responses.[1] Gillis et al[1] reported no significant differences between the Minnesota Multiphasic Personality Inventory (MMPI) means of a group of maxillofacial patients versus the MMPI means of a Mayo Clinic patient control group. It was also reported that most of the maxillofacial patients resumed their normal social habits and that patients in the study seemed to respond to their new clinical situations according to their existing personalities. It has been the authors' experience that optimal facial and oral rehabilitation allows maxillofacial patients to resume their normal social habits, which is consistent with Gillis et al's findings.

It is unlikely that maxillofacial prostheses will exactly duplicate the anatomy of missing or damaged structures. One of the goals associated with maxillofacial treatment is that the physiologic and functional aspects of maxillofacial prosthetic reconstructions will be improved. In some instances, such as replacement of eyes, noses, or ears, the total function of these organs cannot be replaced. Eckert and Desjardins[2] suggested that patients should be provided with prostheses that are comfortable and do not cause irritation. In the past, maxillofacial prosthesis retention has been dependent on frictional contact between prostheses and anatomic structures (skin, mucosa), as well as anatomic undercuts. Frictional contact may result in irritation that cause changes in residual anatomy and increased patient discomfort. These changes generally have negative impacts on overall patient satisfaction. Success of a maxillofacial prosthetic rehabilitation is assessed in terms of prosthesis stability, retention, and support as well as satisfying the patient's expectations of the prostheses approximation of normal contours and anatomy. These goals are similar to goals for success in conventional prosthodontics.

Often, patients experience difficulties with maxillofacial prostheses that use traditional mechanisms of retention. This is especially true when dealing with prosthesis positioning, due to maxillofacial prostheses generally having to be placed in one movement. Otherwise, adhesives, rubber bands, or other retentive elements may lose their retention. Moisture, which occurs by condensation on the interior of nasal prostheses, also reduces retention. Chemical interactions of adhesives with external stains within or on maxillofacial prostheses may cause discoloration. Reactions with prosthetic materials can cause corrosion of materials, and interactions with skin can cause irritation and breakouts.[3]

Parel et al[4] stated that osseointegrated fixtures in the cranial skeleton for retention of facial prostheses marked a revolutionary step in the search for improved soft tissue and maxillofacial replacement. This was later reinforced by Arcuri and Rubenstein.[5] Extraoral maxillofacial prosthetics retained via osseointegrated implants have provided advantages that include improved retention, ease of placement, and retention that is not sensitive to environmental factors such as moisture.[6] Placing implants for predictable osseointegration depends on both osteoinduction and osteoconduction processes for osteosynthesis to be properly stimulated and for recruiting nearby mesenchymal cells to produce bone around embedded implants.

The success of an endosseous implant depends on the level of bone growth around and into the implant. Success is affected by factors that include implant metal material, implant surface roughness, and bone type. Titanium, with a moderately rough surface, is currently the material and surface quality of choice for implants due to the metal's noncorrosive nature and its positive effect on osteosynthesis.[7] Facial bones are classified according to their hardness and density, as described by Lekholm and Zarb.[20] The classifications are Types 1, 2, 3, and 4, with bone density and hardness decreasing in Types 2, 3, and 4. Type 4 bone consists of fine trabecular bone, and it has been described as soft and spongy. Bone Types 1, 2, and 3 have been described as more favorable bone types for implants. When placing implants in Type 4 bone, more time should be allowed for proper osseointegration of the implant.[21]

Endosseous craniofacial implants (CFI's) allow existing elastomer technology to be used to its greatest potential by protecting surface colorations of maxillofacial prostheses, eliminating adhesive-induced base material degeneration, and maintaining long-term fine, thin peripheral margins. Although not all maxillofacial patients are candidates for CFI's, the use of endosseous extraoral implants has proved to be a valuable replacement for available adhesive systems. CFI's and the prosthesis need to withstand the typical forces experienced by the anatomy being replaced without compromising any underlying anatomy. To meet these expectations and to have success with the CFI's, special considerations are necessary for bone depth and type, possibility of future irradiation treatments, and consistent patient hygiene. It has been reported that successful use of dental implants improves retention, and provides a positive impact on patient satisfaction for maxillofacial prosthetics.[7,8]

Implant frameworks for fixed complete dentures were initially waxed around machined gold alloy cylinders, cast with high alloys, and screwed into place with small retaining screws.[13] These prostheses splinted implants together via rigid metallic frameworks that fulfilled the objectives of strength, support, nontissue impingement, and noninterference to obtain the desired results.[14] It was necessary to achieve passive and accurate fitting between restorative components and implants.[15,16] The increased use of computer-assisted design and computer-assisted machining (CAD/CAM) in dentistry has increased the accuracy and improved the biocompatibility of implant frameworks. CAD/CAM frameworks fit more accurately when compared to frameworks cast conventionally with high noble alloys.[17,18]

The factors noted above have resulted in challenging processes, and improved results, for clinical teams dealing with patients with maxillofacial extraoral defects. This report describes the presentation of a patient with a nasal defect and the subsequent fabrication of a nasal prosthesis retained by an implant-retained, titanium alloy, CAD/CAM milled bar.

CLINICAL REPORT

Patient Presentation

A 71-year-old Caucasian man with well-controlled Type 2 diabetes and a history of smoking presented to the prosthodontic clinic at the University of North Carolina–Chapel Hill. He had been treated surgically with total rhinectomy and near-total septomy as a result of a squamous cell carcinoma of the right nasal septum (2005). The medical history revealed that he was diagnosed 3 years previous to the initial presentation to the prosthodontic clinic and had a partial rhinectomy with primary radiation treatment for the recommended period of time. The amount and fields for this radiation therapy were not available for the authors; however, the nasal lesion recurred 5 months later. Due to the recurrence, the patient underwent a total rhinectomy with a left neck dissection. The neck dissection revealed three lymph nodes with involvement and extracapsular extension in the cervical 1–2 regions–49 lymph nodes were removed. The patient was treated with concurrent radiation postoperatively to a total dose of 6300 cGy in 180 cGy fractions. The tumor bed region and contralateral neck received similar doses. The left supraclavicular region received 5040 cGy.

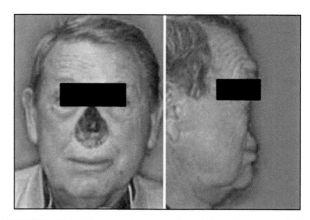

FIGURE 22.1 Preoperative frontal and lateral views of the patient.

At the time of his presentation to the prosthodontic clinic, the clinical extraoral examination revealed resected tissue margins of normal color and shape (Fig 22.1). The nasal mucosa was slightly inflamed. Intraoral examination demonstrated a normal dentition with several missing mandibular molars. A cephalometric radiograph demonstrated adequate bone volume for three extraoral implants surrounding the nasal defect.

Treatment Plan

There was adequate bone volume for the placement of three CFI's in the superior anterior maxilla and glabella regions surrounding the defect. The anterior maxilla was evaluated as Type 3 bone, while the glabella region consisted of hard, compact bone classified as Type 1 or Type 2–these bone types have been described as favorable for successful implant osseointegration.[21] The treatment plan called for implants to be placed with a two-stage surgical protocol. After osseointegration, the implants were to be uncovered; impressions were then to be made to fabricate a titanium alloy framework using a CAD/CAM protocol. Due to the complexity of the framework for the nasal prosthesis, instead of designing a framework with a computer software program, it was thought that a customized wax pattern would be more beneficial. The pattern was to be developed first on the master cast. The wax pattern and master cast (with implant analogs) would then be sent to a milling center for scanning. The scanned data would be transferred to a milling machine for milling the titanium alloy framework. This process is called copy milling, whereby a wax pattern is fabricated by hand and scanned, and a framework is milled from the digitized data. In this instance, magnetic attachments were to be used for retention of the prosthesis. The attachment housings were waxed into the wax pattern prior to scanning, and then subsequently be cemented into the framework for retention of the nasal prosthesis.

Implant Placement

A diagnostic impression was made of the defect and surrounding areas for fabrication of a diagnostic cast. The initial nasal prosthesis was developed in wax, and a clear acrylic resin duplicate of the nasal prosthesis was fabricated for use as a surgical guide and scanning template (Fig 22.2). Radiopaque markers were placed into the surgical guide/scanning appliance. Under general anesthesia, two 4-mm-long CFI's (Vistafix System, Cochlear Corp, Englewood, CO) were placed into the anterior maxilla on either side of the nasal septum and a third implant 3-mm long was placed into the glabella region (Vistafix System). The implants were placed with a two-stage surgical protocol. The implants achieved primary stability. The implants were screwed into position using the handpiece at a 20:1 ratio. When the collars of the implants were against the recessed platform on the outer cortex of the bone, the surgeon discontinued use of the drill unit and used the hand wrench to slowly tighten the implants until resistance was felt. Cover screws were inserted into the

implants and the incisions were closed. The area was covered, and a standard dressing was applied to the area. Six months later the implants were uncovered; all three implants were assessed as clinically stable and considered to be osseointegrated. Three abutments (4 mm cuff height; Vistafix System) were placed and hand tightened. The patient was ready to begin the restorative phase of treatment. During the healing process, the patient decided not to wear any prosthesis. The area was covered with a facial bandage that the patient changed on a daily basis.

Restorative Treatment

Abutment impression copings (Squared #90379, Vistafix System) were placed onto the abutments, and an abutment-level impression was made using a low-viscosity vinylpolysiloxane (VPS) impression material moulage supported by a combination of layers of reinforced high-viscosity VPS impression material.[19] Abutment replicas were attached to the impression copings. The moulage was poured in improved die stone (Hard Rock; WhipMix Corp., Louisville, KY) to generate the master cast. The cast was verified as accurate with a verification index. A nasal prosthesis wax pattern was developed using photographic records provided by the patient as a guide. The nasal prosthesis was sculpted in wax and tried in until the patient was satisfied with the appearance. A framework fabricated from acrylic resin (GC Pattern Resin; CG Corporation, Tokyo, Japan) was designed to fit within the contours of the nasal prosthesis, consistent with the amount of space needed for the nasal prosthesis, as well as satisfying the parameters for framework design relative to strength and attachment locations (Fig 22.3). The pattern was also designed to house the attachments for magnetic retentive elements (Factor II Inc., Lakeside, AZ). The framework and master cast were sent to a dental milling center (Biomet 3i, Palm Beach Gardens, FL) for scanning the resin pattern and milling the CAD/CAM titanium alloy framework using a copy mill technique.

This milling center requires that the clinicians must state that the master cast has been verified to be accurate, which

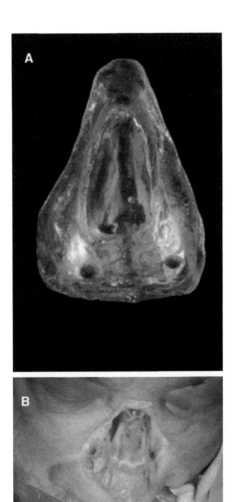

FIGURE 22.2   Clear acrylic resin stent (A) and a coronal view of the patient with the acrylic resin stent in place (B).

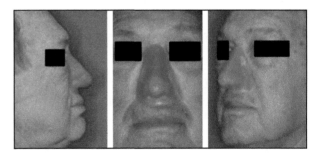

FIGURE 22.3   Lateral, frontal, and left three-fourth views of the patient with the wax prosthesis.

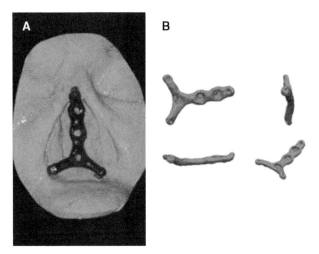

FIGURE 22.4 CAD/CAM framework. (A) Framework in place in the extraoral cast. (B) Various views of the CAD/CAM images of the wax pattern/framework.

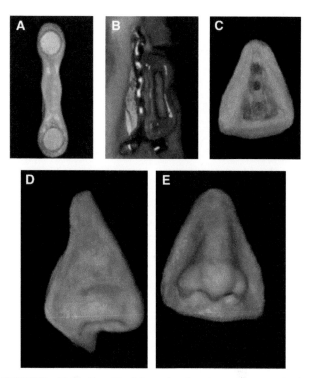

FIGURE 22.5 (A, B) Magnetic housings for prosthesis. (C) Posterior view of the silicone prosthesis. Lateral (D) and frontal (E) views of the finished silicone prosthesis.

was indicated on the work order. At the milling center, the replica analogs were evaluated as to their stability in the stone cast; they were determined to be stable. A tactile scanner was used to map the exact 3-D locations of the analogs in the cast. The resin pattern for the framework was placed onto the analogs with laboratory screws. The tactile scanner mapped the dimensions and contours of the resin pattern. A computer program reformatted the data. The titanium alloy framework was milled, polished, and returned to the authors (Fig 22.4).

The CAD/CAM framework was received at the prosthodontic clinic and evaluated for passive and accurate fit on all the analogs in the master cast. The Sheffield test was used to evaluate the fit on the analogs; the framework passed the laboratory one-screw test. The magnetic attachments were attached to the framework using autopolymerizing acrylic resin (Jet Repair Acrylic P&L Clear; Lang Dental Manufacturing Company, Wheeling, IL). The actual superstructure acrylic resin framework was incorporated directly into the final silicone nasal prosthesis when silicone mass was packed into the flasks. The nasal prosthesis was processed using a combination of Silastic MDX4–4210 and Silastic Medical Adhesive Silicone Type A (Dow Corning, Ayer, MA) with a conventional manual flasking and packing technique (Fig 22.5). The silicone material was intrinsically stained with various artist oils and dry earth pigments prior to packing the material into the flask.

For insertion of the prosthesis, the titanium alloy CAD/CAM framework was placed onto the standard abutments and hand tightened using gold alloy screws (Fig 22.6). The silicone nasal prosthesis went to place on the metal framework retained by the magnets. The nasal prosthesis was characterized based on the patient's skin tone. The patient was very pleased with the results of treatment (Fig 22.7).

Hygiene instructions and demonstrations were given to the patient relative to the silicone and metallic components of the nasal prosthesis. This included instructing the patient on a daily cleaning routine that included cleaning in, under, and around the framework. These efforts would help keep the soft tissues reaction-free and reduce the chance of skin irritation or infection.

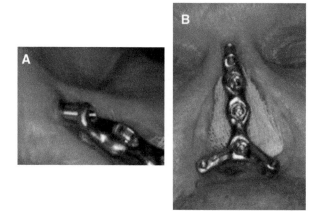

FIGURE 22.6 The framework in place on the patient. (A) Close-up view of the superior abutment screw in the framework. (B) Frontal view of the framework on the patient.

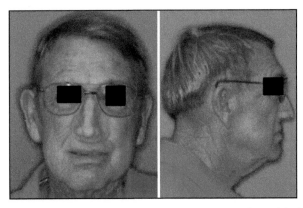

FIGURE 22.7 Frontal and lateral views of the patient with the completed nasal prosthesis in place.

DISCUSSION

In a clinical study published in 1996 with a 6- to 74-month follow-up, Nishimura et al[9] reported implant survival for extraoral endosseous implants used as retention for nasal prostheses at 71.4%. They also noted that implant survival was highly dependent on specific anatomic sites. Implant survival for implants placed into the glabella region was 0% (0/4); however, implant survival for implants placed into the anterior nasal floor was 88.1% (15/17).[9] Nishimura et al[9] also reported that severe soft tissue reactions around implants placed into the anterior nasal floor were rare. In another clinical study published in 2008, Karakoca et al[10] also concluded that anatomic sites into which implants were placed had an effect on implant survival rates; some of the sites also demonstrated peri-implant soft tissue reactions. Peri-implant soft tissue reactions were most commonly associated with lapses in hygiene. They reported that nasal and orbital implants were found to offer promising results in achieving reliable implant survival rates (83.3% and 77.4%, respectively). Regardless of the implant site, decreased survival rates and occasional peri-implant soft tissue reactions were observed in irradiated sites. In 2012, Curi et al[11] published the results of a study of overall implant and prosthesis survival rates. Their 2-year report included variables such as gender, prosthesis location, and radiotherapy. Patients studied had received extraoral implants between the years 2003 and 2010. Curi et al analyzed the long-term (2 years) results of implants used for auricular, nasal,

orbital, and complex midfacial prosthetics. They found that those patients with nasal defects had an overall implant survival rate of 90.9%. This same group had an overall prosthesis survival rate of 90.4%. These survival rates, as well as the overall implant and prosthesis survival rates of other facial areas, allowed Curi et al to conclude that extraoral implants are a safe and reliable method for retention of maxillofacial prostheses. A consensus may be offered based on current literature that extraoral implant survival rates have improved to the point where CFI's may now be routinely considered for use in maxillofacial prosthetics.

Regarding clinical survival rates and associated clinical complications of extraoral prostheses supported by CFI's, Karakoca et al[12] found that average replacement times for original prostheses were as follows: 14.1 months (auricular), 13.4 months (orbital), and 17.6 months (nasal). Survival times for the second replacement prostheses were reported at 14.4, 15.3, and 14.0 months, respectively. They concluded that implant-retained extraoral prostheses had decreased survival rates when compared to the survival rates of intraoral implant-retained or -supported prostheses. They also identified the primary reasons for making new prostheses: discoloration, tearing, and mechanical failures of the acrylic resin substructure or retentive elements. They also reported that the most common complications observed in their study were associated with decreased retention and clip activation, loosening of bar screws and abutments, and loss of attachment between silicone and acrylic resin substructures. Although they reported that implant-retained/-supported prosthetic reconstructions of facial defects had surgical limitations, compromised tissue responses, and lower implant survival rates when compared to intraoral dental implants, CFI's still provided a viable option for improved retention for maxillofacial prostheses. These studies are summarized in Table 22.1.

In this report, efforts were taken to ensure that bone type and depth of the implant sites were sufficient for successful implant osseointegration. The protocols for implant placement were carefully followed, including achieving primary stability during placement and allowing adequate time for implant osseointegration. This was done to minimize many of the common risk factors associated with implant failure, especially for implants placed in the glabella, documented to be an area of high risk for implant failure. The most common risk factors linked to failure with CFI implants are listed in Table 22.2. Also, the patient was very clearly instructed

TABLE 22.1 Prosthesis Cumulative Survival Rates

	Nishimura et al study (1996)[9]	Karakoca et al study (2008)[10]	Curi et al study (2012)[11]
Cumulative survival rates	71.40%	83.30%	90.40%
Type of prosthesis	Nasal	Nasal	Nasal
Study time period	6–74 month follow-up	2 years	7 years

TABLE 22.2   Common Risk Factors Associated with Implant Failure

Common Risk Factors Associated with Craniofacial Implant Failure
Lack of hygiene
Insufficient bone depth or density
Poor bone type or soft tissue type
Insufficient osseointegration
Soft tissue irritation or inflammation
Radiation therapy
Smoking habits

about the importance of hygiene procedures necessary to minimize the risk of soft tissue irritation or infection as well as to report every 6 months to the dental clinic for care and maintenance of his facial prosthesis and milled bar. Since the patient expressed satisfaction with the nasal prosthesis, and the CFI's were appropriately osseointegrated, the nasal prosthesis with copy-milled CAD/CAM framework was deemed successful.

SUMMARY

CFI's have been shown to have lower cumulative survival rates when compared to intraoral endosseous implants; however, when CFI's can be placed and are successful, they can be a tremendous asset to maxillofacial patients for improved retention, stability, support, and function of their maxillofacial prostheses. This clinical report illustrated the use of CFI's and a copy-milled CAD/CAM framework in the successful, short-term treatment of a patient with a nasal prosthesis, secondary to cancer resection of a nasal tumor. Further clinical research is required relative to the longevity of CFI's in maxillofacial prosthetics. In addition to this, further implementation of CAD/CAM technology for more components of the prosthesis, including the prosthesis itself, needs to be explored for feasibility and utility reasons.

ACKNOWLEDGMENTS

The authors thank Ivandario Saldarriaga, research assistant with the UNC-Chapel Hill School of Dentistry Dental Research Labs, for his help in editing the manuscript.

REFERENCES

1. Gillis R, Swenson W, Laney W: Psychological factors involved in maxillofacial prosthetics. *J Prosthet Dent* 1979;41:183–188.

2. Eckert S, Desjardins R: The impact of endosseous implants on maxillofacial prosthetics. In Taylor T (ed): *Clinical Maxillofacial Prosthetics*. Carol Stream, IL, Quintessence, 2000, p. 145.

3. Wilkes GH, Wolfaardt JF: Auricular defect: treatment options. In Branemark PI, Tolman D (eds): *Osseointegration in Craniofacial Reconstruction*. Chicago, Quintessence, 1998, p. 141.

4. Parel S, Branemark P, Tjellstrom A, et al: Osseointegration in maxillofacial prosthetics. Part II: extraoral applications. *J Prosthet Dent* 1986;55:600–606.

5. Arcuri MR, Rubenstein JT: Facial implants. *Dent Clin North Am* 1990;42:161–175.

6. Federspil PA: Implant-retained craniofacial prostheses for facial defects. *GMS Curr Top Otorhinolaryngol Head Neck Surg* 2009;8: Doc03. doi: 10.3205/cto000055. Epub 2011 Mar 10.

7. Van Doorne JM: Extra-oral prosthetics: past and present. *J Invest Surg* 1994;7:267–274.

8. Ismail JY, Zake HS: Osseointegration in maxillofacial prosthetics. *Dent Clin North Am* 1990;34:327–341.

9. Nishimura R, Roumanas E, Moy P, et al: Nasal defects and osseointegrated implants: UCLA experience. *J Prosthet Dent* 1996;76:597–602.

10. Karakoca S, Aydin C, Yilmaz H, et al: Survival rates and periimplant soft tissue evaluation of extraoral implants over a mean follow-up period of three years. *J Prosthet Dent* 2008;100:458–464.

11. Curi MM, Oliveira MF, Molina G, et al: Extraoral implants in the rehabilitation of craniofacial defects: implant and prosthesis survival rates and peri-implant soft tissue evaluation. *J Oral Maxillofac Surg* 2012;70:1551–1557.

12. Karakoca S, Aydin C, Yilmaz H, et al: Retrospective study of treatment outcomes with implant-retained extraoral prostheses: survival rates and prosthetic complications. *J Prosthet Dent* 2010;103:118–126.

13. Zarb GA, Schmitt A: The longitudinal clinical effectiveness of osseointegrated dental implants: the Toronto study. Part III: problems and complications encountered. *J Prosthet Dent* 1990;64:185–194.

14. Zarb GA, Jansson T: Prosthodontic procedures. In Branemark PI, Zarb G, Albrektsson T (eds): *Tissue-Integrated Prostheses: Osseointegration in Clinical Dentistry*. Chicago, Quintessence, 1985, pp. 250–251.

15. Zarb GA, Jansson T: Laboratory procedures and protocol. In Branemark PI, Zarb G, Albrektsson T (eds): *Tissue-Integrated Prostheses: Osseointegration in Clinical Dentistry*. Chicago, Quintessence, 1985, pp. 293–315.

16. Hjalmarsson L, Ortorp A, Smedberg JI, et al: Precision of fit to implants: a comparison of Cresco™ and Procera® implant bridge frameworks. *Clin Implant Dent Relat Res* 2010;12: 271–280.

17. Drago C, Saldarriaga RL, Domagala D, et al: Volumetric determination of the amount of misfit in CAD/CAM and cast implant frameworks: a multicenter laboratory study. *Int J Oral Maxillofac Implants* 2010;25:920–929.

18. Takahashi T, Gunne J: Fit of implant frameworks: an in vitro comparison between two fabrication techniques. *J Prosthet Dent* 2003;89:256–260.

19. Alsiyabi AS, Minsley GE: Facial moulage fabrication using a two-stage poly(vinyl siloxane) impression. *J Prosthodont* 2006;15:195–197.

20. Lekholm U, Zarb GA, Albrektsson T: *Patient Selection and Preparation. Tissue-Integrated Prostheses*. Chicago, Quintessence, 1985, pp. 199–209.

21. Jaffin RA, Berman CL: The excessive loss of Branemark fixtures in type IV bone: a 5-year analysis. *J Periodontol* 1991;62:2–4.

PART IV

IN VITRO STUDIES

23

INFLUENCE OF IMPLANT/ABUTMENT CONNECTION ON STRESS DISTRIBUTION TO IMPLANT-SURROUNDING BONE: A FINITE ELEMENT ANALYSIS

Marcia Hanaoka, dds,[1] Sergio Alexandre Gehrke, dds, phd,[2] Fabio Mardegan, dds,[1] César Roberto Gennari, dds,[1] Silvio Taschieri, md, dds,[3] Massimo Del Fabbro, bsc, phd,[3] and Stefano Corbella, dds, phd[4]

[1]University Paulista, Department of Implantology, São Paulo, Brazil
[2]Catholic University of Uruguay, Montevideo, Uruguay
[3]Università degli Studi di Milano, IRCCS Istituto Ortopedico Galeazzi, Centre for Research in Oral Health, Milan, Italy
[4]Università degli Studi di Milano, IRCCS Istituto Ortopedico Galeazzi, Centre for Research in Oral Implantology, Milan, Italy

Keywords
Finite element analysis; dental implant; internal hexagon; Morse taper.

Correspondence
Dr. Stefano Corbella, IRCCS Istituto Ortopedico Galeazzi, Via R. Galeazzi 4, 20161 Milan, Italy. E-mail: stefano.corbella@gmail.com

The authors deny any conflicts of interest.

Accepted October 5, 2013

Published in *Journal of Prosthodontics* October 2014; Vol. 23, Issue 7

doi: 10.1111/jopr.12150

ABSTRACT

Purpose: The objective of this study was to analyze and compare the stress distribution in the cortical and trabecular bone between the internal hexagon and the Morse taper systems, both with straight abutments.

Materials and Methods: Two implant systems (Morse taper and internal hexagon connections) were simulated in maxillary bone. Loads of 100 N (axial) and 50 N (oblique) in relation to the implant axes were applied. The 3D finite element method was used to simulate and analyze the present study. The analyzed parameters were ultimate tensile strength and Von Mises stress.

Results: Both systems presented stresses below the bone tissue physiological limit as well as a similar distribution in quantitative values, with a higher concentration of tension in the cortical surface near the neck of the implant in the two conditions of applied loads, with higher values for the internal hexagon system. When the groups were evaluated individually, the internal hexagon system showed higher compressive stresses, while in the Morse taper system, the highest values were traction.

Journal of Prosthodontics on Dental Implants, First Edition. Edited by Avinash S. Bidra and Stephen M. Parel.
© 2015 American College of Prosthodontists. Published 2015 by John Wiley & Sons, Inc.

Conclusions: There was a difference in the stress location on the prosthetic components of the systems studied; however, it did not influence trabecular bone stress generation.

Many studies have shown the long-term survival of dental implants placed in both the maxilla and in mandible, supporting partial or full-arch prosthetic rehabilitations.[1-6] However, early and late failures have been reported and clinically evaluated in a significant proportion of the population.[7] These complications can be classified into failures due to peri-implant tissue infections (such as peri-implantitis)[8,9] and others due to occlusal overload, which causes the loss of peri-implant bone and ultimately leads to implant mobility.[10,11]

The transmission of occlusal load to peri-implant bone tissues has widely been studied in vitro and in vivo, recognizing some influencing factors, including patient-dependent factors such as occlusal bite force, parafunctional activities, bone characteristics (bone density and quantity), and implant-prosthesis system-dependent factors such as implant length and width, implant design, texture characteristics, shape and dimensions of implant/abutment connection, materials, and prosthesis characteristics and extension.[12-16] Depending on the characteristics of occlusal load on the implant/abutment structure, the compressive or tensile stress acting at the most coronal portion of crestal bone can cause bone resorption in cases of excessive strength, in response to a microtrauma affecting the bone trabeculae.[17]

When choosing an adequate implant system, one should consider the possibility of minimizing the compressive and tensile forces at the bone-to-implant interface, to lower the risk of peri-implant bone loss due to occlusal load. Finite element analysis (FEA) has been demonstrated to be a valid device to study the distribution of forces in various implant-abutment and prosthesis configurations[12,15,18-20] and can lead to a better understanding of the most efficient implant/abutment system to minimize stress to bone. Several studies have been published analyzing different implant/abutment connections when an experimental occlusal load was applied.[21-23] The design of the implant system, its geometrical characteristics, and the connection type between abutment and implant are important factors in the stability, performance, and longevity of the prosthetic rehabilitation, as long as there is a balance between the force transmission of the bone/implant interface and the abutment/implant interface.[21,24,25]

This objective of this study was to evaluate and compare, through FEA, the generated stresses and load transmission of the abutment/implant connection to the bone tissue in two types of prosthetic connection, internal hexagon (IH) and Morse taper (MT), with the application of different loads, in the posterior region of the maxilla. The hypothesis is that a MT connection can reduce the stresses (both tensile and compressive) to peri-implant bone.

MATERIALS AND METHODS

This study was conducted in the Centro de Tecnologia da Informação Renato Archer-Tridimensional Technologies Division (CTI) in Campinas-São Paulo, Brazil. The 3D meshes used in the study were created from data supplied by the implant manufacturer (Implacil De Bortoli, São Paulo, Brazil), through AutoCAD 2008 software (Autodesk, Mill Valley, CA). Implants were conical, 10 mm long, with a 4-mm diameter. They had either an IH or MT connection. Both systems were fabricated with commercially pure titanium. The intermediate abutments of both systems were straight, made of two pieces for IH (pillar and screw) and of a single piece for MT (Fig 23.1).

No prosthetic crowns were used. The area of interest of this study allowed the abolishment of this component, since the main objective was to create a critical situation for the implant and the prosthetic component, simulating a direct load without the presence of any intermediary between the applied force and the components, excluding the distribution of tensions to adjacent elements through the proximal contact points.

The image from the section of the posterior maxilla corresponds to the first superior molar. This image was given by the CTI database, through 3D CAD software (Rhinoceros 4.0 NURBS Modeling for Windows; Robert McNeel & Associates, Seattle, WA) for the generation of a geometrical

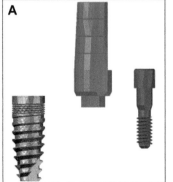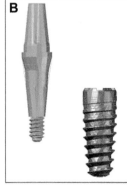

FIGURE 23.1 Components used in the study: (A) internal hexagon and (B) Morse taper.

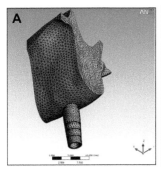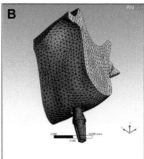

FIGURE 23.2   Model reconstruction.

model. The model of the maxillary bone from this region originated from a patient's CT, with previous approval by the Ethics Committee, being classified as type II, according to the classification proposed by Misch[26] for bone density.

The implant inclination in the 3D model followed the bone anatomy, as well as an ideal clinical hypothetical situation, considering that the IH system was placed at the bone level, and the MT system 1 mm below the cortical bone, according to the manufacturer's instructions. A cortical bone thickness of 2 mm without bone loss on the region of the maxillary sinus represented a hypothetical case of a young patient with recent dental loss in the region of the first molar. It consists of the creation of a mathematical model of the object or system in study, a geometrical phase where the design is made. The solid model is discretized (knots, elements, and mesh visualization), for the model generation of finite elements. It also specifies the properties of the materials involved, loading, and contour conditions.

Two 3D models were transferred to the ANSYS Workbench 12.1 finite element software to generate the nodal points and the mesh (Fig 23.2). These models represent the mathematical models of the implants, internal structures, abutments, and bone tissue. The material proprieties used in this study derived from those presented in the pertinent scientific literature[27–31] (Table 23.1). The Young's modulus of elasticity corresponds to the relation between stress of traction or compression and the corresponding value of elastic deformation (reversible) that a material or structure

TABLE 23.1   Mechanical Proprieties of Materials and Anatomical Structure

Material	Young's Modulus of Elasticity (E) (GPa)	Poisson Ratio (ν)
Implant	110.000	0.33
Cortical bone	13.70	0.30
Trabecular bone	1.37	0.30
Abutment screw	110.000	0.28
Abutment	110.000	0.28

may present. Anybody under action of external forces (traction and compression) presents a longitudinal deformation in the direction these forces are applied, but a deformation in the transverse direction to an axis of axial traction. The ratio between the absolute values of longitudinal and transversal deformation represents the Poisson coefficient.

In this study, a load was applied at the top of the prosthetic pillar of both systems 100 N in the axial direction, and a 50 N oblique force in the buccolingual direction in relation to its long axis at 45°. A static load analysis was performed for both models. Models were restrained at the base of the maxillary first molar in a vise-support to avoid the slipping of the entire model.

The processing step or analysis solution was conducted with the aid of ANSYS Workbench 12.1. The movement of the knots to the elements in function of the applied load was analyzed.[32] In this study, the Von Mises criterion, or theory of maximal distortion, was applied, also analyzing the ultimate tensile strength.

The Von Mises criterion is of special relevance when considering the maximum resistance of a structure when subject to two states of tension (traction and compression). This criterion determines the distortion energy of the structure, that is, the energy related to changes in its shape, as opposed to energy bound to changes in its volume, and may be analyzed in any finite element mesh simultaneously or compared.[33] The Von Mises formula is the most adequate isotropic criterion to predict the flow of ductile materials (any material that may be submitted to great deformations before its rupture), such as metals.

The analyzed parameters were ultimate tensile strength and Von Mises tension. The ultimate tensile strength analysis restricts itself to more fragile materials, which possess little or no flow, such as the bone tissue that suffers compression and traction, and has different characteristics and material coefficients.

A qualitative analysis was performed through ANSYS Workbench 12.1, by means of visual observation of the graphical images of Von Mises stress, generated and printed by the computer program. Additionally, a mathematical or quantitative analysis was conducted through the attributed values in the color columns that accompany the mathematical finite element methods (FEMs). The quantitative results represent the tensions in MPa. The Von Mises values are always positive, as they do not discriminate if the tensions are traction or compression. Further statistical analysis could not be performed because the numerical nature of the experiment would present the same data over a series of observations.

RESULTS

A joint analysis, both qualitative and quantitative, was performed. Both systems presented a transition of movement

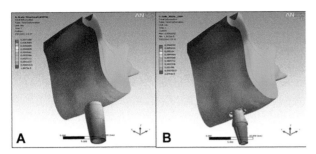

FIGURE 23.3   Image analysis of maximum displacement stress of the HI (A) and MT (B) groups.

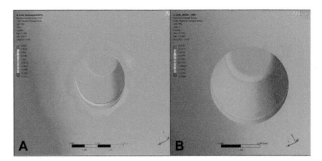

FIGURE 23.5   Stresses on the cortical bone in groups HI (A) and MT (B).

with no jumps, with a gradual decrease in the intensity of tension in the direction of the abutment to the implant and then to the tissues.

In the maximum tension movement analysis of groups IH and MT, with a 100-N load, results of 0.0071958 and 0.0066592 mm, respectively, were observed, which in terms of absolute numbers were of little significance. In the cortical bone, a deformation of 0.005 mm was noted, and this displacement decreased as it moved away from the implant (Fig 23.3).

In the maximum tension movement analysis of groups IH and MT, a 50-N load showed maximum value in the top region of the abutments in both systems; however, in the MT system, the maximum value was 0.037712 mm and in the IH system, it was 0.025065 mm, with a mean difference of 12 μm (Fig 23.4). The results showed a difference in the type of tension on the surface of the cortical bone. Compressive forces could be seen in the IH system with high absolute values. On the contrary, forces observed in the MT system were of tensile nature with a lower value. Still, the MT system presented a compression tension all around the neck of the implant, as seen in the IH, but a little below the cortical bone surface due to its positioning (Fig 23.5).

Considering the IH model, tensions of little expression in the apex of the implant, with a compression tension of −0.46162 MPa, and around its body, a traction tension of

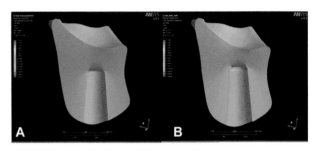

FIGURE 23.6   Stresses in trabecular bone implants HI (A) and MT (B).

0.62349 MPa was observed on both sides in trabecular bone. In the MT system, the apex region of the implant supported a compression of −0.54485 MPa and a traction tension close to the implant body of 0.43573 MPa on both sides (Fig 23.6).

In the region close to the apex of the implants, the results showed a very small difference in relation to the quantitative values presenting a very similar tension compression distribution in both systems. In the 50-N nonaxial load of the IH system, in the buccal side of the cortical bone, traction of 20.436 MPa was observed, and in the lingual side, compression of −5.0485 MPa was observed. In the MT system, the maximum stress was 6.4257 MPa in the buccal side and 3.0648 MPa in the lingual side. In this system, only traction stresses for both sides and of smaller values in relation to the IH system were found (Fig 23.7).

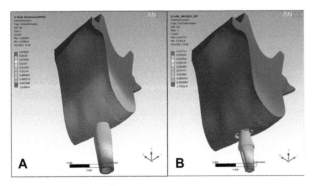

FIGURE 23.4   Maximum displacement stress (A) HI and (B) MT with a 50-N load.

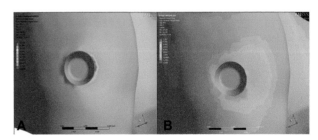

FIGURE 23.7   Stresses generated in the buccal (B) and lingual (l) of the HI (A) and MT (B) systems.

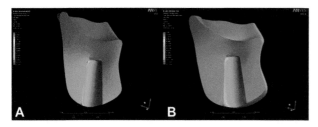

FIGURE 23.8 Stresses in the portion of the buccal and lingual models HI (A) MT (B).

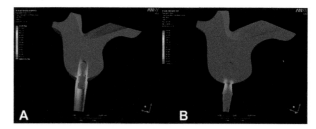

FIGURE 23.10 Von Mises stress of the HI (A) and MT (B) groups, 50 N load.

The results in the trabecular bone of the IH model in the region of the implant apex presented a compression tension of −0.12602 MPa, in the buccal side close to the apex a traction tension of 1.1262 MPa, next to the body of the implant, a traction tension of 0.48559 MPa, and in the lingual face −0.078531 MPa of compression tension. On the implant's apex region, the MT system presented a compression tension of −0.11821 MPa, the buccal side close to the implant apex a traction tension of 0.73736 MPa, next to the body of the implant a tension of 0.41652 MPa, and in the lingual face −0.011266 MPa of compression tension.

A pattern of tension distribution in the region close to the implant apex was observed with little difference in the quantitative values of tensions between the two systems (Fig 23.8). Results of Von Mises tensions with loads of 100 N for the IH system presented a larger concentration of tension on the neck of the implant distributing the tension through the body of the abutment and on its interface with the head of the internal screw of 10.309 MPa. Little tension was observed on the head of the screw, and the tensions were evenly distributed through the body of the implant, diminishing as it directed to the apex. In the MT system, the maximum tension localized more sharply on the neck of the abutment with a value of 18.827 MPa, and little tension was seen on the body of the implant (Fig 23.9). The Von Mises stress location presented itself differently between both systems, with higher quantitative values for the MT system. However, there was little tension transmission to the implant and the surrounding bone tissue.

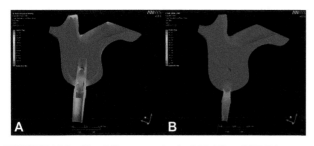

FIGURE 23.9 Von Mises stress in the MT (A) and HI (B) groups with a 100 N load.

The results of Von Mises stress for groups IH and MT (50 N load) have shown that the higher Von Mises stress of the IH system was located in the neck, and that in the buccal face, the stress was 49.278 MPa, while in the lingual face, it was 41.065 MPa. The stresses distributed along the body of the middle part of the implant were of 16.427 MPa, being the response of the tension flow coming from the abutment wall. In the MT system, the higher Von Mises stress was concentrated on the region of the abutment neck, with a value of 250.6 MPa on the buccal side and 188.37 MPa on the lingual side, being distributed almost symmetrically on the abutment and with very little stress present on the body of the implant (Fig 23.10).

DISCUSSION

The biomechanical interactions between the implants and the supported structures supply us with the knowledge of the load transmission process. The load direction, type of abutment/implant connection, implant length and diameter, and bone quality and quantity are key factors influencing the distribution of stresses to the bone tissue.[12–16] For the study of these stresses, FEM is a valuable mathematical tool used to predict the effects of stress after occlusal loading. The material shape and physical properties are built through computation, and physical interaction of several components of the model is calculated in terms of tension and deformation occurring on the tissues.[34]

In this study, the bone structure was modeled through a CT that can provide results closer to a real scenario, because there is a difference in the behavior of stresses in work conducted with elliptical models, cobblestones, and CT scan data.[35] Most of the literature[24,25,36–38] has used cylindrical bone models, blocks, or segments of maxilla with straight lines; however, we cannot dismiss the obtained results, since the FEM methodology allowed such simplification.

In the present study, the model properties were considered homogeneous, isotropic, and linearly elastic. We assumed a condition of 100% bone/implant contact and the application of static loads, which may not necessarily be a real situation, but gives an idea of what occurs clinically, since several variables are unable to be reproduced. These simplifications corroborate previous FEM studies that also used such methodology.[37,38]

Comparing the two models of implant systems, it was observed that in the ultimate tensile strength analysis, desirable biomechanical results were achieved, since the distribution was harmonious, presenting a higher stress close to the load application point (abutment), decreasing gradually toward the bone tissue. It supplies us a global view of the analysis, showing that the tested models, IH and MT, are cohesive and follow the same pattern of stress distribution, which is, higher stress around the neck of the implant, decreasing distribution toward the distal direction as well as in the vestibulo-lingual direction. This owes to the fact that in both models, conical implants of the same length and diameter were used in the same bone base. Stresses in the cortical bone surface along the neck of the implant were found in both implant systems, with a 100 N axial load as well as with a 50 N oblique load. These findings corroborate the results found in other works,[25] showing that the cortical bone participates effectively in absorbing loads transmitted through the abutment. This confirms that stresses distributed on the most coronal bone can have important clinical implications, for example, when placing short implants. In fact, it can be assumed that implant length has a minimal impact on reducing the overall stresses to the marginal bone, without affecting clinical outcomes.

In the 100 N load in the MT model, more traction than compression stresses on the cortical surface were observed, being the same quantitative values lower than the IH system with a different distribution in a smooth and diffuse fashion. Similar results have also been found in other works[15,27,39–41] when these authors compared the taper cone system with internal and external hexagon systems. The conical interface of the abutment/implant system can resist great axial tensions transmitting to the internal walls of the implant, providing a location closer to the apex. Besides, this type of connection can improve the stress distribution on the alveolar bone crest, diminishing the marginal reabsorption originating from the stress accumulation.[25,41]

The MT system presented a compression stress located below the cortical bone surface and had a behavior similar to the IH system. This can be explained by the fact of the implant being installed a little bit below the surface of the cortical bone and because of the design of the abutment geometry. In the apex region of the implant (in simulated trabecular bone) observed on two systems, the tensions are distributed evenly and with low intensity with quantitative differences of little significance and with values below the physiological values accepted by cortical and medullary bone.[15]

In the present study, the load direction influenced the intensity of the generated stresses, in the ultimate tensile strength as well as in the Von Mises stress analysis, with an increase of the stresses of both models in the oblique loading

system. Several authors reported the influence on load direction in their studies with increases in tension values of bone tissue.[24,42,43] Moreover, in the 50 N oblique load, the stress distribution occurred differently on the surface of the cortical bone close to the cervical region of the implant. In the IH system, the stresses presented in a well-defined and balanced form on both faces, while in the MT system, it occurred in a smooth and diffuse fashion; however, the stresses in the MT system were arranged similarly, but with a lower quantitative value than the IH system, where they were located a little below and on the internal face of the cortical bone, demonstrating the same behavior on stress distribution in this system. Analyzing the Von Mises stress, the IH system concentrated the higher stresses on the cervical region of the implant, and in the MT system, there was a larger concentration in the cervical region of the abutment, similar to results found by other authors.[24,25,27,36,38,40]

In this work, little tension was observed in the internal screw of the IH system with both types of loading, a positive factor in terms of fractures or looseness of this prosthetic component, which is one of the most frequent complications.[44] It can be linked to the protection granted by the larger contact area with the walls of the abutment, working as a shield protecting the screw and avoiding its loss in this connection.

Following the findings in this work, the assumption that the saucerization phenomenon is more related to the stress field than to other factors should be reviewed, because the MT system as well as the IH system presented stresses below the physiological limit of the bone. Weng et al demonstrated that saucerization can be more related to the location of the microgap between the abutment/implant than by microbiological and micromechanical factors.[45]

CONCLUSION

Based on the findings of this study, it can be concluded that both types of implants presented a similar stress distribution in the cortical and trabecular bone and below the physiological limit allowed by the bone, with an increase in the stress value when an oblique load was applied. Still, the abutment geometry of the MT system and the fact that it is more submerged in the cortical bone favored the decrease in the stress value on the surface, presenting traction stress on both types of loading.

REFERENCES

1. Adell R, Eriksson B, Lekholm U, et al: Long-term follow-up study of osseointegrated implants in the treatment of totally edentulous jaws. *Int J Oral Maxillofac Implants* 1990;5: 347–359.

2. Astrand P, Ahlqvist J, Gunne J, et al: Implant treatment of patients with edentulous jaws: a 20-year follow-up. *Clin Implant Dent Relat Res* 2008;10:207–217.

3. Jemt T, Johansson J: Implant treatment in the edentulous maxillae: a 15-year follow-up study on 76 consecutive patients provided with fixed prostheses. *Clin Implant Dent Relat Res* 2006;8:61–69.

4. Francetti L, Azzola F, Corbella S, et al: Evaluation of clinical outcomes and bone loss around titanium implants with oxidized surface: six-year follow-up results from a prospective case series study. *Clin Implant Dent Relat Res* 2014;16:81–88.

5. Mamalis A, Markopoulou K, Kaloumenos K, et al: Splinting osseointegrated implants and natural teeth in partially edentulous patients: a systematic review of the literature. *J Oral Implantol* 2012;38:424–434.

6. Nissan J, Narobai D, Gross O, et al: Long-term outcome of cemented versus screw-retained implant-supported partial restorations. *Int J Oral Maxillofac Implants* 2011;26:1102–1107.

7. Manor Y, Oubaid S, Mardinger O, et al: Characteristics of early versus late implant failure: a retrospective study. *J Oral Maxillofac Surg* 2009;67:2649–2652.

8. Lindhe J, Meyle J: Peri-implant diseases: Consensus Report of the Sixth European Workshop on Periodontology. *J Clin Periodontol* 2008;35:282–285.

9. Quirynen M, De Soete M, van Steenberghe D: Infectious risks for oral implants: a review of the literature. *Clin Oral Implant Res* 2002;13:1–19.

10. Chambrone L, Chambrone LA, Lima LA: Effects of occlusal overload on peri-implant tissue health: a systematic review of animal-model studies. *J Periodontol* 2010;81:1367–1378.

11. Tawil G: Peri-implant bone loss caused by occlusal overload: repair of the peri-implant defect following correction of the traumatic occlusion. A case report. *Int J Oral Maxillofac Implants* 2008;23:153–157.

12. Chang SH, Lin CL, Hsue SS, et al: Biomechanical analysis of the effects of implant diameter and bone quality in short implants placed in the atrophic posterior maxilla. *Med Eng Phys* 2012;34:153–160.

13. Rungsiyakull C, Rungsiyakull P, Li Q, et al: Effects of occlusal inclination and loading on mandibular bone remodeling: a finite element study. *Int J Oral Maxillofac Implants* 2011;26:527–537.

14. Jiao T, Chang T, Caputo AA: Load transfer characteristics of unilateral distal extension removable partial dentures with polyacetal resin supporting components. *Aust Dent J* 2009;54:31–37.

15. Baggi L, Cappelloni I, Di Girolamo M, et al: The influence of implant diameter and length on stress distribution of osseointegrated implants related to crestal bone geometry: a three-dimensional finite element analysis. *J Prosthet Dent* 2008;100:422–431.

16. Tabata LF, Rocha EP, Barao VA, et al: Platform switching: biomechanical evaluation using three-dimensional finite element analysis. *Int J Oral Maxillofac Implants* 2011;26:482–491.

17. Garetto LP, Chen J, Parr JA, et al: Remodeling dynamics of bone supporting rigidly fixed titanium implants: a histomorphometric comparison in four species including humans. *Implant Dent* 1995;4:235–243.

18. Lewis MB, Klineberg I: Prosthodontic considerations designed to optimize outcomes for single-tooth implants. A review of the literature. *Aust Dent J* 2011;56:181–192.

19. Assuncao WG, Barao VA, Tabata LF, et al: Biomechanics studies in dentistry: bioengineering applied in oral implantology. *J Craniofac Surg* 2009;20:1173–1177.

20. Wakabayashi N, Ona M, Suzuki T, et al: Nonlinear finite element analyses: advances and challenges in dental applications. *J Dent* 2008;36:463–471.

21. Yamanishi Y, Yamaguchi S, Imazato S, et al: Influences of implant neck design and implant-abutment joint type on peri-implant bone stress and abutment micromovement: three-dimensional finite element analysis. *Dent Mater* 2012;28:1126–1133.

22. Tang CB, Liul SY, Zhou GX, et al: Nonlinear finite element analysis of three implant-abutment interface designs. *Int J Oral Sci* 2012;4:101–108.

23. Freitas-Junior AC, Rocha EP, Bonfante EA, et al: Biomechanical evaluation of internal and external hexagon platform switched implant-abutment connections: an in vitro laboratory and three-dimensional finite element analysis. *Dent Mater* 2012;28:e218–e228.

24. Cehreli MC, Akca K, Iplikcioglu H: Force transmission of one- and two-piece Morse-taper oral implants: a nonlinear finite element analysis. *Clin Oral Implants Res* 2004;15:481–489.

25. Chun HJ, Shin HS, Han CH, et al: Influence of implant abutment type on stress distribution in bone under various loading conditions using finite element analysis. *Int J Oral Maxillofac Implants* 2006;21:195–202.

26. Misch CE: Bone classification, training keys to implant success. *Dent Today* 1989;8:39–44.

27. Quaresma SE, Cury PR, Sendyk WR, et al: A finite element analysis of two different dental implants: stress distribution in the prosthesis, abutment, implant, and supporting bone. *J Oral Implantol* 2008;34:1–6.

28. Ichim I, Swain MV, Kieser JA: Mandibular stiffness in humans: numerical predictions. *J Biomech* 2006;39:1903–1913.

29. Carter DR, Spengler DM: Mechanical properties and composition of cortical bone. *Clin Orthopaed Relat Res* 1978;135:192–217.

30. Steinemann S: The properties of titanium. In Schroeder A, Sutter F, Buser D (eds): *Oral Implantology Basics, ITI Hollow Cylinder System* (ed 2). Stuttgart, Thieme, 1996.

31. Zysset PK, Guo XE, Hoffler CE, et al: Elastic modulus and hardness of cortical and trabecular bone lamellae measured by nanoindentation in the human femur. *J Biomech* 1999;32:1005–1012.

32. Holmgren EP, Seckinger RJ, Kilgren LM, et al: Evaluating parameters of osseointegrated dental implants using finite element analysis—a two-dimensional comparative study examining the effects of implant diameter, implant shape, and load direction. *J Oral Implantol* 1998;24:80–88.

33. Mori S, Burr DB: Increased intracortical remodeling following fatigue damage. *Bone* 1993;14:103–109.

34. Bystrov VS, Paramonova E, Dekhtyar Y, et al: Computational and experimental studies of size and shape related physical properties of hydroxyapatite nanoparticles. *J Phys Condens Matter* 2011;23:065302.

35. Lambrecht JT, Berndt DC, Schumacher R, et al: Generation of three-dimensional prototype models based on cone beam computed tomography. *Int J Comput Assist Radiol Surg* 2009;4:175–180.

36. Akca K, Cehreli MC, Iplikcioglu H: Evaluation of the mechanical characteristics of the implant-abutment complex of a reduced-diameter Morse-taper implant. A nonlinear finite element stress analysis. *Clin Oral Implants Res* 2003;14:444–454.

37. Anitua E, Tapia R, Luzuriaga F, et al: Influence of implant length, diameter, and geometry on stress distribution: a finite element analysis. *Int J Periodont Res Dent* 2010;30:89–95.

38. Li T, Kong L, Wang Y, et al: Selection of optimal dental implant diameter and length in type IV bone: a three-dimensional finite element analysis. *Int J Oral Maxillofac Surg* 2009;38:1077–1083.

39. Merz BR, Hunenbart S, Belser UC: Mechanics of the implant-abutment connection: an 8-degree taper compared to a butt joint connection. *Int J Oral Maxillofac Implants* 2000;15:519–526.

40. Pessoa RS, Muraru L, Junior EM, et al: Influence of implant connection type on the biomechanical environment of immediately placed implants – CT-based nonlinear, three-dimensional finite element analysis. *Clin Implant Dent Relat Res* 2010;12:219–234.

41. Hansson S: Implant-abutment interface: biomechanical study of flat top versus conical. *Clin Implant Dent Relat Res* 2000;2:33–41.

42. Kitamura E, Stegaroiu R, Nomura S, et al: Influence of marginal bone resorption on stress around an implant–a three-dimensional finite element analysis. *J Oral Rehabil* 2005;32:279–286.

43. Lin CL, Wang JC, Ramp LC, et al: Biomechanical response of implant systems placed in the maxillary posterior region under various conditions of angulation, bone density, and loading. *Int J Oral Maxillofac* 2008;23:57–64.

44. Papaspyridakos P, Chen CJ, Chuang SK, et al: A systematic review of biologic and technical complications with fixed implant rehabilitations for edentulous patients. *Int J Oral Maxillofac Implants* 2012;27:102–110.

45. Weng D, Nagata MJ, Bell M, et al: Influence of microgap location and configuration on peri-implant bone morphology in nonsubmerged implants: an experimental study in dogs. *Int J Oral Maxillofac Implants* 2010;25:540–547.

24

AN IN VITRO COMPARISON OF FRACTURE LOAD OF ZIRCONIA CUSTOM ABUTMENTS WITH INTERNAL CONNECTION AND DIFFERENT ANGULATIONS AND THICKNESS: PART I

Abdalah Albosefi, bdt, msc,[1] Matthew Finkelman, phd,[2] and Roya Zandparsa, dds, msc, dmd[3]

[1]Former resident, Prosthodontic Division and Advanced Education in Esthetic Dentistry, Department of Prosthodontics and Operative Dentistry, Tufts University School of Dental Medicine, Boston, MA
[2]Assistant Professor, Department of Public Health and Community Service, Tufts University School of Dental Medicine, Boston, MA
[3]Clinical Professor, Prosthodontic Division and Advanced Education in Esthetic Dentistry, Department of Prosthodontics and Operative Dentistry, Tufts University School of Dental Medicine, Boston, MA

Keywords
Ceramic abutment stability; shear stress; implant/abutment connection; ceramics.

Correspondence
Dr. Roya Zandparsa, Prosthodontic Division and Advanced Education in Esthetic Dentistry, Department of Prosthodontics and Operative Dentistry, Tufts University School of Dental Medicine, 1 Kneeland St., Boston, MA 02111.
E-mail: roya.zandparsa@tufts.edu

Presented at the American College of Prosthodontists local meeting, Boston, MA, April 2012.

Research sponsored by Straumann USA LLC, Andover, MA.

Accepted August 12, 2013

Published in Journal of Prosthodontics June 2014; Vol. 23, Issue 4

doi: 10.1111/jopr.12118

ABSTRACT

Purpose: The purpose of this in vitro study was to compare the fracture load of one-piece zirconia custom abutments with different thicknesses and angulations.

Materials and Methods: Forty zirconia custom abutments were divided into four groups. Group A-1 and group B-1 simulated a clinical situation with an ideal implant position, which allows for the use of straight zirconia custom abutments with two thicknesses (0.7 and 1 mm). Groups A-2 and B-2 simulated a situation with a compromised implant position requiring 15° angulated abutments with different thicknesses (0.7 and 1 mm). Implant replicas were mounted in self-cure acrylic jigs to support the abutments in all groups. The zirconia custom abutments were engaged in the implant replicas using a manual torque wrench. Each jig was secured and mounted in a metallic vice 30° relative to a mechanical indenter. All groups were subjected to shear stress until failure using a universal testing machine with a 0.5 mm/min crosshead speed with the force transferred to the lingual surface of the zirconia custom abutments 2 mm below the top surface. The universal testing machine was controlled via a computer software system that also completed the stress-strain diagram and recorded the breaking fracture load. The fracture loads were recorded for comparison among the groups and subjected to statistical analysis (two-way ANOVA).

Results: The mean fracture load of zirconia custom abutments across the groups (A-1 through B-2) ranged from 160 ± 60 to 230 ± 95 N. The straight zirconia custom abutment exhibited the highest fracture load among the groups ($p = 0.009$); however, the thickness of the zirconia custom abutment had no influence on the strength of any of the specimens ($p = 0.827$).

Conclusions: There was no statistically significant difference in fracture strength between the 0.7 and 1.0 mm groups; however, angulated zirconia custom abutments had the lowest fracture load.

Clinical Implication: The results of this in vitro study will help dental practitioners with their decision-making process in selecting the type of custom abutment to be used clinically.

The influence of connection type on the long-term stability of the abutment/implant complex has been analyzed for metallic abutments in several studies.[1,2] In contrast, to date, the stability of one-piece internally connected zirconia abutments has not been specifically investigated. It might be expected that one-piece zirconia abutments exhibit different resistance to loading as a result of different thicknesses and angulations. Following the functional and biological success of implant-supported restorations, esthetic aspects gain primary importance. Standardized titanium abutments exhibit high survival rates because of their excellent physical properties.[3] However, their application can impair the esthetic result. In the case of soft tissue recession, exposure of the gray titanium abutment can lead to failure of the reconstruction in highly visible anterior regions.[4] Furthermore, when titanium abutments are used in patients with a thin labial mucosa, a grayish discoloration of the mucosa can occur, owing to the gray metal color showing through.[4,5] The esthetic shortcomings of titanium led to the development of ceramic materials as an alternative for esthetically demanding patients.[5]

In the search for ceramic abutment material with improved physical properties, yttria-stabilized zirconia was introduced in 1996.[6] The bending strength of zirconia is 900 MPa, and its fractural toughness reaches 9 MPa/m^2.[7] Zirconia abutments showed resistance to a high load of up to 730 N in one in vitro study.[8] In comparison, the naturally occurring mean inciso-occlusal loads in anterior regions amount to 110 N for teeth and 370 N for implants.[9,10] With these data from in vitro studies, zirconia was expected to reduce the risk of fracture; however, the type and architecture of the implant/abutment connection, thickness, and angulations might have a substantial influence on the stability and fixation of brittle ceramic abutments.

Implants are designed with different types of implant/abutment connections. The abutments can either be fixed onto an external connecting part of the implant or internally into the implant.[11] The internal connection of zirconia

abutments can be accomplished either by the abutment itself (one-piece) or by means of secondary components (two-piece). One-piece abutments are made entirely of ceramic, whereas for two-piece abutments the internal connecting part can be either a secondary titanium abutment or separate metallic insert mounted on the implant together with the abutment and fixed by means of one abutment screw.[11] The aim of this in vitro study was to compare the fracture load of one-piece zirconia custom abutments with different thicknesses and angulations.

MATERIALS AND METHODS

Sample Size and Power Calculation

For the sample size calculation, some studies related to this study were reviewed, and the closest study was chosen to measure the strength of the relationship between variables (effect size).[1,12] With a sample size of 40 (10 per group) 90% power was achieved to detect a difference among the groups. Statistical software (R 2.11.1) was used to calculate the sample size required to achieve an $\alpha = 0.05$ and a power of 90%.

Experimental Design

This in vitro study measured and compared the fracture load of one-piece zirconia custom abutments made in two angulations (0°, 15°) and two thicknesses (0.7 and 1 mm; Fig 24.1). Forty zirconia custom abutments (Cares Bone level regular cross-fit [RC] 4.1 mm × 12 mm; Straumann LLC, Andover, MA) were divided into four groups. Groups A-1 and B-1 simulated a clinical situation with an ideal implant position from a prosthetic point of view, which allows for the use of straight zirconia custom abutments with two thicknesses (0.7 and 1 mm). Groups A-2 and B-2 simulated a situation with a compromised implant position

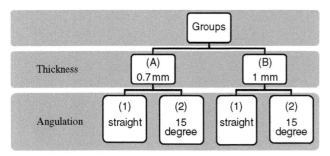

FIGURE 24.1   Group distribution.

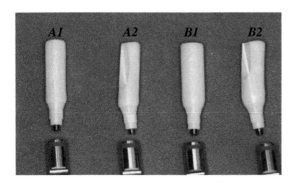

FIGURE 24.2   Cares regular cross-fit zirconia custom abutments connected to regular platform lab analog 4.1 mm × 12 mm, A1 = straight (0° angle) zirconia custom abutment (0.7-mm thick), A2 = angulated (15° angle) zirconia custom abutment (0.7-mm thick), B1 = straight (0° angle) zirconia custom abutment (1-mm thick), B2 = angulated (15° angle) zirconia custom abutment (1-mm thick).

requiring 15° angulated abutments with different thicknesses (0.7 and 1 mm; Fig 24.2).

Specimen Preparation

Forty implant replicas (10 for each subgroup) (Straumann implant replica, 4.1 mm × 12 mm RC octagon restorative platform; Straumann LLC) were placed in cubic self-cure acrylic jigs (Caulk® Orthodontic Resin; Dentsply Caulk, York, PA). The acrylic jigs were standardized with 2.5 × 2.5 × 2.5 cm³ dimensions. To make sure that the implant replicas were adjusted to be perpendicular to the jig's surface (90°), each replica was attached to a laboratory surveyor (Dentsply Neytech, Yucaipa, CA) by using a guide pin (Impression Post RC4.1 mm; Straumann LLC). A water scale was used to adjust the implant replicas with the surveyor's pen.

The implant replicas placed in cubic acrylic jigs were scanned to design custom abutments digitally at the manufacturer's facility by a single operator using a surface scanner (Straumann® Cares® Scan CS2; Straumann LLC). This scanner uses a laser beam to trace a polymer scan-body and render a digitized image of the implant analog; it then designed the custom abutments digitally.[13] The finish line was set and adjusted as necessary using 3D imaging design

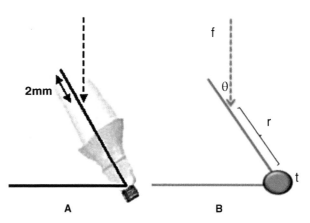

FIGURE 24.3   (A and B) Direction of load applied to the specimens using Instron machine. Note that, t = torque vector (implant/abutment connection), r = length of the lever arm vector = 7.1 mm (the distance between the force being applied on the abutment's surface and the implant abutment connection), f = force vector (the force applied by the Instron machine), θ = angle between the force vector and the lever arm vector.

software (Straumann® Cares® Visual 6.0; Straumann LLC). The scanned information was transferred electronically to the production facility.

After zirconia custom abutments were made by the manufacturer, they were engaged to the implant replicas into the cubic acrylic jig, using a manual torque wrench based on manufacturer's recommendations (35 N cm).[13] The acrylic jigs were mounted and adjusted at 30° relative to the mechanical indenter for all groups. The indenter was covered by a resilient material (Durasoft; Scheu Dental GmbH, Iserlohn, Germany). The indenter contacts the entire mesio-distal-occluding surface in a contact width of approximately 2 to 4 mm. The resilient material is a coextrusion compound material consisting of a hard polycarbonate base and soft polyester urethane, which was used to reduce localized contact stress intensities and to distribute stress over the complete testing unit, including screws and abutments. Then, the shear stress was measured by loading the specimens to failure with a 0.5 mm/min crosshead speed with the force transferred to the lingual surface of the zirconia custom abutments, 2 mm below the top surface using a universal testing machine (Model 5566; Instron, Canton, MA; Fig 24.3). The universal testing machine was controlled via a computer software system (Bluehill®2 Software, Canton, MA), which also completed the stress-strain diagram and recorded the breaking loads.

Statistical Analysis

Descriptive statistics were reported for each group (means, standard deviations, minimum, and maximum values). A two-way ANOVA was performed to assess the statistical significance of each factor. A Kolmogorov-Smirnov test was also performed to check the normal distribution of residuals across the groups.

RESULTS

The mean fracture load of one-piece zirconia custom abutments across the groups (A-1 through B-2) ranged from 160 ± 60 to 230 ± 95 N where the numbers were rounded to the nearest 10. The p-value of the Kolmogorov-Smirnov test was $p = 0.301$, meaning there was no evidence that the assumption of normal distribution of the residuals is violated. On the basis of this, a two-way ANOVA was performed for this group.

Straight abutments showed a higher fracture load than angulated abutments. The mean fracture load from a highest to lowest was 230 ± 95 (B-1), 227 ± 70 (A-1), 168 ± 59 (B-2), 160 ± 60 (A-2). When the test was conducted for the first time, the interaction was not significant between the variables ($p = 0.981$), so the test was performed for a second time without the interaction, and it was found that the straight zirconia custom abutments exhibited a significantly higher fracture load than angulated zirconia custom abutments ($p = 0.009$; Table 24.1). No statistically significant difference was found between groups with different thicknesses (group A-1/group A-2; group B-1/group B-2; $p = 0.827$).

DISCUSSION

Researchers highlighted the importance of whether the evaluated specimens are zirconia dioxide abutments with a metallic insertion or all-ceramic components.[14–17] The majority of published investigations on all-ceramic implant abutments made from zirconia dioxide examined simulated single incisor replacements.[8,18–20] These papers reported fracture load between 429 and 793 N under load angles that range from 30° to 60°. It seems that there is a strong correlation between measured fracture load and the type of

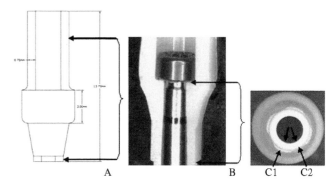

FIGURE 24.4 The relation between the lever arm vector and the fracture behavior of zirconia custom abutments. (A) The length of the lever arm vector = 12.6 mm. (B) The length of the implant/abutment connection = 5.5 mm. (C) The thickness of implant abutment connection (C1 = 0.6 mm and C2 = 0.4 mm).

implant/abutment connection.[11] In this study, the mean fracture load for 0° and 15° in one-piece zirconia custom abutments ranged from 160 ± 60 to 230 ± 95 N. It is difficult to compare our fracture load values with results from other studies, due to the various ranges of angles, difference in force application, and different study designs.

The moment of force (torque moment) played an important role in this study and had an important effect on the fracture load of the zirconia custom abutments. The strength of the specimens might be affected by three quantities: the force applied to the specimens, the length of the lever arm connecting the axis to the point of force application, and the angle between the force vector and the lever arm[21] (Fig 24.3).

For one-piece zirconia custom abutments, the length of the lever arm vector was 12.6 mm, with 0.4 and 0.6 mm thicknesses in the area of implant/abutment connection (Fig 24.4). This thickness is designed by the manufacturer and is standard and unchangeable. The thinnest part in one-piece zirconia custom abutments is in the implant/abutment connection area (0.4 and 0.6 mm). In addition, this area is the most critical area in the abutments because of the force concentration that might be one of the reasons for failures in this area. This finding might mean that the thickness of zirconia custom abutments in this design had no influence on the fracture load, since the thickness of implant/abutment connection is standard; however, the angulation had a negative influence on the fracture load, because when the force was applied on angulated abutments, the angle (θ) between the force vector (f) and the lever arm (r) increased, decreasing the force required to break the specimens. This could have been one of the reasons for failure in this design.

To estimate the failure risk associated with implant-supported restorative concepts consistent with their fracture loads as determined in an in vitro setting, it is important to separately consider the forces expected in actual clinical situations. Ferrario et al measured single-tooth occlusion forces in healthy young adults and reported results of 150

TABLE 24.1 Fracture Load Means, SDs, Minimum, and Maximum Values ($n = 10$/Group)

	Groups			
	A1	A2	B1	B2
Thickness	0.7 mm	0.7 mm	1 mm	1 mm
Angulations	0°	15°	0°	15°
Mean	227 N	160 N	230 N	168 N
SD	70	60	95	59
Min	141 N	104 N	111 N	109 N
Max	360 N	314 N	406 N	308 N

$p = 0.827$ between A1 and A2, B1 and B2.
$p = 0.009$ between A1 and B1, A2 and B2.

and 140 N for men in the central and lateral incisors, respectively.[22] Higher occlusion forces are to be expected in individuals with functional disorders such as bruxism.[23] In this study, static loading was applied, and the force was applied slowly with a 0.5 mm/min crosshead speed. This corresponds to the load in a parafunctional situation rather than during chewing. In this study, the mean fracture load for all of the zirconia custom abutments exceeded the abovementioned occlusion forces; however, we note continued uncertainty in predicting the performance of one-piece zirconia custom abutments in individuals with functional disorders. Special attention might need to be paid to the occlusal relationship of the lower and upper jaw whenever possible. It was recommended that keeping such abutments free from dynamic occlusion might extend the lifespan of such abutments.[24–26] The straight zirconia custom abutments exhibited statistically significantly higher mean fracture loads than angulated abutments did. These findings lead us to reject our original null hypothesis. It is possible that in one-piece zirconia custom abutments, loading forces are higher in the area of the apical hexagon, colocalized with the thinnest portion of the abutment.[24–27]

In this study, artificial dynamic thermal aging was not applied to the specimens due to the failure to exert a statistically significant influence on the fracture load of either straight or angulated abutments in previous studies.[28,29] Static loading was performed at an angle of 30° to the long axis of the abutments to simulate a parafunctional situation. In this study, the most typical fracture pattern (95% of the specimens among the groups) was an oblique fracture line below the implant shoulder (Fig 24.5). This finding confirmed Adatia et al's observations, which indicate

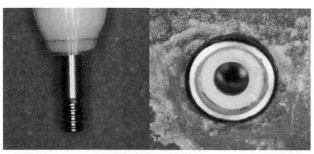
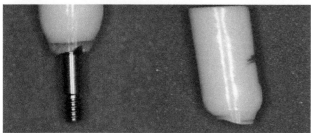

FIGURE 24.5 Views of the fracture pattern of the zirconia custom abutments, appearing as an oblique line below the abutment's shoulder.

that certain grinding procedures above the level of the implant shoulder for the purpose of abutment individualization have no impact on fracture load.[20]

It is difficult to compare data between studies on the fractural stability of zirconia custom abutments because of different study designs. In this study, the implants and abutments were embedded in orthodontic acrylic resin jigs, simulating horizontal bone loss, whereas in the other investigations the implant-supported restorations were embedded up to the implant shoulder.[8] As a result, the loads were applied with different lever arms. Furthermore, variations in the angle of the applied load, static or dynamic testing methods, and the size and shape of the abutments and restoration can have an important influence on the results. A variation in the fracture pattern was also observed in other studies reporting on alumina, zirconia, and titanium abutments with internal connections.[12,16] In only one of those studies, however, an implant neck distortion was found in a specimen bearing a titanium abutment.[16] In another investigation testing alumina and zirconia abutments, fracture of the abutment, and/or fracture of both the abutment and crown were the main reasons for failure.[12] In contrast to these results, zirconia custom abutment components failed by fracture in both groups with different thicknesses and angulations, but the fracture was significantly higher in the groups with 15° angulations.

CONCLUSIONS

Within the limitations of this in vitro study, the following conclusions can be drawn:

1. Angulated zirconia custom abutments had the lowest fracture load of the present investigations; however, there was no statistically significant difference in the thicknesses between the 0.7 and 1.0 mm group.
2. The thickness of one-piece zirconia custom abutments had no influence on the fracture load.

ACKNOWLEDGMENTS

The authors extend sincere thanks to the Straumann USA, LLC for their generous materials support and Ms. Jennifer Jackson and Ms. Kelly Jork for all their help and support.

REFERENCES

1. Sailer I, Sailer T, Stawarczyk B: In vitro study of the influence of the type of connection on the fracture load of zirconia abutments with internal and external implant abutment connection. *Int J Oral Maxillofac Implants* 2009;24:850–858.

2. Buser D, Mericske R, Bernard JP: Long term evaluation of non-submerged ITI implants. *Clin Oral Implants Res* 1997;8: 161–172.

3. Anderson B, Odman P, Lindvall AM, et al: Cemented single crowns on osseointegrated implants after 5 years. *Int J Prosthodont* 1998;11:212–218.

4. Prestipino V, Ingber A: All ceramic implant abutments: esthetic indications. *J Esthet Dent* 1996;8:255–262.

5. Jung RE, Sailer I, Hammerle CHF: In vitro color changes of soft tissue caused by restorative materials. *Int J Periodontics Restorative Dent* 2007;27:251–257.

6. Wohlwend A, Studer S, Schaere P: Zirconia oxide abutments. *Quintessence Dent Tech* 1996;22:364–381.

7. Riger W: *Medical Applications of Ceramics*. London, Academic Press, 1989.

8. Yildirim M, Fischer H, Marx R, et al: In vivo fracture resistance of implant-supported all-ceramic restorations. *J Prosthet Dent* 2003;90:325–331.

9. Haraldson T, Carlsson GE, Ingervall B: Functional state bite force and postural muscle activity in patients with osseointegrated oral implant bridges. *Acta Odontol Scand* 1979;37: 195–206.

10. Paphangkorakit J, Osborn JW: The effect of pressure on maximum incisal bite force in men. *Arch Oral Biol* 1997;42: 11–17.

11. Sailer I, Philipp A, Zembic A, et al: A systematic review of the performance of ceramic and metal implant abutments supporting fixed implant reconstructions. *Clin Oral Implants Res* 2009;20:4–31.

12. Att W, Kurun S, Gerds T: Fracture resistance of single tooth implant supported all ceramic restorations. *J Prosthet Dent* 2006;95:111–116.

13. Straumann Product Catalog, 2013: 80, www.straumann.us.

14. Butz F, Heydecke G, Okutan M, et al: Survival rate, fracture strength and failure mode of ceramic implant abutments after chewing simulation. *J Oral Rehabil* 2005;32:838–843.

15. Kolbeck C, Behr M, Rosentritt M, et al: Fracture force of tooth–tooth- and implant–tooth-supported all-ceramic fixed partial dentures using titanium vs. customised zirconia implant abutments. *Clin Oral Implants Res* 2008;19:1049–1053.

16. Canullo L, Morgia P, Marinotti F: Preliminary laboratory evaluation of bicomponent customized zirconia abutments. *Int J Prosthodont* 2007;20:486–488.

17. Att W, Kurun S, Gerds T, et al: Fracture resistance of single-tooth implant-supported all-ceramic restorations after exposure to the artificial mouth. *J Oral Rehabil* 2006;33: 380–386.

18. Gehrke P, Dhom G, Brunner J, et al: Zirconium implant abutments: fracture strength and influence of cyclic loading on retaining-screw loosening. *Quintessence Int* 2006;37:19–26.

19. Aramouni P, Zebouni E, Tashkandi E, et al: Fracture resistance and failure location of zirconium and metallic implant abutments. *J Contemp Dent Pract* 2008;9:41–48.

20. Adatia ND, Bayne SC, Cooper LF, et al: Fracture resistance of yttria-stabilized zirconia dental implant abutments. *J Prosthodont* 2009;18:17–22.

21. Hall AS, Archer FE, Gilbert RI: *Engineering Statics* (ed 2). Sydney, Australia, UNSW Press, 2005, pp. 39–227.

22. Ferrario VF, Sforza C, Serrao G, et al: Single tooth bite forces in healthy young adults. *J Oral Rehabil* 2004;31:18–22.

23. Nishigawa K, Bando E, Nakano M: Quantitative study of bite force during sleep associated bruxism. *J Oral Rehabil* 2001;28:485–491.

24. Balshi TJ, Ekfeldt A, Stenberg T, et al: Three-year evaluation of Branemark implants connected to angulated abutments. *Int J Oral Maxillofac Implants* 1997;12:52–58.

25. Sethi A, Kaus T, Sochor P: The use of angulated abutments in implant dentistry: five-year clinical results of an ongoing prospective study. *Int J Oral Maxillofac Implants* 2000;15: 801–810.

26. Sethi A, Kaus T, Sochor P, et al: Evolution of the concept of angulated abutments in implant dentistry: 14-year clinical data. *Implant Dent* 2002;11:41–51.

27. Torbjorner A, Fransson B: A literature review on the prosthetic treatment of structurally compromised teeth. *Int J Prosthodont* 2004;17:369–376.

28. Heydecke G, Butz F, Hussein A, et al: Fracture strength after dynamic loading of endodontically treated teeth restored with different post-and-core systems. *J Prosthet Dent* 2002;87: 438–445.

29. Nothdurft FP, Doppler KE, Erdelt KJ, et al: Fracture behavior of straight or angulated zirconia implant abutments supporting anterior single crowns. *Clin Oral Investig* 2011;15: 157–163.

25

SURFACE CHARACTERISTICS AND CELL ADHESION: A COMPARATIVE STUDY OF FOUR COMMERCIAL DENTAL IMPLANTS

Ruohong Liu, dds, ms,[1,*] Tianhua Lei,[2] Vladimir Dusevich, phd,[2] Xiamei Yao, phd,[2] Ying Liu, phd,[2] Mary P. Walker, dds, phd,[1,2] Yong Wang, phd,[2] and Ling Ye, dds, phd[2,*]

[1]Department of Restorative Dentistry, University of Missouri-Kansas City School of Dentistry, Kansas City, MO
[2]Department of Oral Biology, University of Missouri-Kansas City School of Dentistry, Kansas City, MO

> The article is associated with the American College of Prosthodontists' journal-based continuing education program. It is accompanied by an online continuing education activity worth 1 credit. Please visit www.wileyhealthlearning .com/jopr to complete the activity and earn credit.

Keywords
Dental implants; MicroSpy profiler; scanning electron microscopy; energy dispersive X-ray spectroscopy; Raman microspectroscopy; primary osteoblastic cell; cell adhesion.

Correspondence
Ling Ye, 3650 Chambers Pass, Building 3610, Fort Sam Houston, TX 78234–6315. E-mail: ling.ye.mil@mail.mil

*Current address: Naval Medical Research Unit San Antonio, Fort Sam Houston, TX

Supported by NIH/NIDCR DE016977, and Rinehart Foundation, School of Dentistry, University of Missouri-Kansas City.

The work from this manuscript was given as an oral presentation (Abstract No. 52) at the General Session & Exhibition of IADR/AADR/CADR Annual Meeting, San Diego, CA, March 2011, and an oral presentation (Abstract No. 724) at the Annual Meeting & Exhibition of the AADR/CADR, Tampa, FL, March 2012.

The authors deny any conflicts of interest.

Accepted February 24, 2013

Published in *Journal of Prosthodontics* December 2013; Vol. 22, Issue 8

doi: 10.1111/jopr.12063

ABSTRACT

Purpose: The aims of this study were to compare surface properties of four commercial dental implants and to compare those implant systems' cell adhesion, which may be affected by the surface properties, and to provide scientific information on the selection of implants for clinicians.

Materials and Methods: The surface properties of four commonly used dental implants (3i Nanotite™, Astra OsseoSpeed™, Nobel Biocare TiUnite®, and Straumann SLActive®) were studied using MicroSpy profiler, scanning electron microscopy (SEM), energy dispersive X-ray spectroscopy, and Raman microspectroscopy. Primary mouse alveolar bone cells were cultured on the surface of implants from the four companies. After 48-hour culture, SEM in combination with a quantitative analysis of SEM images was used to examine the cell adhesion. Cell adhesion rates (ratios of cell surface to implant surface) among different systems were compared.

Results: Distinct differences were found among these implants. Comparisons of roughness among three locations: flank, top, and valley within the same implant system, or in the same location among different implants were made. Generally Astra and Straumann systems showed the roughest surface, whereas 3i showed the smoothest surface. Multiple cracks were found on the surface of the Nobel Biocare system, which also had a dramatically lower level of titanium. In addition, rutile phase of titanium oxide was found in 3i, Astra, and Straumann systems, and anatase phase of titanium oxide was only detected in the Nobel Biocare system. After 48-hour culture, Astra and Straumann systems displayed the highest cell adhesion at the areas of flank, top, and valley of the implant surface. Primary cells also reached confluence on the valley, but significantly less in the 3i system. Nobel Biocare showed the least cell adhesion on the flank and valley.

Conclusion: Implant systems have distinct differences in surface properties, leading to different cell adhesion results. Further in vivo study is needed to study the impact of the surface characteristics and different cell adhesion on the osseointegration between implant and bone.

The concept of osseointegration was first introduced by Per-Ingvar Brånemark in the 1950s.[1] Since then, dental implants have evolved tremendously in all aspects: material, design, surface treatment, abutment connection, restoration options, and techniques. In North America as well as around the world, dental implants have become a routine treatment in dental offices and well known to patients. Theoretically, dentists now can choose from more than 2000 implants from close to 100 implant companies for any particular restoration requirements.[2] However, there is no guideline for selection of a specific implant system other than commercial marketing, personal preferences, or anecdotal experiences. Almost all dental implant companies claim some kind of superiority of their products in their marketing materials; however, except for the information from marketing brochures, it is difficult for clinicians to decide which system should be used and which system is better than other systems. Although many implant companies allege the superiority of their products, it seems that those claims are not based on sound and long-term clinical scientific research.[2,3]

Currently no evidence or criteria support the products from one particular implant company producing more reliable clinical results. Eckert et al reviewed the clinical evidence of the performance of six dental implant systems (Astra, Centerpulse, Dentsply/Friadent, Implant Innovations, Nobel Biocare, Straumann) certified by the American Dental Association. A total of 69 references were provided by those six implant manufacturers, and none directly compared one implant system with another system.[4] Esposito et al systematically reviewed randomized controlled clinical trials (RCT) comparing different implant systems with a follow-up of 5 years, and found only four RCTs with sufficient data met the inclusion criteria. None were conducted in North America, and all received support from the industry.[5] Bhatavadekar examined publications from 1970 to 2006 using implants from Astra Tech, Straumann, 3i, and Nobel Biocare, and found the studies were extremely heterogeneous, making comparisons difficult.[6] Although many studies focused on the surface of implants, very few compared the surface properties and osseointegration of current commercially available dental implants or provided guidance for the clinical selection of dental implants.

Immediately following implant placement, the interaction between the cells and implant surface will define the cell/implant interface and may eventually affect the final bone/implant interface.[7] From the perspective of the host, the initial healing phase and subsequent osseointegration depend on the availability of osteogenic cells and their capability of adhesion and proliferation onto the implant surface.[8] From the implant perspective, surface properties play a more crucial role in cell-surface interaction, because surface properties can be modified to promote cell adhesion, proliferation, and differentiation through a variety of modifications or improvements, including grit blasting, acid-etching, anodization, calcium phosphate coating, and plasma-spraying.[9–12] Consequently, different implants from different companies present a variety of implant surfaces with different characteristics of topographic and physicochemical properties,[13–17] and all implant companies claim their products provide excellent osseointegration. Currently, there is a lack of information regarding the direct comparison of cell culture or in vivo comparison among those dental implant systems. One recent publication compared the cell adhesion on the actual implant surface; however, the study only selected implants from one company, and the products are not internationally recognized.[18]

In this study, we compared the four most popular dental implants from four major dental implant companies (Biomet 3i, Astra Tech, Nobel Biocare, Straumann), which in total make up ~85% of the world market of dental implants.[19] All four systems had positive in vivo data.[20–24] Surface properties of implants from those companies were analyzed with MicroSpy Profiler, scanning electron microscopy (SEM), energy dispersive X-ray spectroscopy (EDS), and Raman microspectroscopy. In addition, we studied the interaction of implant surface and bone cells in those implants. To the best of our knowledge, our study is the first to directly compare cell adhesion on the actual implant surface of different implant systems. Moreover, instead of using cell lines, we used the primary osteoblastic cells from mouse alveolar bone, which may be more similar to the phenotype of in vivo cells. Interestingly, our preliminary data showed that different implant systems displayed different cell adhesion capability, which may be connected with their characteristic surface properties.

MATERIALS AND METHODS

Implants

Commercially available implants from four implant companies were purchased directly from the supplier: 3i Nanotite™ (4 × 10 mm, Biomet 3i, Palm Beach Gardens, FL), Astra OsseoSpeed™ (3.1 × 11 mm, Astra Tech, Molndal, Sweden), Nobel Biocare TiUnite® (3.5 × 10 mm, Nobel Biocare, Goteborg, Sweden), and Straumann SLActive® (3.3 × 10 mm, Straumann, Waldenburg, Switzerland; Table 25.1). The sizes of implants from different implant companies are not standard, and for the purpose of comparability implants close to each other in dimensions were selected.

Optical Profiler

The 3D roughness was measured by an Optical Profilometer (FRT MicroProf 100, Fries Research & Technology, Bergisch Gladbach, Germany). The optical profilometer quantifies the roughness and scans the surface topography in 3D. The implants were transferred in their storage boxes as delivered to FRT of America, LLC (San Jose, CA) to measure the surface roughness. There were nine measurements on each implant (three for top, three for threaded valley, and three for flank). Three implants from each company were used to obtain reliable mean values.[25] To

calculate the sample number for the roughness measurement, power analysis was performed and showed that a sample size of three would generate enough power (>0.9) for the statistical analysis. The roughness is expressed as Sa, which is the arithmetic average of the 3D roughness. After one-way ANOVA *F*-test, to keep nominal type I error rate, Ryan-Einot-Gabriel-Welsch Multiple Range Test (REGWQ; SAS 9.3, Cary, NC) was used to compare the roughness among different systems at different locations. A *p*-value of <0.05 was considered statistically significant.

SEM and EDS

The surface morphology and elemental composition were analyzed with SEM and EDS, respectively. Three specimens from each type of implant were analyzed by the same instrumentation protocol. All dental implants were taken from their original package directly from the supplier. To avoid scratching the implant surface with instruments, those implants were handled with a plastic plier and plastic gloves. Each implant was attached on an aluminum stub with sticky conductive carbon tape. The surface of each implant was examined with a field emission environmental scanning electron microscope (Philips XL30; FEI Co., Hillsboro, OR). Pictures were taken in both secondary and backscattered electrons. For EDS analysis, 7 kV accelerating voltage was used to improve peak/background ratio for light elements. Three spectra from different locations on each implant were acquired and were proved to be similar. So for further analysis, spectra for each implant were summarized.

Raman Microspectroscopy

The chemical structure of surface coatings was determined from the corresponding peaks using a Raman spectrometer (LabRam HR800, Jobin Yvon Inc., Edison, NJ). An He-Ne laser (632.8 nm) was used through the 100× objective of an optical microscope, and the scattered signal was analyzed by a high resolution spectrometer coupled to an air-cooled CCD system. The Raman spectra were acquired in the range of 100 to 1000 cm^{-1}. At least three spots per specimen were examined.

TABLE 25.1 **Dental Implants Used in the Study**

Company	Surface	Description	Length (mm)	Width (mm)	Item No.
Biomet 3i	NanoTite™	Tapered certain PREVAIL	10.0	4/3 mm(P)	NIITP4310
Nobel Biocare	TiUnite™	NobelReplace Tapered groovy	10.0	3.5	32,212
Astra Tech Dental	OsseoSpeed®	Tapered, MicroThread	11.0	3.0	24,882
Straumann	SLActive®	Straumann bone level implant	10	3.3	021.2110

Primary Osteoblastic Cell Isolation

With the modified protocol,[26] primary osteoblastic cells from mouse alveolar bone were collected as follows. Mouse mandibular bodies from 9- to 11-day-old mouse pups were dissected to remove teeth, dental follicles, and other soft tissue, such as muscle, gingiva, and skin. Dissected mandibles were minced and further digested with digestion solution (0.2% collagenase/0.05% trypsin in alpha-MEM) for 15 minutes on a shaker plate at 225 rpm at 37°C. The first digestion, usually full of fibroblastic cells from the periosteal layers, was discarded. The next three sequential collagenase/trypsin digestions for 15 minutes at 37°C were collected and pooled together. The cell suspension then was filtered through a 70-μm strainer to break up clumps and cultivated for further use.

Cell Culture on Implants

All the implants were taken from their original package directly and handled with plastic pliers and plastic gloves in a cell culture hood. To calculate the sample number for the cell attachment, power analysis was performed and showed that a sample size of four would generate enough power (>0.8) for the statistical analysis. Implants from each company were placed in a semi-solid medium containing 0.5% agar.[27,28] The primary osteoblastic cell suspension (3×10^5 cell/ml) was applied to the respective implants.[29] Following 48 hours of cell cultivation on the implants in 5% CO_2, the implants were fixed in 2% glutaraldehyde in 0.1 M cacodylate buffer for 10 minutes. After fixation, implants with adherent cells were dehydrated through serial ethanol (30% to 100%). The samples were then sputter-coated with gold and platinum, and examined with field emission environmental SEM (Philips XL30).

Quantitative Analysis of Cell Culture

Cell adhesion on the implant surface was examined under SEM. Because of different morphologies of flanks and valleys in different implant systems, the cell adhesion on flank and valley were combined, and cell adhesion on the top was examined separately. The cell adhesion rate (%) was calculated as the ratio of cell adhesion area to total area. The quantitative analysis was performed blindly using the Image Analysis System (AnalySIS, Lakewood, CO). At least three locations in each implant were randomly selected and measured for statistical analysis. Using GraphPad InStat version 3.01 (La Jolla, CA), the cell adhesion rates in different systems were analyzed with one-way ANOVA. Then, the differences between groups were compared with Tukey-Kramer Multiple Comparison test. A p-value of <0.05 was considered statistically significant.

RESULTS

Roughness was examined by an Optical Profilometer (FRT MicroProf 100), as shown in Figure 25.1. Nine measurements on each implant (3 for flank, 3 for top, 3 for threaded valley), three implants from each company, were examined.

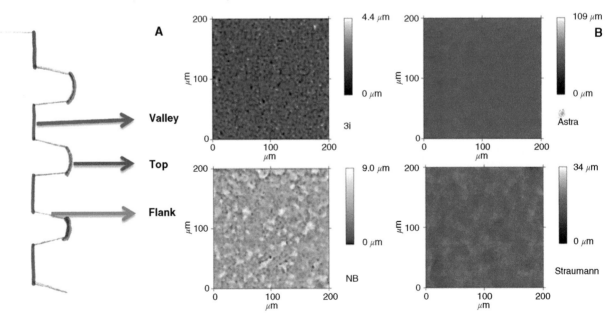

FIGURE 25.1 Roughness measurements from optical profilometer. (A) Threaded flank, top, and valley were measured and compared separately. (B) Examples of scanning images, filter size 34.286 μm. NB: Nobel Biocare.

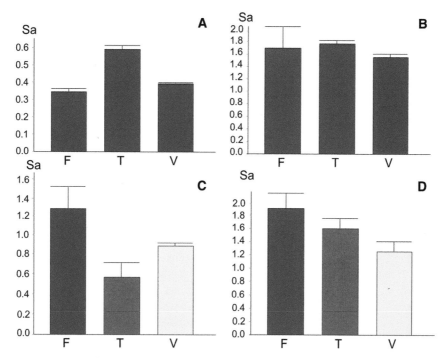

FIGURE 25.2 Comparison of roughness (Sa) among flank (F), top (T), and valley (V) in different implant systems. Sa is the arithmetic average of the 3D roughness. (A and B) Roughness measurement bars of the same color indicate no statistical difference; (C and D) the bars with different colors indicate statistical difference. (A) Roughness in 3i implant system, no statistically significant difference at the three locations; (B) roughness in Astra system, no significant difference; (C) roughness in Nobel Biocare system, significant differences were found, flank > valley > top; (D) roughness in Straumann system, flank > top > valley. Data shown as mean + standard deviation.

REGWQ was used to compare the roughness among different locations (flank, top, valley) within the same systems (Fig 25.2) and among different systems at different locations (Fig 25.3). For the 3i and Astra systems, there were no significant differences in roughness among flank, top, and valley (Figs 25.2A and 25.2B). Meanwhile, significant differences in roughness were found in Nobel Biocare and Straumann systems. For the Nobel Biocare system, the order of roughness from high to low was flank > valley > top (Fig 25.2C). On the other hand, the order of roughness from high to low for Straumann was flank > top > valley (Fig 25.2D). Further comparisons were made on the same locations among different systems. REGWQ indicated that 3i had the lowest measurements of roughness on all three locations; Astra and/or Straumann had the highest roughness measurements on the different locations (Fig 25.3). For the flank, the order of roughness from high to low was Straumann > Astra, Nobel Biocare > 3i (Fig 25.3A). For the top, the order from high to low was Astra, Straumann > Nobel Biocare, 3i (Fig 25.3B). For the valley, the order of roughness from high to low was Astra > Straumann > Nobel Biocare > 3i (Fig 25.3C).

SEM was used to examine the surfaces among different implant systems. No dramatic differences were found in the same system among the flank, top, and valley locations. Therefore, only images from the valley were displayed and discussed. SEM revealed distinct surface characteristics among different systems. Consistent with the results of the roughness measurement, 3i had the smoothest surface with the least elevations and depressions among the four systems (Figs 25.4A and 25.4a). Astra showed a two-phase "rock in the gravel" type of microstructure (Figs 25.4B and 25.4b). Nobel Biocare demonstrated a relatively regularly organized elevated "figure 8" microstructure (Figs 25.4C and 25.4c). Straumann showed an irregular honeycomb structure similar to the mark made by pulling shoes off a fresh muddy surface (Figs 25.4D and 25.4d). One interesting point identified only in the Nobel Biocare implant but not in the other three systems was the presence of multiple cracks in the surface layer (Fig 25.4e). Similar cracks can even be observed in the picture from Nobel Biocare official website http://www.nobelbiocare.com/en/about-nobel-biocare/research-development/tiunite/ (as of 1/27/2013).

The superimposed EDS spectra for four implants revealed the presence of titanium in all four systems (Fig 25.5). Straumann showed the highest amount, and Nobel Biocare showed the sharply lowest titanium content (about half of the Straumann system). The closest to Straumann in the titanium

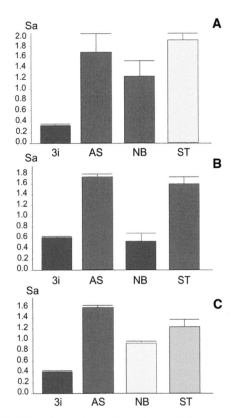

FIGURE 25.3 Comparison of roughness (Sa) among different implant systems in (A) flank, (B) top, and (C) valley. Same color roughness measurement bars indicate no statistical difference; the bars with different colors indicate statistical difference. (A) for the flank area, Straumann has the roughest, and 3i has the smoothest flank, no difference between Astra and Nobel Biocare; (B) for the top area, Astra = Straumann > 3i = Nobel Biocare; (C) for the valley area, Astra > Straumann > Nobel Biocare > 3i. AS: Astra; NB: Nobel Biocare; ST: Straumann. Data shown as mean + standard deviation.

content was 3i. The spectrum for 3i also showed small amounts of calcium and phosphate, suggesting a thin coating of calcium phosphate. In addition, the 3i system showed the

presence of vanadium and aluminum, indicating the presence of titanium alloy. Next to 3i in amount of titanium was Astra, which contained an elevated amount of oxygen, possibly covered with a thicker titanium oxide layer. A sharply lower amount of titanium than other implants was observed in Nobel Biocare, whose spectrum also showed relatively large amounts of phosphate and oxygen (Fig 25.5).

In addition, surface coating structural information, such as relative titanium and oxygen bonds, was determined from the corresponding peaks using Raman microspectroscopy. Nobel Biocare implant showed the typical spectrum of the anatase phase of titanium oxide, whereas the other systems showed that titanium oxide was in rutile phase (Fig 25.6).

For the purpose of comparison, one implant from each company was used to show implant surfaces without cell culture (Fig 25.7). Four implants from each company were used for the cell adhesion study. In comparison with implants after cell culture or ones without cell culture, dramatic differences of primary osteoblastic cell adhesion were revealed with SEM examination (Fig 25.7). After 48-hour culture, primary osteoblastic cells attached and proliferated on the surface of different systems; however, the extent of attachment and proliferation were not the same among implants systems. In the 3i system, cells mainly attached and proliferated in the valley of the thread (Fig 25.7a). For both Astra and Straumann systems, the cellular behavior was similar, with primary osteoblastic cells reaching confluence and covering almost all the threads (Figs 25.7b and 25.7d) or microthreads (Fig 25.7b). On the other hand, cells did not grow well on the surfaces of Nobel Biocare implant and only covered a partial surface of threads (Fig 25.7c).

To better illustrate the cell adhesion patterns in different implant systems, enlarged lateral view and frontal view pictures from different systems are shown in Figures 25.8 and 25.9. Although all four systems are screw-thread type implants with flank, top, and valley, the morphology of the screw is not the same in those systems. Generally, two types of screws can be observed from the lateral view pictures. Nobel Biocare and 3i have flat valleys and tops with steep

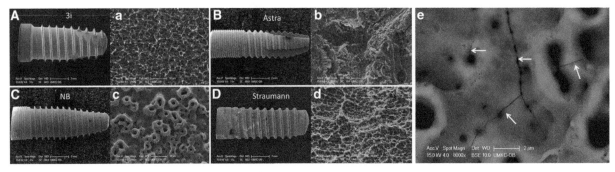

FIGURE 25.4 Lower (11×) and higher magnification (2000×) SEM images of implants from (A and a) 3i, (B and b) Astra, (C and c) Nobel Biocare, and (D and d) Straumann. (e) Cracks (white arrows) on the surface layer of Nobel Biocare implants.

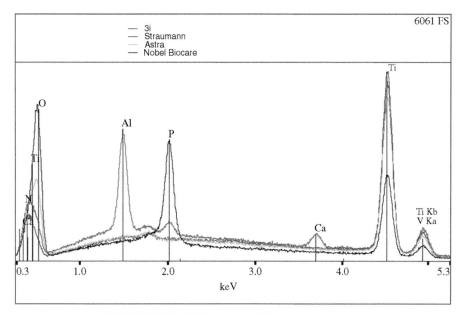

FIGURE 25.5   EDS analysis of four implant systems.

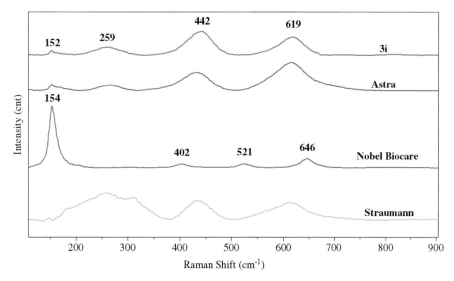

FIGURE 25.6   Raman microspectroscopy analysis showed spectra of rutile or anatase phase of titanium oxide in the four implant systems. Rutile phase of titanium oxide was found in 3i, Astra, and Straumann systems, whereas the anatase phase, with the characteristic scatterings at $154\,\mathrm{cm}^{-1}$, was present only in Nobel Biocare.

flanks (Figs 25.8A and 25.8C), whereas curved valleys and tops with shallow flanks are seen in Astra and Straumann (Figs 25.8B and 25.8D). After 48-hour cell culture, Astra and Straumann systems display a similar cell adhesion pattern. Cells grew well to cover most of the flank, top, and valley (Figs 25.8b and 25.8d). For the 3i system, the cells reached confluence, but only with a thin layer of cells to cover the valley area, which is not comparable with the multiple layers of cells in Astra and Straumann. In addition, many fewer cells

were found at the flank and top areas (Fig 25.8a). For the Nobel Biocare system, there were even fewer at the valley area, also not attached to the valley surface; however, the cells grew more at the top compared with the 3i system (Fig 25.8c).

Similar cell adhesion patterns as shown in the lateral view (Fig 25.8) were confirmed by the frontal view (Fig 25.9), which is better suited for quantitative analysis. Due the different screw patterns shown in Figures 25.8A to 25.8D,

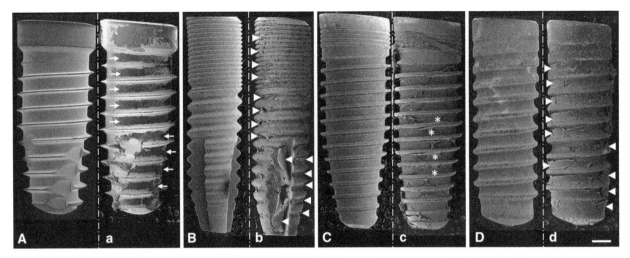

FIGURE 25.7   Low magnification (11×) comparison of different systems, (A and a) 3i, (B and b) Astra, (C and c) Nobel Biocare, and (D and d) Straumann in the without cell (A, B, C, and D) or after cell culture (a, b, c, d). After 48 hours of culture, primary osteoblastic cells reached confluence in all four systems. (a) Cells grew mainly at the valley area in 3i system (a: arrows); (b) cells covered microthreads, threads, and the notch in Astra (b: arrowheads); (c) cells grew less and only covered part of the thread in Nobel Biocare (c, stars); (d) similar to Astra, cells covered almost all the threads in Straumann system (d, arrowheads). Bar = 1 mm.

it would be difficult to separate the attached cells between the flank and valley areas, especially for the Astra and Straumann systems. Therefore, the cell adhesion for flank and valley was combined. By using the implant without cell culture as reference, the flank and valley areas were combined and calculated together (Fig 25.9, white rectangular boxes). ANOVA showed the significant difference of cell adhesion rates among the four implant systems (Fig 25.10). Astra and Straumann systems displayed the highest cell adhesion rate, followed by 3i. Nobel Biocare showed the lowest cell adhesion rate.

Higher magnification (500×) frontal view pictures (Fig 25.11) had to be used to perform the quantitative analysis for the top area among Astra, Nobel Biocare, and Straumann systems. Compared with the other systems, a rather narrow top can be seen in the 3i system, which may result in the mixed adhesion data at this area (Figs 25.8a and 25.9A). Therefore, cell adhesion rate on the top of 3i was not measured or compared with the other systems. Statistical analysis showed no significant difference on the top between the Astra and Straumann; however, the cell adhesion rate on the top of Nobel Biocare was significantly lower than Astra and Straumann (Fig 25.12).

DISCUSSION

The surface quality of implants determines the tissue reaction at the implant/tissue interface from the moment an implant is placed, hence playing a pivotal role in the osseointegration

process. Many methods have been introduced and used to improve the surface properties of dental implants to optimize the osseointegration and overall success rate, such as blasting, anodic oxidation, and coating.[9–12] As defined by Albrektsson and Wennerberg, there are three properties regarding the implant surface quality: mechanical properties, topographic properties, and physicochemical properties.[30] These surface modifications not only change the topographic properties, but also the physicochemical properties of the implant surface.[13–17] In this study, four widely used dental implant systems were examined with Optical Profilometer, SEM, EDS, and Raman microspectroscopy. Together, the four implant systems studied cover ~85% of the world market (Nobel Biocare 30%; Straumann 25%; 3i 15% to 20%; Astra 12%).[19] Each one of the four implant systems has shown positive clinical results.[20–24] However, there is limited information regarding the direct comparison among these implant systems.

Surface topography, especially roughness, affects the implant-bone response, and there is a positive relationship between bone-to-implant contact and surface roughness.[31,32] Recently 3D evaluation of roughness (Sa) was introduced and considered as a more important and reliable method than the 2D roughness measurement, Ra.[19] In addition, to avoid confusion, the surface evaluation of screw-type implants should be based on the flank, top, and valley locations.[19] In this study, the 3D surface roughness in flanks, tops, and valleys were measured and compared separately. For the first time, significant differences of the surface roughness among flank, top, and valley in Nobel Biocare and Straumann

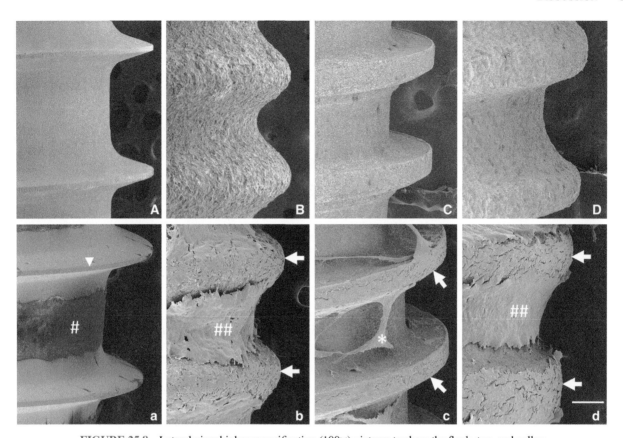

FIGURE 25.8 Lateral view higher magnification (100×) pictures to show the flank, top, and valley in different systems. (A and a) 3i, (B and b) Astra, (C and c) Nobel Biocare, and (D and d) Straumann in the conditions of without cell (A, B, C, and D) or after cell culture (a, b, c, d). Flat valley and top with steep flank in 3i and Nobel Biocare (A and C), whereas curved valley and top with shallow flank in Astra and Straumann (B and D). Cells reached confluence in part of the valley in 3i (a, #), almost no cells on the very thin top (a, arrowhead); multiple layers of confluent cells covered most of the valley and flank in Astra and Straumann (b and d, ##), with cell-covered top (b and d, arrows). Cells did not grow well on the Nobel Biocare, and did not attach to the valley (c, star); however, the flat top was covered with many cells (c, arrows). Bar = 200 μm.

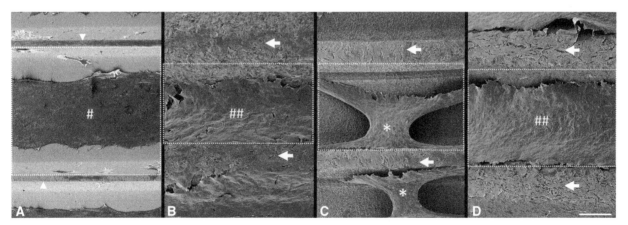

FIGURE 25.9 Higher magnification (100×) frontal view pictures from different systems after cell culture: (A) 3i, (B) Astra, (C) Nobel Biocare, and (D) Straumann. Cells reached confluence at the valley area in 3i (A, #), with mixed cell adhesion pattern on the thin top (A, arrowheads); multiple layers of confluent cells covered most of the valley and flank in Astra and Straumann (B and D, ##), with cell-covered top (B and D, arrows). Cells did not attach to the valley in Nobel Biocare (c, star); however, the flat top was covered with many cells (c, arrows). Bar = 200 μm. Using the implants without cell culture as reference, the flank and valley areas were marked by white rectangular boxes.

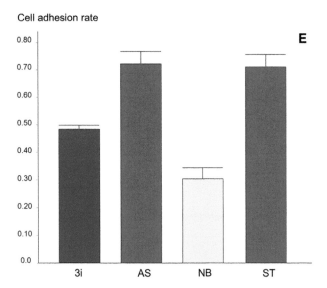

FIGURE 25.10   ANOVA showed significantly different cell adhesion rates: the ratio of cell surface/total surface (Y-axis) among different systems (AS: Astra; NB: Nobel Biocare; ST: Straumann). Cell adhesion rates shown in the same color indicate no statistical difference; the bars with different colors indicate statistical difference ($p < 0.05$). For the cell adhesion rates at the area of flank and valley, Astra = Straumann > 3i > Nobel Biocare; data shown as mean + standard deviation.

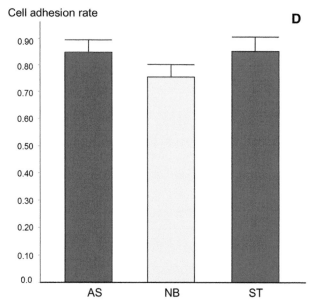

FIGURE 25.12   ANOVA showed significantly different cell adhesion rates (Y-axis) on the top among different systems (AS: Astra; NB: Nobel Biocare; ST: Straumann). Cell adhesion rates shown in the same color indicate no statistical difference; the bars with different colors indicate statistical difference ($p < 0.05$). For the cell adhesion rates at the top area, Astra = Straumann > Nobel Biocare, data shown as mean + standard deviation.

implants were shown. When roughness was compared among different implant systems at the same location, statistically significant differences were also found. Biomet 3i has the smoothest surface at all three locations (flank, top, valley). Generally, Astra and Straumann have the roughest surfaces, and Nobel Biocare followed. It was suggested that a roughness value between 1 and 1.5 μm provides optimal surface for bone integration.[25] The roughness in Astra and

Straumann on all three locations falls closer to this range than 3i and Nobel Biocare, which may explain our cell adhesion data, and may further differentiate the performance of the implants when it comes to osseointegration.

The distinct surface characteristics among these implant systems have been reported by others. One interesting observation of Nobel Biocare was the existence of multiple cracks. The existence of cracks in Nobel Biocare implants was

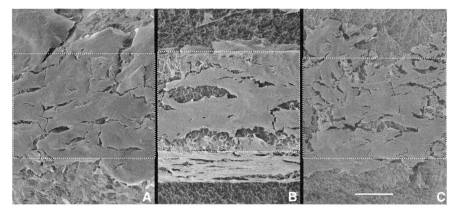

FIGURE 25.11   Higher magnification (500×) frontal view pictures from the top area in (A) Astra, (B) Nobel Biocare, and (C) Straumann. 3i was not quantified because of much lower and mixed cell adhesion on the thin top. Cells reached confluence at the top area of all three systems. Bar = 50 μm. Using the implants without cell culture as reference, the top areas were marked by white rectangular boxes.

reported in several recent SEM studies,[33–35] but not in others.[36,37] In our study, those thin and long cracks can be seen in all three flank, top, and valley locations, and can also be observed at all different SEM examining modes. Therefore, we suspect that the cracks are generated by the manufacturing process, rather than by an artifact from our examination. Another interesting point not reported before in Nobel Biocare implants is the sharp decrease of titanium, based on the EDS analysis. Currently there is no report regarding the effects of those cracks or low titanium level on the biocompatibility or osseointegration.

Raman microspectroscopy revealed both the typical rutile phase and anatase phase of titanium oxide in these implant systems.[38–40] The rutile phase of titanium oxide dominated in the 3i, Astra, and Straumann systems, whereas the anatase phase, the natural form of titanium oxide,[41] is found in Nobel Biocare. Interestingly, the rutile phase has been shown either to enhance osteoblast response[41,42] or to be less prone to initiate an inflammatory response.[43] In addition, it has been suggested that the dissolution of titanium metal ions from rutile is one order of magnitude lower than that from anatase.[44] Therefore, the rutile phase in 3i, Astra, and Straumann may be more biocompatible than the anatase phase in Nobel Biocare.

The interaction of implant surface and bone cells is critical for the clinical success of implants. The topographic modification of implant surface through specific treatments, such as sand-blasting, acid-etching, and titanium plasma-spraying, has been shown to affect the biological response of bone cells in vitro.[30,45–47] However, most of those in vitro cell culture experiments were performed on specially made titanium disks, instead of on the dental implants used in clinical practices. Although the titanium disks tried to mimic the dental implant surfaces, the topographic characterization of a flat disk is not the same as that of the implant surface. The titanium disks have the flat surface, whereas the real screw-type implants have different locations, such as flank, top, and valley, and our study has shown that roughness measurements may vary based on different locations.

Currently no cell adhesion study compares implants from different companies. One study to compare the cell adhesion on the actual implant surface examined implants from only one company, which was not internationally recognized.[18] To the best of our knowledge, our study is the first cell adhesion study to directly compare commonly used implants from different companies. In addition, we used primary osteoblastic cells harvested from alveolar bone, which may present a similar phenotype as the osteogenic cells right after in vivo implant placement. Cell lines, especially those from a tumor, should not be used to study the surface topography.[7]

Interestingly, our study found different cell adhesion rates not only among different implant systems, but also at different areas (flank, top, and valley) in the same system.

Generally, primary osteoblastic cells grew and proliferated well on both Astra and Straumann systems, which exhibited similar morphology at flank, top, and valley areas. After Astra and Straumann, cells reached confluence in the 3i system, but only to form a rather thin layer of cell and to cover the valley area. The cell adhesion in the flank and top was much less in the 3i system. For the Nobel Biocare system, primary osteoblastic cells did not attach as well as other systems, especially at the valley area, and quantitative analysis showed the least adhesion rate at the flank and valley areas.

The cell adhesion data were supported and correlated with the data from the comparison on the surface characteristics among those implant systems. Astra and Straumann have the roughest surfaces and also displayed the highest cell adhesion rate on all three locations (flank, top, valley). Although Nobel Biocare has a rougher surface than 3i, the multiple cracks on the surface and anatase phase of titanium dioxide[44] may explain the negative cell adhesion results for the Nobel Biocare system. One interesting point for the Nobel Biocare system is the improved cell adhesion at the top area, when compared with flank and valley. Our data currently cannot render an explanation for this, which needs further investigation.

Although osteoblastic cells play a more direct role in the process of osseointegration, which is reflected by more published studies using osteoblastic cell lines or primary cells,[45,47,48] the in vivo implant-bone interaction may be affected by other factors, such as blood cell reaction and platelet activation, because early blood cell reaction and platelet activation may eventually affect the migration and differentiation of osteogenic cells in the healing process.[8,49,50] In addition, it is not clear whether those differences from the cell adhesion experiment will have any impact on the osseointegration between implant and bone in vivo, because all four implant systems have shown positive clinical results.[20–24] Indeed, to answer the question if those different surface characteristics will have any impact or correlation on the osseointegration between implant and bone, further in vivo animal study or human studies will be necessary.

CONCLUSION

Our preliminary data indicated that the four implant systems displayed distinct surface characteristics. Astra and Straumann systems showed the roughest surface, whereas 3i showed the smoothest surface. Multiple cracks were found on the surface of the Nobel Biocare system. In addition, the rutile phase of titanium oxide was found in 3i, Astra, and Straumann. The anatase phase of titanium oxide was detected in Nobel Biocare. Correspondingly, Astra and Straumann displayed the highest primary cell adhesion at the flank, top, and valley areas. Primary cells also reached confluence on the valley, but significantly less than in the 3i system. Nobel Biocare showed the least cell adhesion on the flank and valley. Further in vivo study is needed to study the impact of the surface characteristics and different cell adhesion on the osseointegration between implant and bone.

REFERENCES

1. Branemark R, Branemark PI, Rydevik B, et al: Osseointegration in skeletal reconstruction and rehabilitation: a review. *J Rehabil Res Dev* 2001;38:175–181.

2. Jokstad A, Braegger U, Brunski JB, et al: Quality of dental implants. *Int Dent J* 2003;53:409–443.

3. Albrektsson T, Wennerberg A: Oral implant surfaces: Part 2—review focusing on clinical knowledge of different surfaces. *Int J Prosthodont* 2004;17:544–564.

4. Eckert SE, Choi YG, Sanchez AR, et al: Comparison of dental implant systems: quality of clinical evidence and prediction of 5-year survival. *Int J Oral Maxillofac Implants* 2005;20:406–415.

5. Esposito M, Grusovin MG, Coulthard P, et al: A 5-year follow-up comparative analysis of the efficacy of various osseointegrated dental implant systems: a systematic review of randomized controlled clinical trials. *Int J Oral Maxillofac Implants* 2005;20:557–568.

6. Bhatavadekar N: Assessing the evidence supporting the claims of select dental implant surfaces: a systematic review. *Int Dent J* 2008;58:363–370.

7. Anselme K, Ponche A, Bigerelle M: Relative influence of surface topography and surface chemistry on cell response to bone implant materials. Part 2: biological aspects. *Proc Inst Mech Eng H* 2010;224:1487–1507.

8. Davies JE: Understanding peri-implant endosseous healing. *J Dent Educ* 2003;67:932–949.

9. Cochran DL: A comparison of endosseous dental implant surfaces. *J Periodontol* 1999;70:1523–1539.

10. Yeo IS, Han JS, Yang JH: Biomechanical and histomorphometric study of dental implants with different surface characteristics. *J Biomed Mater Res B Appl Biomater* 2008;87:303–311.

11. Le Guehennec L, Soueidan A, Layrolle P, et al: Surface treatments of titanium dental implants for rapid osseointegration. *Dent Mater* 2007;23:844–854.

12. Schliephake H, Aref A, Scharnweber D, et al: Effect of modifications of dual acid-etched implant surfaces on peri-implant bone formation. Part I: organic coatings. *Clin Oral Implants Res* 2009;20:31–37.

13. Stanford CM: Surface modifications of dental implants. *Aust Dent J* 2008;53(Suppl 1):S26–S33.

14. Albrektsson T: Hard tissue implant interface. *Aust Dent J* 2008;53(Suppl 1):S34–S38.

15. Duyck J, Slaets E, Sasaguri K, et al: Effect of intermittent loading and surface roughness on peri-implant bone formation in a bone chamber model. *J Clin Periodontol* 2007;34:998–1006.

16. Ferguson SJ, Langhoff JD, Voelter K, et al: Biomechanical comparison of different surface modifications for dental implants. *Int J Oral Maxillofac Implants* 2008;23:1037–1046.

17. Coelho PG, Granjeiro JM, Romanos GE, et al: Basic research methods and current trends of dental implant surfaces. *J Biomed Mater Res B Appl Biomater* 2009;88:579–596.

18. Alves SF, Wassall T: In vitro evaluation of osteoblastic cell adhesion on machined osseointegrated implants. *Braz Oral Res* 2009;23:131–136.

19. Wennerberg A, Albrektsson T: On implant surfaces: a review of current knowledge and opinions. *Int J Oral Maxillofac Implants* 2010;25:63–74.

20. Bergkvist G, Koh KJ, Sahlholm S, et al: Bone density at implant sites and its relationship to assessment of bone quality and treatment outcome. *Int J Oral Maxillofac Implants* 2010;25:321–328.

21. Ostman PO, Wennerberg A, Albrektsson T: Immediate occlusal loading of NanoTite PREVAIL implants: a prospective 1-year clinical and radiographic study. *Clin Implant Dent Relat Res* 2010;12:39–47.

22. Glauser R, Ruhstaller P, Windisch S, et al: Immediate occlusal loading of Branemark System TiUnite implants placed predominantly in soft bone: 4-year results of a prospective clinical study. *Clin Implant Dent Relat Res* 2005;7(Suppl 1):S52–S59.

23. Palmer RM, Howe LC, Palmer PJ, et al: A prospective clinical trial of single Astra Tech 4.0 or 5.0 diameter implants used to support two-unit cantilever bridges: results after 3 years. *Clin Oral Implants Res* 2012;23:35–40.

24. Barbier L, Abeloos J, De Clercq C, et al: Peri-implant bone changes following tooth extraction, immediate placement and loading of implants in the edentulous maxilla. *Clin Oral Investig* 2012;16:1061–1070.

25. Wennerberg A, Albrektsson T: Suggested guidelines for the topographic evaluation of implant surfaces. *Int J Oral Maxillofac Implants* 2000;15:331–344.

26. Suda N, Kitahara Y, Hammond VE, et al: Development of a novel mouse osteoclast culture system including cells of mandibular body and erupting teeth. *Bone* 2003;33:38–45.

27. Fanchon S, Bourd K, Septier D, et al: Involvement of matrix metalloproteinases in the onset of dentin mineralization. *Eur J Oral Sci* 2004;112:171–176.

28. Torres-Quintana MA, Lecolle S, Septier D, et al: Inositol hexasulphate, a casein kinase inhibitor, alters enamel formation in cultured embryonic mouse tooth germs. *J Dent Res* 2000;79:1794–1801.

29. Klein MO, Bijelic A, Toyoshima T, et al: Long-term response of osteogenic cells on micron and submicron-scale-structured hydrophilic titanium surfaces: sequence of cell proliferation and cell differentiation. *Clin Oral Implants Res* 2010;21:642–649.

30. Albrektsson T, Wennerberg A: Oral implant surfaces: Part 1—review focusing on topographic and chemical properties of different surfaces and in vivo responses to them. *Int J Prosthodont* 2004;17:536–543.

31. Shalabi MM, Gortemaker A, Van't Hof MA, et al: Implant surface roughness and bone healing: a systematic review. *J Dent Res* 2006;85:496–500.

32. Vandamme K, Naert I, Vander Sloten J, et al: Effect of implant surface roughness and loading on peri-implant bone formation. *J Periodontol* 2008;79:150–157.

33. Dohan Ehrenfest DM, Coelho PG, Kang BS, et al: Classification of osseointegrated implant surfaces: materials, chemistry and topography. *Trends Biotechnol* 2010;28:198–206.

34. Kang BS, Sul YT, Oh SJ, et al: XPS, AES and SEM analysis of recent dental implants. *Acta Biomater* 2009;5:2222–2229.

35. Dohan Ehrenfest DM, Vazquez L, Park YJ, et al: Identification card and codification of the chemical and morphological characteristics of 14 dental implant surfaces. *J Oral Implantol* 2011;37:525–542.

36. Sul YT, Byon E, Wennerberg A: Surface characteristics of electrochemically oxidized implants and acid-etched implants: surface chemistry, morphology, pore configurations, oxide thickness, crystal structure, and roughness. *Int J Oral Maxillofac Implants* 2008;23:631–640.

37. Jarmar T, Palmquist A, Branemark R, et al: Characterization of the surface properties of commercially available dental implants using scanning electron microscopy, focused ion beam, and high-resolution transmission electron microscopy. *Clin Implant Dent Relat Res* 2008;10:11–22.

38. Li J-G, Ishigaki T, Sun X: Anatase, brookite, and rutile nanocrystals via redox reactions under mild hydrothermal conditions: phase-selective synthesis and physicochemical properties. *J Phys Chem C* 2007;111:4969–4976.

39. Busquim TdP, Elias CN, May JE, et al: Titanium oxide layer on the surface of anodized dental implants. In Gilbert J (ed): *Medical Device Materials V; Proceedings from the Materials & Processes for Medical Devices Conference 2009*. Novelty, OH, ASM International, 2010, pp. 60–65.

40. Felske A, Plieth WJ: Raman spectroscopy of titanium dioxide layers. *Electrochimica Acta* 1989;34:75–77.

41. Feng B, Weng J, Yang BC, et al: Characterization of surface oxide films on titanium and adhesion of osteoblast. *Biomaterials* 2003;24:4663–4670.

42. Saldana L, Barranco V, Garcia-Alonso MC, et al: Concentration-dependent effects of titanium and aluminum ions released from thermally oxidized Ti6Al4V alloy on human osteoblasts. *J Biomed Mater Res A* 2006;77:220–229.

43. Valles G, Gonzalez-Melendi P, Gonzalez-Carrasco JL, et al: Differential inflammatory macrophage response to rutile and titanium particles. *Biomaterials* 2006;27:5199–5211.

44. Huang N, Chen YR, Luo JM, et al: In vitro investigation of blood compatibility of Ti with oxide layers of rutile structure. *J Biomater Appl* 1994;8:404–412.

45. Goto T, Yoshinari M, Kobayashi S, et al: The initial attachment and subsequent behavior of osteoblastic cells and oral epithelial cells on titanium. *Biomed Mater Eng* 2004;14:537–544.

46. Wennerberg A, Albrektsson T: Effects of titanium surface topography on bone integration: a systematic review. *Clin Oral Implants Res* 2009;20(Suppl 4):172–184.

47. Guida L, Annunziata M, Rocci A, et al: Biological response of human bone marrow mesenchymal stem cells to fluoride-modified titanium surfaces. *Clin Oral Implants Res* 2010;21: 1234–1241.

48. Yamashita D, Machigashira M, Miyamoto M, et al: Effect of surface roughness on initial responses of osteoblast-like cells on two types of zirconia. *Dent Mater J* 2009;28:461–470.

49. Park JY, Davies JE: Red blood cell and platelet interactions with titanium implant surfaces. *Clin Oral Implants Res* 2000;11:530–539.

50. Park JY, Gemmell CH, Davies JE: Platelet interactions with titanium: modulation of platelet activity by surface topography. *Biomaterials* 2001;22:2671–2682.

PART V

GENERAL CONSIDERATIONS

26

OUTCOMES OF DENTAL IMPLANTS IN OSTEOPOROTIC PATIENTS. A LITERATURE REVIEW

Ioanna N. Tsolaki, dds,[1] Phoebus N. Madianos, dds, phd,[2] and John A. Vrotsos, dds, dr dent, ficd[2]

[1]Private Practice, Athens, Greece
[2]Department of Periodontology, School of Dentistry, University of Athens, Greece

Keywords

Osteoporosis; dental implants; osseointegration; jaw bone; biphosphonates; bone quality; gender; age.

Correspondence

Ioanna N. Tsolaki, Papadiamantopoulou 44, Zografou, Athens 15771, Greece. E-mail: itsolaki@yahoo.com

Accepted April 10, 2008

Published in *Journal of Prosthodontics* June 2009; Vol. 18, Issue 4

doi: 10.1111/j.1532-849X.2008.00433.x

ABSTRACT

Purpose: This article reviews available data on the outcome of dental implants in osteoporotic patients.

Materials and Methods: A search was performed in PubMed and completed in July 2007. The keywords "dental AND implants AND osteoporosis," "dental AND implants AND age," "dental AND implants AND gender," and "dental AND implants AND bone AND quality," with no limitations for language or year of publication, resulted in 82, 598, 94, and 541 articles, respectively. After abstract scanning (in case of doubt the article was read), 39 nonreview articles studying dental implant outcomes in osteoporotic/osteopenic subjects remained for our review. The bibliographies of the 39 articles were also inspected, but no additional studies were identified.

Results: Thirteen of 16 animal studies found lower osseointegration rates in osteoporotic/osteopenic bone than in normal bone. Six in nine clinical reports mention success. Eight of 12 studies in humans support the applicability of dental implants in osteoporotic patients.

Conclusions: There are no data to contraindicate the use of dental implants in osteoporotic patients; however, a proper adjustment of the surgical technique and a longer healing period may be considered in order to achieve osseointegration. Data on the use of biphosphonates in osteoporotic patients and implant outcomes are very limited, and no conclusions can be drawn. In addition, large prospective studies investigating the long-term success of dental implants in osteoporotic individuals are required.

Dental implants constitute a well-documented treatment modality.[1-3] Osteoporosis is the most common human metabolic bone disease.[4] The influence of this disease on the jawbone is still a matter of controversy. The outcome of dental implants in patients with osteoporosis in the jaws or in other skeletal sites will be the subject of this article.

Definition of Osteoporosis

Osteoporosis has been defined as a systemic skeletal disease characterized by low bone mass and microarchitectural deterioration of bone tissue, with consequent increase in bone fragility and susceptibility to fracture.[5]

According to the World Health Organization (WHO), subjects with a T-score value 2.5 standard deviations (SDs) or more below the mean bone mineral density (BMD) value of the young (20 to 29 years old) sex-matched reference population at the total hip, femoral neck, or lumbar spine are classed as osteoporotic.[6] Osteoporosis is divided into osteoporosis with pathologic fracture, without pathologic fracture, and osteoporosis caused by other diseases (multiple myelomatosis, endocrine disorders, etc.). When a fragility fracture is present, the condition is defined as "established osteoporosis."[7]

Subjects with a T-score value 1 to 2.5 SDs below the mean BMD value of the young sex-matched reference population in the prementioned skeletal sites are classed as osteopenic.[6]

Bone mineral content (BMC) is the amount of mineral in the specific site scanned, and when divided by the area measured, it can be used to derive a value for BMD[8] (mg/cm^2). When quantitative computed tomography (QCT) is used, BMD is not an areal but a volumetric density measurement (mg/cm^3).[9]

Epidemiology of Osteoporosis

Osteoporosis occurs in about one-third of the Western female population above the age of 65 years.[10] Currently, it is estimated that over 200 million people worldwide suffer from this disease.[11] Because the distribution of values for the BMD in the young healthy population is Gaussian, the incidence of osteoporosis increases exponentially after the age of 50 years.[12]

According to others, at some point in their lives, 40% of women[13-15] or 50% of women over the age of 50[16] and up to 29% of men[17] may sustain an osteoporotic fracture.

A higher prevalence of fragility fractures has been described in white populations,[18] especially in non-Hispanic Caucasians;[19] lower rates have been found among black populations.[18] In Europe, the Scandinavian countries have the highest prevalence of fragility fractures.[20]

Pathophysiology of Osteoporosis

Sex-hormone deficiency seems to be an important causal factor of primary osteoporosis in both men and women. Estrogen deficiency in women causes bone loss both through the loss of the direct action of estrogen on bone cells (that restrain bone turnover) and through the loss of the action of estrogen on the intestine and kidney (that maintain extra-skeletal calcium fluxes).[21] It leads to increased numbers of bone multicellular units and to uncoupling of bone formation and bone resorption.[22]

Men exhibit only a slow phase of bone loss during which increased levels of sex-hormone-binding globulin (SHBG) bind sex steroids in an inactive complex.[23]

Cancellous bone is much more richly vascularized by osseous vascular complexes that pass between the less dense trabeculae. This arrangement produces a much higher surface-to-volume ratio to bone extracellular fluids. Therefore, cancellous bone responds more quickly to metabolic alterations and for this reason, skeletal sites such as vertebral bodies, the forearm, and hip are more susceptible to processes that increase bone resorption, such as osteoporosis.[24] Similarly, it can be expected that any osteoporosis influence should be greater in the maxilla rather than in the mandible, because of the presence of a higher percentage of trabecular bone in the former.[25]

Osteoporosis risk factors[4,8,26-29] are presented in Table 26.1.

Systemic Complications of Osteoporosis

There is no evidence that bone loss itself causes any symptoms. Progressive bone loss has therefore been called "the silent thief."[16] Fractures among the elderly may occur after a moderate trauma or even spontaneously. The most common fractures associated with osteoporosis occur at the hip, spine, and wrist.[16,30]

Dental Implants and Osteoporosis

Osteoporosis in other skeletal sites seems to be associated with a decrease of BMD in the jaw. The authors agree that the correlation is not strong enough to be used for proper predictions in the jaw.[31] In addition, a majority of relevant studies suggest that postmenopausal osteoporosis may be important for the progression of bone loss in periodontitis.[22] This may reduce bone quantity at implantation sites. Finally, a correlation of periodontitis with peri-implantitis has been suggested,[32] and therefore a question arises concerning peri-implantitis in osteoporotic patients.

TABLE 26.1   Osteoporosis Risk Factors

▪ Female sex	° Athletic amenorrhea
▪ Age	° Hyperprolactinemia
▪ Asian or white ethnic origin	° Panhypopituitarism
▪ Genetic disorders	° Premature menopause
▪ 1st-degree relative with low trauma fracture	● Gastrointestinal diseases
▪ Thin habitus	● Hematological diseases
▪ Deficiency states:	● Idiopathic hypercalciuria
● Calcium	● Idiopathic scoliosis
● Magnesium	● Multiple sclerosis
● Vitamin D	● Neuromuscular disorders
▪ Diseases:	● Post-transplant bone disease
● Amyloidosis	● Rheumatologic diseases
● Chronic metabolic acidosis	● Sarcoidosis
● Chronic obstructive pulmonary disease	● Stroke
● Cystic fibrosis	▪ Drugs:
● Depression	● Anticoagulants
● Emphysema	● Anticonvulsants
● End-stage renal disease	● Antiepileptics
● Endocrine disorders:	● Cyclosporines
° Acromegaly	● Cytotoxic drugs
° Addison's disease	● Excessive thyroxine dose
° Cushing's syndrome	● Glucocorticoids
° Diabetes mellitus	● Gonadotropin-releasing hormone agonists
° Hyperparathyroidism	● Lithium
° Thyrotoxicosis	● Tacrolimus
● Hypogonadal states:	▪ Immobilization
° Androgen insensitivity	▪ Cigarette smoking
° Anorexia nervosa/bulimia	▪ Alcoholism
	▪ Parenteral nutrition

MATERIALS AND METHODS

A search was performed in PubMed and completed in July 2007. The main keywords of the search were "dental AND implants AND osteoporosis." The search yielded 82 articles. No limitations were set for language or year of publication. The inclusion criteria were nonreview articles dealing with the possible relation between osteoporosis and dental implants. After scanning abstracts, 38 articles, including 9 clinical reports and 18 animal and 11 human studies, remained for our review.

To identify additional studies that were not returned in the first search even though they study the possible relation between dental implants outcome and osteoporosis, three more keywords were used:

(1) "dental AND implants AND age" → 598 articles
(2) "dental AND implants AND gender" → 94 articles
(3) "dental AND implants AND bone AND quality" → 541 articles.

Inclusion and exclusion criteria remained the same, and the studies' abstracts were scanned (in cases of doubt the article was read), but only one that had not been included in our first search directly referred to the osteoporosis condition. In other words, the use of the last three keywords added one study directly addressing the question of osteoporosis effect on dental implants outcome. Finally, 39 articles were included in the results of the present review; however, the rest of the second group studies were not totally excluded from our article. We reconsidered the second group articles, excluding this time not only reviews but also clinical reports and animal studies. We are focusing now on the final conclusions of the already sufficiently studied age, gender, and bone-quality effect on dental implants outcome. The reason is that the strong relation of the above three parameters with osteoporosis offers important indirect information suiting well to our discussion.

The bibliographies of the 39 reviewed articles were also inspected, but no additional studies were identified.

RESULTS

Thirteen of 16 animal studies found lower osseointegration rates in osteopenic/osteoporotic bone than in normal bone.[33–45] It is suggested that there is a biphasic effect of female gonadal hormone deficiency that may temporarily interfere in the early implant-tissue integration process, and which may be associated with a failure to upregulate a select set of bone extracellular matrix genes.[43] It is also suggested that osseointegration in osteoporotic animals is 50% slower than that of normal experiment animals.[38,43] Only three[46–48] out of 16 animal studies found no difference (Table 26.2).

Three animal studies (two of them are not included in Table 26.2, because they did not compare healthy to osteoporotic animals but only treated to untreated osteoporotic animals) addressed the question of whether therapies used in osteoporotic animals affect osseointegration. Two of them suggested that estrogen replacement therapy may promote bone healing around titanium implants in osteoporotic bone.[40,49] The third study supported that local administration of growth hormone at the point of surgery could enhance osteoid synthesis and mineralization around titanium sheets in an osteoporotic animal.[50]

Six in nine clinical reports mention success,[51–56] even after immediate loading[54] of dental implants in osteoporotic patients. Two of the three [57–59] clinical reports that mention failure of dental implants either just hypothesize the presence of osteoporosis[58] or refer to mandible fractures.[59]

Twelve studies in humans directly address the question of systemic osteoporosis effect on dental implants outcome[60–71] (Table 26.3). Eight of the studies[60–67] reveal a rather optimistic opinion concerning the applicability of dental implants

TABLE 26.2 Animal Studies Reviewed

Study	Animal Model	Nr. of Animals	Postimplantation Period	OP-Like Conditions	Results	Type of Examination
Keller et al, 2004[42]	Rabbit	4 groups of 10	4 weeks	By daily intramuscular injections of glucocorticoids	Altered and compromised ECM expression in all animals with OP-like conditions, reduced bone-implant interface when OP-like conditions were present prior to the establishment of osseointegration, no significant differences in pull-out strength	Histologic, mechanical property testing
Cho et al, 2004[36]	Rats	5 groups of 7	12 weeks	OVE	Osseointegration achieved, surrounding bone stabilized	Histologic and histomorphometric analysis
Okamura et al, 2004[48]	Rats	4 groups of 5	1 month	OVE	High turnover situation is more favorable for implantation than low-turnover one	Biochemical, histological, and histometrical analysis
Narai and Nagahata, 2003[40]	Rats	25	1 month	OVE	Reduced removal torque in OP animals compared to healthy or alendronate-administered OP animals	Removal torque, histologic, histometric evaluation
Duarte et al, 2003[33]	Rats	15 OVE, 15 sham-OVE	60 days	OVE	No significant differences in cortical bone but lower bone-implant contact in cancellous regions of OP bone	Histometric analysis, biochemical serum analysis
Fini et al, 2002[35]	Rats, sheep	9 OVE and 9 sham-OVE rats, 3 OVE and 3 sham-OVE sheep	Rats: 8 weeks Sheep: 12 weeks	OVE	Delay of peri-implant bone formation and maturation in OP animals	Histomorphometric examination, bone-implant interface microhardness
Ozawa et al, 2002[43]	Rats	28 OVE, 28 sham surgery	2 and 4 weeks	OVE	Delay of osseointegration in OVE rats, differences diminished at 4 weeks postimplantation	Histomorphometric analysis, biomechanical push-in test, RT-PCR
Jung et al, 2001[39]	Rabbit	14 OVE, 13 sham surgery	12 weeks	OVE	Lower bone volume but no statistically significant lower bone-to-metal contact in OVE versus sham-operated rabbits	Histomorphometric analysis, removal torque, osteoblast culturing
Pan et al, 2000[41]	Rats	18 OVE and 18 sham-OVE 168 days postimplantation	28, 84, 168 days post-OVE or post-sham-OVE	OVE	Significant decrease in the bone volume around the implant and implant-bone contact in the cancellous bone area in OVE compared to sham-operated rats	Histologic and histomorphometric measurements
Lugero et al, 2000[37]	Rabbits	8 controls and 12 OP	8 weeks	OVE	Less bone formation in OP cases, improved bone formation with screw-type implants in cases and controls	Histomorphometry

Reference	Animal	Number	Duration	Intervention	Results	Examination
Yamazaki et al, 1999[45]	Rats	30 test and 30 controls	7 to 56 days	OVE	Lower rate of bone contact and relative bone mass around the implant in cancellous bone of OVE rats	Histologic and histomorphometric examination
Fujimoto et al, 1998[47]	Rabbit	6 steroid-treated and 6 controls	3 months	Prednisolone treatment	Steroid administration effects less osseointegration in the mandibles than in the skeletal bone	Removal torque of implants in the mandible and the tibia and microdensitometry measurements in the left femur
Nasu et al, 1998[46]	Rats	2 groups of 6 test animals and 6 controls	7 to 42 days	Ca-deficient diet	No differences in osseointegration between cases and controls	Microradiographs and autoradiographs
Mori et al, 1997[38]	Rabbit	2 groups of 12 animals each and 12 controls	2, 4, 8, or 12 weeks	OVE or OVE + low-Ca diet	Osseointegration is achieved in OP animals, but a longer healing period is needed	Histologic and microradiographic examination of the bone-implant interface in the tibia
Martin et al, 1988[44]	Beagle dogs	5 OVE, 5 sham-OVE	2 months	OVE	OVE caused no difference in the amount of ingrowth of bone, significant increase in the amount of fibrous connective tissue	Mechanical tests, histological study
Hayashi et al, 1994[34]	Rats	3 models	24 weeks	OVE, OVE + neurectomy	Significant decrease of affinity index bone-implant in OP-like cases	Histological study

OVE = ovariectomy/ovariectomized; ECM = extracellular matrix; HRT = hormone replacement therapy; OP = osteoporosis/osteoporotic; BMC% = BMD percentage of age-matched (describes the mean value matched for age and sex and is normally 100%); B = biphosphonates; PTV = Periotest values.

TABLE 26.3 Human Studies Reviewed

Study	Patients	OP Patients	Sites with Diagnosed OP	BMD Measurement	Implant Receiving Jaw	Nr. of Implants in the OP Group	Nr. of Implants in the Control Group	Bone Quality Assessment	Experimental Period	Osseointegration Assessment	Results
Alsaadi et al, 2007[71]	1212 females, 792 males				Mandible, Maxilla		6946 implants totally in OP + non-OP		Up to abutment connection	Intraoral radiography, PTV ≥5, subjective signs of pain or infection that required implant removal	Osteoporosis significantly related to early implant failures
Amorim et al, 2006[64]	39 women/48 to 70 years old	19	Lumbar spine, femoral neck	DXA	Mandible	39	43	Panoramic X-rays, histomorphometric, bone biopsy	9 months	Clinical and X-ray examination	No association
Jeffcoat, 2006[63]	25 postmenopausal women receiving B + 25 postmenopausal women without B	50				102	108		3 years	Clinical and X-ray examination	Success: 99.2% without, 100% with oral biphosphonates
Smolka et al, 2006[67]	10 females + 5 males, 18 to 68 years old, mean age 52 years, patients, only 5 in 1-year follow-up	9 females	Generalized osteoporosis	Bone densitometry	8 mandibles, 8 maxillas			CT scanning	Maximum 1 year	CT scanning for grafts bone density measurements	Generalized osteoporosis did not increase the resorption rate of calvarial transplants
Moyet al, 2005[70]	1140 patients, 12 to 94 years, 59.4% females, 161 on PMHRT, 304 on no PMHRT, median age = 58 years				Mandible, maxilla				Retrospective cohort study, 1982–2003	Implant survival	Lower success rate for postmenopausal women on HRT
van Steenberghe et al, 2002[65]	399, 15 to 80, mean age 50, SD ± 14 years					2		Clinical and panoramic examination, CT scanning when needed	Up to the abutment connection		No increased percentage of early failures in OP
Friberg et al, 2001[60]	11 females + 2 males, 55 to 79 years, mean age 68 years	13	Lumbar spine, hip	DXA	Mandible, maxilla	70	No control group	Clinical and X-rays examination	6 months to 11 years, mean 3.3 years	Clinical and X-ray examination	Maxilla: 97%, mandible: 97.3% success
von Wowern et al, 2001[66]	22 patients, 18 postmenopausal women, 54 to 78 years, mean age 65 years	7 women with OP in the mandible, 8 with OP in the forearm	Forearm, mandible	Dual-photon scanner for BMC in the jaws	Mandibles	7 × 2 and 8 × 2	No control group	Clinical and X-rays examination	5 years	Clinical and X-ray examination	Load-related bone formation minimizing mandibular BMC loss

Study	Patients	OP already diagnosed	BMD site measured	BMD method	Implant location	Bone assessment	No. implants	No.	Maximum follow-up	Outcome measure	Conclusion
August et al, 2001[68]	No treatment for OP. Maxilla: 78, 36 cases, 60, 41, 60 controls. Mandible: 90, 39 cases, 54, 18, 50 controls (mean ages: 66.3, 61.7, 36, 34.5, 64.2)				Mandible, maxilla		Maxilla: 302, 111. Mandible: 268, 130	Maxilla: 112, 64, 172. Mandible: 101, 32, 121	Maximum 5 years	Stability at stage II uncovering surgery by manual torque and X-ray	Estrogen deficiency may be a risk factor for dental implant failure in the maxilla
Becker et al, 2000[61]	49 cases, 49 controls (19 males + 30 females in each group), 44 to 85 years	7 controls and 10 cases already diagnosed OP	Proximal and distal radius and ulna	pDEXA at the distal and proximal radius and ulna	Mandible, maxilla	Visual assessment of local bone	184	180	Average 3 years and 10 months	Implant survival	No association
Minsk and Polson, 1998[62]	116 (25 on HRT + 91 without HRT) women, older than 50 years				Mandible, maxilla					Implant survival	HRT may not improve implants success
Blomqvist et al, 1996[69]	11 (7 females + 4 males) cases, 11 controls, 46 to 75, mean age 59 years			Single-photon gamma absorptiometry of forearm	Maxilla + bone grafting	Osteometry, hematologic, urinary tests	74	71	14 to 58 months, mean of 30 months	Implant survival	Significantly different BMD% in successful and failure cases

OVE = ovariectomy/ovariectomized; ECM = extracellular matrix; HRT = hormone replacement therapy; OP = osteoporosis/osteoporotic; BMC% = BMD percentage of age-matched (describes the mean value matched for age and sex and is normally 100%); B = biphosphonates; PTV = Periotest values.

in osteoporotic patients. Hormone replacement therapy (HRT) may not be related to significantly increased implant success,[62,68] although previously mentioned animal studies implied the opposite. It is suggested that simple visual assessment of local bone quality has a moderately sized relationship to implant failure.[61] Only four of 12 studies relate osteoporosis to increased failure rates of dental implants,[68–71] especially in the maxilla.[68] But one of these three studies found statistically insignificant results.[68]

DISCUSSION

The following parameters have to be discussed in our attempt to sufficiently analyze the present subject:

(1) WHO definition of osteoporosis,
(2) animal studies deficiencies,
(3) human studies deficiencies,
(4) indirect information from studies on dental implants and age, gender, and jawbone quality, and
(5) implication of biphosphonate therapy in dental implants outcomes.

WHO Definition of Osteoporosis

The WHO criteria are aimed at providing a quantitative definition that would separate individuals having the disease, even if no osteoporotic fracture had occurred yet, from those at risk of becoming osteoporotic, and those who are still normal. Since BMD is continuously distributed in the population, and the risk of fracture is also continuous, in the absence of fracture, there is no absolute criterion that can be made to delineate an individual with the disease from one without. For this reason, there is an overlap between BMD in populations with and without fracture.[72] The estimation of fracture risk by BMD measurements is similar to the assessment of the risk of stroke by blood pressure readings. Despite the decision of a cutoff threshold value that separates individuals with recognized high risk for osteoporotic fracture or stroke from the rest, there is no threshold of BMD/blood pressure that discriminates absolutely between those who will or will not have a clinical event.[8] BMD is one of the main, but not the only, factor determining the risk of fracture.[72] It has been shown that the loss of connectivity within the network of trabecular bone is independent from BMD risk factor for fractures.[73] Additionally, bone geometry features such as bone size, the distribution of bone mass around its bending axis (moments of inertia), and some derivative functions, such as the hip axis length, affect bone strength and fracture risk.[74]

BMD measures at various sites have given discordant results.[72] So, individuals may be deemed osteoporotic at one specific site and not at another. The WHO criteria for the diagnosis of osteoporosis were defined for DXA (dual X-ray absorptiometry) of the forearm, spine, and hip, and selected at a level that would identify as osteoporotic 30% of the population of postmenopausal women. The definition did not originally intend to be applied to other patient groups, or to BMD measurements made by different methods and at other skeletal sites.[74,75] This is important when considering the impact of systemic osteoporosis in the jawbone.

The normative data against which BMD comparisons are most often made have been determined for Caucasian men and women, and do not necessarily apply to other ethnic groups.

Although BMD is clearly related to body weight, routine clinical bone mass assessments are not weight adjusted.[74]

Animal Studies Deficiencies

It must be underlined that in 14 of the 16 prementioned animal studies implants were not placed in the jaws.[33–45,48] They were inserted in the tibia[33–39,42–45,48] (11 studies) or the femur[35,40,43] (three studies). Only two studies[46,47] tested dental implants in the mandible of experiment animals and, interestingly enough, they both found no significant difference of osseointegration rate between osteoporotic/osteopenic animals and controls. Particularly, Fujimoto et al[47] found that rabbits' systemic osteoporosis-like condition had less effect on osseointegration of titanium implants in the mandible than in skeletal bone; however, this study refers to steroid-induced osteoporosis, and its pathogenetic mechanisms are different from those of postmenopausal osteoporosis.[22]

Besides the already mentioned implantation site, there are several other important factors involved in the final results of these studies:

(a) *Animal model:* The rat was used in 10[33–36,40,41,43,45,46,48] of 16 animal studies; however, it may not provide the best model for the analogous condition in humans because of the failure to achieve true skeletal maturity and the normal inhibition of intracortical remodeling.[76] On the contrary, the rabbit, used in five studies,[37–39,42,47] achieves skeletal maturity shortly after reaching sexual development at approximately six months and shows significant intracortical remodeling.[77] Regarding dogs, used in one study,[44] data are controversial. Some studies,[78] but not all,[79–83] have shown insignificant bone loss in dogs after cessation of ovarian function. Last, the sheep, used in one study,[35] is considered a good animal model, although seasonal fluctuations of bone mass and biochemical markers must be addressed as a potential variable when studying osteoporosis.[76,84]

(b) *Method used for the creation of osteoporosis-like condition:* In 13[33–41,43–45,48] of the 16 animal studies, ovariectomy is used for the creation of osteoporosis-like conditions; however, according to Mori et al, ovariectomy did not result in adequate reduction of BMD in rabbits unless it was combined with a low-Ca diet.[38] Two studies were based on corticosteroid-induced osteoporosis[42,47] and one in calcium-deficient diet.[46] In addition, there is a variety of experiment animal ages, diets, and intervening time between ovariectomy and implant surgery.

(c) *Evaluation of the obtained level of osteopenia/osteoporosis:* As already mentioned, a variety of protocols have been used for the induction of osteoporosis. In addition, bone changes in ovariectomized rats are considered as osteopenia rather than osteoporosis.[84] Despite these two facts, 10[33,35,36,39,41–43,45–47] of the 16 studies do not mention any assessment of BMD prior to implantation so that the level of the provoked osteopenia/osteoporosis could be clarified.

(d) *Osseointegration assessment criteria:* There are a variety of measurements used for the assessment of osseointegration. Some of them (mechanical test values) evaluate osseointegration indirectly and may be affected by other parameters such as implant fixation mainly in cortical bone,[40] implant surface, length, width, composition, shape, and healing period.[47] Keller et al found a statistically significant decrease in implant-bone contact in osteoporotic rabbits compared to controls, although interfacial strength was not affected.[42]

(e) *Postimplantation observation period:* Postimplantation observation period varies from 7 days to 168 days in the rat model, from 2 weeks to 3 months in the rabbit model, 12 weeks for the sheep model, and 2 months for beagle dogs. The relatively short observation period is one of the shortcomings of these studies. Additionally, dental implants in clinical practice are differently loaded from animal models. Thus, short-term animal studies offer no information concerning the long-term response of the osteoporotic bone to the presence of functionally loaded dental implants.

Human Studies Deficiencies

Various study design characteristics perplex the comparison of the existing human studies and limit their contribution to the clarification of dental implant outcomes in osteoporotic patients. A quick presentation of limiting factors follows.

In a total of 12 studies in humans, six retrospective[61,62,65,69–71] and six prospective,[60,63,64,66–68] control groups are not included in three,[60,62,66] implants are not divided according to site of implantation in three of them,[62,63,67] and osteoporosis is not diagnosed in any skeletal site in four studies.[62,68–70] It is interesting that three of the last four studies are the ones that mention osteoporosis as a risk factor for dental implant failure.

None of the studies stratified patients for the number of postmenopausal years. One study presented relative information that controls had nine fewer postmenopausal years than osteoporotic patients.[69]

In addition, sample size was usually small. Ten studies had 0 to 19 osteoporotic patients,[60–62,64–70] one study did not clarify the number,[71] and only one study[63] included 50 osteoporotic women. Follow-up periods were usually short. One study followed patients up to stage II uncovering surgery,[68] and two to the abutment connection.[65,71] Only two studies had a mean follow-up period of five or more years.[66,70] As expected, the initially small sample size is furthermore reduced in the long-term evaluation.

Success criterion of osseointegration is another factor of major importance. Five of the 12 studies refer to implant survival as the only success criteria.[61,62,65,69,70]

Osteoporosis is a site-specific disease. There is a tendency to support that jawbone is also affected in osteoporotic patients.[20,31] Still, jawbone is not one of the main skeletal sites affected by osteoporosis. The fact that some studies examined osseointegration of dental implants in osteoporotic patients without clarifying the existence of osteoporosis in the jaws[60–62,65,68–70] and the severity of the existing osteopenia/osteoporosis,[63] or having already proved that osteoporosis has not affected implantation sites of the certain subjects,[64,67] maintains confusion.

After having discussed the limiting factors of the available human studies, it is now obvious that the ideal study about dental implants in osteoporotic patients is not among them. Two main issues of research existed.

The first one was whether osseointegration may be obtained in osteoporotic patients. A majority of studies appear positive. According to Friberg et al, implant placement in patients in whom the average bone density showed osteoporosis in both lumbar spine and hip as well as poor local bone texture may be successful over a period of many years (mean follow-up period 3 years and 4 months, ranging from 6 months to 11 years).[60] The mean healing periods were extended to 8.5 months in the maxilla and 4.5 months in the mandible. Extending the healing period by 50% agrees with prementioned animal study results.[38,43]

The second issue is the long-term results of dental implants in osteoporotic patients. In this case, a better study design may be recognized in the study of von Wowern and Gotfredsen,[66] mainly because of the estimation of mandibular osteoporosis by mandibular BMC measures at baseline, just after attachment insertion, and at 2- and 5-year visits. In addition, this study has the longest follow-up period, long-term edentulous patients, all implants placed in both mandibular canine regions, and clinical and radiographic assessment of dental implants. Unfortunately, there is no control group, and only seven women out of 22 patients showed mandibular osteoporosis at the start of trial. No implant failures were observed. BMC measures at implantation sites showed a load-related, positive bone remodeling that minimizes or in some cases counteracts age-related changes in bone remodeling processes. Simultaneously, a significantly larger bone height loss occurred in women with mandibular osteoporosis and dental implants than in the remaining women with dental implants after the 5-year follow-up (not earlier), despite the high level of oral hygiene and the prementioned positive functional stimulus.

Therefore, further research on the long-term outcomes of dental implants in patients with osteoporosis in the jawbone is needed. Larger sample sizes are required to sufficiently document the relationship between dental implant outcomes and osteoporosis, especially since the severity of osteoporosis may influence the strength of the studied relationship. Clear evidence that osteoporosis has affected the jawbone of tested patients is of major importance. Finally, to our knowledge, there are no studies dealing with the previously mentioned question of peri-implantitis in osteoporotic patients.

Dental Implants and Age, Gender, and Jawbone Quality

The analysis of existing data about the impact of age and sex on dental implant success may offer indirect information about the outcome of dental implants in osteoporotic patients. This is because age and gender are risk factors for osteoporosis. If osteoporosis was a risk factor for dental implant osseointegration, then relevant studies might have found a positive relationship between aging and gender and implant failure. There is a general consensus that there is no impact of age or gender on implant failure.[25,60,64,68–69,85–119] Some studies[120–125] found even better results for women than men. Others found higher bone loss for the first year[108] or lower initial stability[126,127] in the female population, but these facts were not followed by increased long-term failure rates.[126] Some articles more or less clearly support the opposite without sufficient documentation.[68,128–133] These results support the opinion that osteoporosis is not a contraindication to dental implants, despite the fact that several confounding factors are involved in these studies. Site-specific factors have a greater impact on dental implant outcome than age and gender.[90] There is a positive, although rough, estimation of long-term[91] dental implants outcome in osteoporotic patients.

The osteoporotic bone is characterized as type IV according to the Lekholm and Zarb classification,[134] that is, soft bone. Soft bone, not necessarily osteoporotic, has been related to low success rates of dental implants in some studies, because of its reduced potential to offer initial implant stability.[63,86,135–145] On the contrary, other studies did not find such differences.[99,100,146–162]

Bone quality is a significant factor, but not the only one determining result. Implant design,[138,141,144,158,163,174] length,[163,165] surface characteristics,[138,151–153,155,158,159,164–177] surgical technique,[154,163,165,178,179] prosthodontic rehabilitation,[148,165,180] and patient hygiene[148,164] are some of the factors involved. Smedberg et al[181] reported 100% implant success in type 3 or 4 quality combined with type A, B, or C bone quantity in maxillary overdentures followed for two years, in comparison to 77% for implants in type 3 or 4 bone quality combined with type D or E bone quantity.

Friberg et al,[182] studying the frequency of early and late failures of Branemark System implants, related this outcome to differences in the surgical protocol, as well as to various patient and implant characteristics. Regarding jawbone quality, type 4 showed the highest failure rate in maxilla (40.4%) and type 1 in the mandible (13%). After proper adjustment of the surgical technique (omitting the threading procedure, using wide diameter implants in standard diameter bone sites, and extending the healing period in low-density bone), type 2 bone showed a failure rate of 4.7%, and type 4 a failure rate of 2.8%. It can be concluded that proper adjustment of the surgical preparation is a major factor in the determination of dental implant outcome.

Biphosphonate Therapy

Biphosphonate drugs are used as an alternative of HRT for the prevention and treatment of osteoporosis. The long-term application of these drugs may induce osteonecrosis of the jaws (ONJ), due to decreased osteoclast numbers and activity resulting in decreased bone resorption. Although the precipitating event that produces this complication may be spontaneous, biphosphonate therapy is considered a contraindication to implants;[183–187] however, it is recognized that oral biphosphonates are a low-risk group versus the high-risk intravenous biphosphonates[63,183] used in cancer therapy. This was confirmed by Jeffcoat's[63] recent randomized, placebo-controlled study; however, the two- to three-year follow-up period of this study is not sufficient to determine the long-term effects of long half-life biphosphonates. Data on the use of biphosphonates in osteoporotic patients and implant outcomes are very limited. Therefore, no conclusions can be drawn.

PRACTICAL MEASURES AIMED AT THE IMPROVEMENT OF DENTAL IMPLANT OUTCOMES IN OSTEOPOROTIC PATIENTS

In cases of treatment with dental implants, osteoporotic patients may be candidates for surgical techniques used to overcome the disadvantages of reduced bone quantity and deteriorated bone quality.[89,146,153,188–200]

The detailed analysis of such techniques is beyond the scope of this article, because they are not a special treatment for osteoporotic patients. Briefly we are mentioning the following:

Reduced bone quantity may be an indication for:

(1) A reduction of number of implants. According to Branemark et al,[198] a reduced jawbone volume was the major reason for limiting the number of implants to four in mandibles and maxillae of fully edentulous patients. It is interesting that although a tendency existed for an increased failure rate in patients with four implants, the survival rate for both implants and prostheses at the end of the 10-year observation period was the same with the six implants-per-jaw-patients group.

(2) Bone augmentation techniques.[195–197]

(3) Osteotome sinus floor elevation.[195]

(4) Zygomatic implants.[199]

Poor bone quality is considered a relative problem because of the lack of primary implant stability. The following have been proposed:

(1) A longer healing period. This seems to be needed if osteoporosis is exhibited in the jawbone. There are no studies to give the exact time needed, but a healing period 50% longer than normal has proved sufficient.[60] There are studies supporting immediate and early loading in soft bone;[146,153] nevertheless, the conservative approach is at present considered safer.

(2) The relation between the last used drill and the diameter of the implant chosen may be altered, which means that a smaller drill or an implant with larger than normal diameter may be used.[88,190–194]

(3) The osteotome technique, which may improve bone density around the implant, since the implant is placed without drilling.[195]

(4) Root-shaped implants.[192]

(5) Penetration in cortical layers to a higher extent;[45] however, regarding bicortical implant anchorage, the available data are controversial.[200]

CONCLUSION

There are no data to contraindicate the use of dental implants in osteoporotic patients; however, a proper adjustment of the surgical technique and a longer healing period may be considered in order to achieve osseointegration. Data on the use of biphosphonates in osteoporotic patients and implant outcomes are very limited, and no conclusions can be drawn. In addition, large prospective studies investigating the long-term success of dental implants in osteoporotic individuals are required.

ACKNOWLEDGMENT

Ioanna N. Tsolaki would like to thank Prof. Ulf Lekholm for his contribution to her initial involvement with the present subject.

REFERENCES

1. Lindquist LW, Carlson GE, Jemt T: A prospective 15-year follow-up study of mandibular fixed prostheses supported by osseointegrated implants. Clinical results and marginal bone loss. *Clin Oral Impl Res* 1996;7:329–336.

2. Lazzara R, Siddiqui AA, Binon P, et al: Retrospective multi-center analysis of 3i endosseous dental implants placed over a five-year period. *Clin Oral Impl Res* 1996;7:73–83.

3. Buser D, Mericske-Stern R, Bernard JP, et al: Long-term evaluation of non-submerged ITI implants. Part 1: 8-year life table analysis of a prospective multicenter study with 2359 implants. *Clin Oral Impl Res* 1997;8:161–172.

4. Lerner UH: Bone remodeling in post-menopausal osteoporosis. *J Dent Res* 2006;85:584–595.

5. Consensus Development Conference: Diagnosis, prophylaxis and treatment of osteoporosis. *Am J Med* 1993;94:646–650.

6. WHO Study Group: Assessment of Fracture Risk and Its Implications to Screening for Postmenopausal Osteoporosis. WHO Technical Report, Vol. 843. Geneva, World Health Organization, 1984.

7. The WHO Family of International Classifications. http://www.who.int/classifications, accessed October 28, 2008.

8. Kanis JA: Diagnosis of osteoporosis and assessment of fracture risk. *Lancet* 2002;359:1929–1936.

9. Faulkner KG: Clinical use of bone densitometry. In Marcus R, Feldman D, Kelsey J (eds): *Osteoporosis*, Vol 2 (ed 2). St. Louis, MO, Academic Press, 2001, pp. 433–458.

10. Eddy DM, Johnston CC, Cummings SR, et al: Osteoporosis: review of the evidence for prevention, diagnosis, and treatment and cost-effectiveness analysis. Status report. *Osteoporos Int* 1998;4 (Suppl):1–80.

11. Cooper C: Epidemiology of osteoporosis. *Osteoporosis Int* 1999;9(Suppl 2):S2–S8.

12. Kanis JA: Assessment of bone mass. In Kanis JA (ed): *Textbook of Osteoporosis*. Ames, IA, Blackwell, 1996, pp. 71–85.

13. Geelhoed EA, Prince RL: The epidemiology of osteoporotic fracture and its causative factors. *Clin Biochem Rev* 1994;15:173–178.

14. Melton LJ, III, Chrischilles EA, Cooper C, et al: Perspective: how many women have osteoporosis? *J Bone Miner Res* 1992;7:1005–1010.

15. Prince RL, Knuiman MW, Gulland L: Fracture prevalence in Australian population. *Aust Public Health* 1993;17:124–128.

16. National Osteoporosis Foundation. http://www.nof.org, accessed October 28, 2008.

17. Jones G, Nguyen T, Sambrook PN, et al: Symptomatic fracture incidence in elderly men and women: the Dubbo Osteoporosis Epidemiology Study (DOES). *Osteoporos Int* 1994;4:277–282.

18. Solomon L: Osteoporosis and fracture of the femoral neck in the South African Bantu. *J Bone Joint Surg* 1986;50-B:2–13.

19. Villa ML, Nelson L, Nelson D: Race, ethnicity, and osteoporosis. In Marcus R, Feldman D, Kelsey J (eds): *Osteoporosis*, Vol 2 (ed 2). St. Louis, MO, Academic Press, 2001, pp. 569–584.

20. Melton LJ, Kan SH, Wahner HW, et al: Lifetime fracture risk: an approach to hip fracture risk assessment based on bone mineral density and age. *J Clin Epidemiol* 1988;41:985–994.

21. Riggs BL, Melton LJ, III: A unitary model for involutional osteoporosis: estrogen deficiency causes both type I and type II osteoporosis in postmenopausal women and contributes to bone loss in aging men. *J Bone Miner Res* 1998;13:763–773.

22. Lerner UH: Inflammation-induced bone remodeling in periodontal disease and the influence of post-menopausal osteoporosis. *J Dent Res* 2006;85:596–607.

23. Riggs BL, Khosla S, Melton LJ, III: The type I/type II model for involutional osteoporosis: update and modifications based on new observations. In Marcus R, Feldman D, Kelsey J (eds): *Osteoporosis*, Vol 2 (ed 2). St. Louis, MO, Academic Press, 2001, pp. 49–58.

24. Bono CM, Einhorn TA: Overview of osteoporosis: pathophysiology and determinants of bone strength. *Eur Spine* 2003;12(Suppl 2):S90–S96.

25. von Wowern N, Kollerup G: Symptomatic osteoporosis: a risk factor for residual ridge reduction of the jaws. *J Prosthet Dent* 1992;67:656–660.

26. von Wowern N: General and oral aspects of osteoporosis: a review. *Clin Oral Invest* 2001;5:71–82.

27. Lewiecki EM, Kendler DL, Kiebzak GM, et al: Special report of the official positions of the International Society of Clinical Densitometry. *Osteoporos Int* 2004;15:779–784.

28. Schneider A, Shane E: Osteoporosis secondary to illnesses and medications. In Marcus R, Feldman D, Kelsey J (eds): *Osteoporosis*, Vol 2 (ed 2). St. Louis, MO, Academic Press, 2001, pp. 303–326.

29. Abstracts of Seventh International Symposium on Osteoporosis: Translating research into clinical practice. *Osteoporos Int* 2007;18(Suppl 2):S193–S244.

30. International Osteoporosis Foundation/Health Professionals. http://www.iofbonehealth.org/health-professionals.html, accessed October 28, 2008.

31. Hohlweg-Majert B, Schmelzeisen R, Pfeiffer BM, et al: Significance of osteoporosis in craniomaxillofacial surgery: a review of the literature. *Osteoporos Int* 2006;17:167–179.

32. Schou S, Holmstrup P, Worthington HV, et al: Outcome of implant therapy in patients with previous tooth loss due to periodontitis. *Clin Oral Implants Res* 2006;17(Suppl 2):104–123.

33. Duarte PM, Cesar Neto JB, Gonclaves PF, et al: Estrogen deficiency affects bone healing around titanium implants: a histomorphometric study in rats. *Implant Dent* 2003;12:340–346.

34. Hayashi K, Uenoyama K, Mashima T, et al: Remodeling of bone around hydroxyapatite and titanium in experimental osteoporosis. *Biomaterials* 1994;15:11–16.

35. Fini M, Giavaresi G, Rimondini L, et al: Titanium alloy osseointegration in cancellous and cortical bone of ovariectomized animals: histomorphometric and bone hardness measurements. *Int J Oral Maxillofac Implants* 2002;17:28–37.

36. Cho P, Schneider GB, Krizan K, et al: Examination of the bone-implant interface in experimentally induced osteoporotic bone. *Implant Dent* 2004;13:79–87.

37. Lugero GG, de Falco Caparbo V, Guzzo ML, et al: Histomorphometric evaluation of titanium implants in osteoporotic rabbits. *Implant Dent* 2000;9:303–309.

38. Mori H, Manabe M, Kurachi Y, et al: Osseointegration of dental implants in rabbit bone with low mineral density. *J Oral Maxillofac Surg* 1997;55:351–361.

39. Jung Y-C, Han C-H, Lee I-S: Effects of ion beam-assisted deposition of hydroxyapatite on the osseointegration of endosseous implants in rabbit tibiae. *Int J Oral Maxillofac Implants* 2001;16:809–818.

40. Narai S, Nagahata S: Effects of alendronate on the removal torque of implants in rats with induced osteoporosis. *Int J Oral Maxillofac Implants* 2003;18:218–223.

41. Pan J, Shirota T, Ohno K, et al: Effect of ovariectomy on bone remodeling adjacent to hydroxyapatite-coated implants in the tibia of mature rats. *J Oral Maxillofac Surg* 2000;58:877–882.

42. Keller JC, Stewart M, Roehm M, et al: Osteoporosis-like bone conditions affect osseointegration of implants. *Int J Oral Maxillofac Implants* 2004;19:687–694.

43. Ozawa S, Ogawa T, Iida K, et al: Ovariectomy hinders the early stage of bone-implant integration: histomorphometric, biomechanical, and molecular analyses. *Bone* 2002;30:137–143.

44. Martin RB, Paul HA, Bargar WL, et al: Effects of estrogen deficiency on the growth tissue into porous titanium implants. *J Bone Joint Surg Am* 1988;70:540–547.

45. Yamazaki M, Shirota T, Tokugawa Y, et al: Bone reactions to titanium screw implants in ovariectomized animals. *Oral Surg Oral Med Oral Pathol Oral Radiol Endod* 1999;87:411–418.

46. Nasu M, Amano Y, Kurita A, et al: Osseointegration in implant-embedded mandible in rats fed calcium-deficient diet: a radiological study. *Oral Diseases* 1998;4:84–89.

47. Fujimoto T, Niimi A, Sawai T, et al: Effects of steroid-induced osteoporosis on osseointegration of titanium implants. *Int J Oral Maxillofac Implants* 1998;13:183–189.

48. Okamura A, Ayukawa Y, Iyama S, et al: Effect of the difference of bone turnover on peri-titanium implant osteogenesis in ovariectomized rats. *J Biomed Mater Res* 2004;70A:497–505.

49. Qi M-C, Zhou X-Q, Hu J, et al: Oestrogen replacement therapy promotes bone healing around dental implants in

osteoporotic rats. *Int J Oral Maxillofac Surg* 2004;33: 279–285.

50. Tresguerres I, Clemente C, Donado M, et al: Local administration of growth hormone enhances periimplant bone reaction in an osteoporotic rabbit model. A histologic, histomorphometric and densitometric study. *Clin Oral Impl Res* 2002;13: 631–636.

51. Fujimoto T, Niimi A, Nakai H, et al: Osseointegrated implants in a patient with osteoporosis: a case report. *Int J Oral Maxillofac Implants* 1996;11:539–542.

52. Eder A, Watzek G: Treatment of a patient with severe osteoporosis and chronic polyarthritis with fixed implant-supported prosthesis: a case report. *Int J Oral Maxillofac Implants* 1999;14:587–590.

53. Friberg B: Treatment with dental implants in patients with severe osteoporosis: a case report. *Int J Periodont Rest Dent* 1994;14:349–353.

54. Degidi M, Piatelli A: Immediately loaded bar-connected implants with an anodized surface inserted in the anterior mandible in a patient treated with biphosphonates for osteoporosis: a case report with a 12-month follow-up. *Clin Implant Dent Relat Res* 2003;5:269–272.

55. Cranin AN: Endosteal implants in a patient with corticosteroid dependence. *J Oral Implantol* 1991;17:414–417.

56. Steiner M, Ramp WK: Endosseous dental implants and the glucocorticoid-dependent patient. *J Oral Implantol* 1990;16: 211–217.

57. Starck W, Epker BN: Failure of osseointegrated dental implants after biphosphonate therapy for osteoporosis: a case report. *Int J Oral Maxillofac Implants* 1995;10:74–78.

58. Davenport WL, Heldt L, Bump RL: Salvage of the mandibular staple bone plate following bone infection. *J Oral Maxillofac Surg* 1985;43:981–986.

59. Rothman SL, Schwartz MS, Chafetz NI: High-resolution computerized tomography and nuclear bone scanning in the diagnosis of postoperative stress fractures of the mandible: a clinical report. *Int J Oral Maxillofac Implants* 1995;10:765–768.

60. Friberg B, Ekestubbe A, Mellstrom D, et al: Branemark implants and osteoporosis: a clinical exploratory study. *Clin Implant Dent Relat Res* 2001;3:50–56.

61. Becker W, Hujoel P, Becker B, et al: Osteoporosis and implant failure: an exploratory case-control study. *J Periodontol* 2000;71:625–631.

62. Minsk L, Polson AM: Dental implant outcomes in postmenopausal women undergoing hormone replacement. *Compend Contin Educ Dent* 1998;19:859–862, 864.

63. Jeffcoat MK: Safety of oral biphosphonates: controlled studies on alveolar bone. *Int J Oral Maxillofac Implants* 2006;21: 349–353.

64. Amorim MA, Takayama L, Jorgetti V, et al: Comparative study of axial and femoral bone mineral density and parameters of mandibular bone quality in patients receiving dental implants. *Osteoporos Int* 2007;18:703–709.

65. van Steenberghe D, Jacobs R, Desnyder M, et al: The relative impact of local and endogenous patient-related factors on implant failure up to the abutment stage. *Clin Oral Impl Res* 2002;13:617–622.

66. von Wowern N, Gotfredsen K: Implant-supported overdentures, a prevention of bone loss in edentulous mandibles? A 5-year follow-up study. *Clin Oral Impl Res* 2001;12:19–25.

67. Smolka W, Eggensperger N, Carollo V, et al: Changes in the volume and density of calvarial split bone grafts after alveolar ridge augmentation. *Clin Oral Implants Res* 2006;17: 149–155.

68. August M, Chung K, Chang Y, et al: Influence of estrogen status on endosseous implant osseointegration. *J Oral Maxillofac Surg* 2001;59:1285–1289.

69. Blomqvist JE, Alberius P, Isakson S, et al: Factors in implant integration failure after bone grafting. An osteometric and endocrinologic matched analysis. *Int J Oral Maxillofac Surg* 1996;25:63–68.

70. Moy PK, Medina D, Shetty V, et al: Dental implant failure rates and associated risk factors. *Int J Oral Maxillofac Implants* 2005;20:569–577.

71. Alsaadi G, Quirynen M, Komarek A, et al: Impact of local and systemic factors on the incidence of oral implant failures, up to abutment connection. *J Clin Periodontol* 2007;34:610–617.

72. Lofman O: *Osteoporosis in Women. Epidemiological and Diagnostic Perspectives*. Linkoping, Sweden, Linkoping University Press, 2002.

73. Legrand E, Chappard D, Pascaretti C, et al: Trabecular bone microarchitecture, bone mineral density, and vertebral fractures in male osteoporosis. *J Bone Miner Res* 2000;15: 13–19.

74. Marcus R, Majumder SH: The nature of osteoporosis. In Marcus R, Feldman D, Kelsey J (eds): *Osteoporosis*, Vol 2 (ed 2). St. Louis, MO, Academic Press, 2001, pp. 3–17.

75. Pacheco EMB, Harrison EJ, Ward KA, et al: Detection of osteoporosis by dual energy X-ray absorptiometry (DXA) of the calcaneus: is the WHO criterion applicable? *Calcif Tissue Int* 2002;70:475–482.

76. Yamazaki I, Yamaguchi H: Characteristics of an ovariectomised osteopenic rat model. *J Bone Miner Res* 1989;4:13–22.

77. Kimmel DB: Animal models for in vivo experimentation in osteoporosis research. In Marcus R, Feldman D, Kelsey J (eds): *Osteoporosis*, Vol 2 (ed 2). St. Louis, MO, Academic Press, 2001, pp. 29–47.

78. Boyce RW, Franks AF, Jankowsky ML, et al: Sequential histomorphometric changes in cancellous bone from ovariohysterectomized dogs. *J Bone Miner Res* 1990;5:947–953.

79. Martin RB, Butcher RL, Sherwood LL, et al: Effects of ovariectomy in beagle dogs. *Bone* 1987;8:23–31.

80. Malluche HH, Faugere MC, Rush M, et al: Osteoblastic insufficiency is responsible for maintenance of osteopenia after loss of ovarian function in experimental beagle dogs. *Endocrinology* 1986;119:2649–2654.

81. Faugere MC, Friedler RM, Fanti P, et al: Bone changes occurring early after cessation of ovarian function in beagle dogs: a histomorphometric study employing sequential biopsies. *J Bone Miner Res* 1990;5:263–372.

82. Monier-Faugere MC, Geng Z, Qi Q, et al: Calcitonin prevents bone loss but decreases osteoblastic activity in ovariohysterectomized beagle dogs. *J Bone Miner Res* 1996;11:446–455.

83. Monier-Faugere MC, Friedler RM, Bauss F, et al: A new biphosphonate, BM 21.0955, prevents bone loss associated with cessation of ovarian function in experimental dogs. *J Bone Miner Res* 1993;8:1345–1355.

84. Turner AS: Animal models of osteoporosis-necessity and limitations. *Eur Cells and Materials* 2001;1:66–81.

85. Kondell PA, Nordenram A, Landt H: Titanium implants in the treatment of edentulousness: influence of patient's age on prognosis. *Gerodontics* 1988;4:280–284.

86. Bass SL, Triplett RG: The effects of preoperative resorption and jaw anatomy on implant success. A report of 303 cases. *Clin Oral Implant Res* 1991;2:193–198.

87. Jemt T: The implant-supported prostheses in the edentulous maxilla. *Clin Oral Implant Res* 1993;6:456–461.

88. Zarb GA, Schmitt A: The longitudinal clinical effectiveness of osseointegrated dental implants in anterior partially edentulous patients. *Int J Prosthodont* 1993;6:180–188.

89. Ochi S, Morris HF, Winkler S: The influence of implant type, material, coating, diameter, and length on Periotest values at 2nd stage surgery: Dental Implant Clinical Research Group Interim Report No 4. *Implant Dent* 1994;3:159–162.

90. Bryant SR: Osseointegration of oral implants in older and younger adults. *Int J Oral Maxillofac Implants* 1998;13: 492–499.

91. Bryant SR, Zarb GA: Crestal bone loss proximal to oral implants in older and younger adults. *J Prosthet Dent* 2003;89:589–597.

92. Smith RA, Berger R, Dodson TB: Risk factors associated with dental implants in healthy and medically compromised patients. *Int J Oral Maxillofac Implants* 1992;7:367–372.

93. Jones JD, Lupori J, Van Sickels JE, et al: A 5-year comparison of hydroxyapatite-coated titanium plasma-sprayed and titanium plasma-sprayed cylinder dental implants. *Oral Surg Oral Med Oral Pathol Radiol Endod* 1999;87:649–652.

94. den Dunnen AC, Slagter AP, de Baat C, et al: Adjustments and complications of mandibular overdentures retained by four implants. A comparison between superstructures with and without cantilever extensions. *Int J Prosthodont* 1998;11:307–311.

95. Cune MS, de Putter C: A single dimension statistical evaluation of predictors in implant-overdenture treatment. *J Clin Periodontol* 1996;23:425–431.

96. Versteegh PA, van Beek GJ, Slagter AP, et al: Clinical evaluation of mandibular overdentures supported by multiple-bar fabrication: a follow-up study of two implant systems. *Int J Oral Maxillofac Implants* 1995;10:595–603.

97. Ochi S, Morris HF, Winkler S: Patient demographics and implant survival at uncovering: Dental Implant Clinical Research Group Interim Report No 6. *Implant Dent* 1994;3: 247–251.

98. Yerit KC, Posch M, Seeman M, et al: Implant survival in mandibles of irradiated oral cancer patients. *Clin Oral Implants Res* 2006;17:337–344.

99. Hall JA, Payne AG, Purton DG, et al: A randomized controlled clinical trial of conventional and immediately loaded tapered implants with screw-retained crowns. *Int J Prosthodont* 2006;19:17–19.

100. Aalam AA, Nowzari H: Clinical evaluation of dental implants with surfaces roughened by anodic oxidation, dual acid-etched implants, and machined implants. *Int J Oral Maxillofac Implants* 2005;20:793–798.

101. Lemmerman KJ, Lemmermen NE: Osseointegrated dental implants in private practice: a long-term case series study. *J Periodontol* 2005;76:310–319.

102. Granstrom G: Osseointegration in irradiated cancer patients: an analysis with respect to implant failures. *J Oral Maxillofac Surg* 2005;63:579–585.

103. Chou CT, Morris HF, Ochi S, et al: AICRG, part II: crestal bone loss associated with the Ankylos implant: loading to 36 months. *J Oral Implantol* 2004;30:134–143.

104. Naert I, Koutsikakis G, Quirynen M, et al: Biologic outcome of implant-supported restorations in the treatment of partial edentulism. Part 2: a longitudinal radiographic study. *Clin Oral Implants Res* 2002;13:390–395.

105. van Steenberghe D, Quirynen M, Naert I, et al: Marginal bone loss around implants retaining hinging mandibular overdentures, at 4-, 8- and 12-years follow-up. *J Clin Periodontol* 2001;28:628–633.

106. Hurzeler MB, Kirsch A, Ackermann KL, et al: Reconstruction of the severely resorbed maxilla with dental implants in the augmented maxillary sinus: a 5-year clinical investigation. *Int J Oral Maxillofac Implants* 1996;11:466–475.

107. Meijer HJ, Batenburg RH, Raghoebar GM: Influence of patient age on the success rate of dental implants supporting an overdenture in an edentulous mandible: a 3-year prospective study. *Int J Oral Maxillofac Implants* 2001;16:522–526.

108. Attard NJ, Zarb GA: Long-term treatment outcomes in edentulous patients with overdentures: the Toronto study. *Int J Prosthodont* 2004;17:425–433.

109. Engfors I, Ortorp A, Jemt T: Fixed implant-supported prosthesis in elderly patients: a 5-year retrospective study of 133 edentulous patients older than 79 years. *Clin Implant Dent Relat Res* 2004;6:190–198.

110. Elkhoury JS, McGlumphy EA, Tatakis DN, et al: Clinical parameters associated with success and failure of single-tooth titanium plasma-sprayed cylindric implants under stricter criteria: a 5-year retrospective study. *Int J Oral Maxillofac Implants* 2005;20:687–694.

111. Neukam FW, Hausamen JE, Scheller H: Moglichkeiten und Grenzen der Implantologie beim altern Patienten. *Dtsch Zahnarztl Z* 1989;44:490–492.

112. Doyle SL, Hodges JS, Pesun IJ, et al: Factors affecting outcomes for single-tooth implants and endodontic restorations. *J Endod* 2007;33:399–402.

113. Snauwaert K, Duyck J, van Steenberghe D, et al: Time dependent failure rate and marginal bone loss of implant supported prostheses: a 15-year follow-up study. *Clin Oral Investig* 2000;4:13–20.

114. Hall JA, Payne AG, Purton DG, et al: Immediately restored, single-tapered implants in the anterior maxilla: prosthodontic and aesthetic outcomes after 1 year. *Clin Implant Dent Relat Res* 2007;9:34–45.

115. Balshi SF, Wolfinger GJ, Balshi TJ: A retrospective analysis of 44 implants with no rotational primary stability used for fixed prosthesis anchorage. *Int J Oral Maxillofac Implants* 2007;22:467–471.

116. Friberg B, Ekestubbe A, Sennerby L: Clinical outcome of Brånemark system implants of various diameters: a retrospective study. *Int J Oral Maxillofac Implants* 2002;17:671–677.

117. Mericske-Stern R, Zarb GA: Overdentures: an alternative implant methodology for edentulous patients. *Int J Prosthodont* 1993;6:203–208.

118. Penarrocha M, Guarinos J, Sanchis JM, et al: A retrospective study (1994–1999) of 441 ITI® implants in 114 patients followed-up during an average of 2.3 years. *Med Oral* 2002;7:144–155.

119. Wang IC, Reddy MS, Geurs NC, et al: Risk factors in dental implant failure. *J Long Term Eff Med Implants* 1996;6:103–117.

120. Wagenberg B, Froum SJ: A retrospective study of 1925 consecutively placed immediate implants from 1988 to 2004. *Int J Oral Maxillofac Implants* 2006;21:71–80.

121. Brochu JF, Anderson JD, Zarb GA: The influence of early loading on bony crest height and stability: a pilot study. *Int J Prosthodont* 2005;18:506–512.

122. Degidi M, Piattelli A, Felice P, et al: Immediate functional loading of edentulous maxilla: a 5-year retrospective study of 388 titanium implants. *J Periodontol* 2005;76:1016–1024.

123. Schwartz-Arad D, Grossman Y, Chaushu G: The clinical effectiveness of implants placed immediately into fresh extraction sites of molar teeth. *J Periodontol* 2000;71:839–844.

124. Jebreen SE, Khraisat A: Multicenter retrospective study of ITI implant-supported posterior partial prosthesis in Jordan. *Clin Implant Dent Relat Res* 2007;9:89–93.

125. Wyatt CC, Zarb GA: Bone level changes proximal to oral implants supporting fixed partial prostheses. *Clin Oral Implants Res* 2002;13:162–168.

126. Balshi SF, Allen FD, Wolfinger GJ, et al: A resonance frequency analysis assessment of maxillary and mandibular immediately loaded implants. *Int J Oral Maxillofac Implants* 2005;20:584–594.

127. Ostman PO, Hellman M, Wendelhag I, et al: Resonance frequency analysis measurements of implants at placement surgery. *Int J Prosthodont* 2006;19:77–83, discussion 84.

128. Salonen MA, Oikarinen K, Virtanen K, et al: Failures in the osseointegration of endosseous implants. *Int J Oral Maxillofac Implants* 1993;8:92–97.

129. Strietzel FP, Lange KP, Svegar M, et al: Retrospective evaluation of the success of oral rehabilitation using the Frialit-2 implant system. Part I: influence of topographic and surgical parameters. *Int J Prosthodont* 2004;17:187–194.

130. Schliephake H, Neukam FW, Wichmann M: Survival analysis of endosseous implants in bone grafts used for the treatment of severe alveolar ridge atrophy. *J Oral Maxillofac Surg* 1997;55:1227–1233, discussion 1233–1234.

131. Brocard D, Barthet P, Baysse E, et al: A multicenter report on 1022 consecutively placed ITI implants: a 7-year longitudinal study. *Int J Oral Maxillofac Impl* 2000;15:691–700.

132. Zix J, Kessler-Liechti G, Mericske-Stern R: Stability measurements of 1-stage implants in the maxilla by means of resonance frequency analysis: a pilot study. *Int J Maxillofac Implants* 2005;20:747–752.

133. Kordatzis K, Wright PS, Meijer HJ: Posterior mandibular residual ridge resorption in patients with conventional dentures and implant overdentures. *Int J Oral Maxillofac Implants* 2003;18:447–452.

134. Lekholm U, Zarb GA: Patient selection and preparation. In Brånemark P-I, Zarb GA, Albrektsson T (eds): *Tissue-Integrated Prostheses: Osseointegration in Clinical Dentistry*. Chicago, IL, Quintessence, 1985, pp. 199–209.

135. Jaffin RA, Berman CL: The excessive loss of Branemark fixtures in type IV bone: a 5 year analysis. *J Periodontol* 1991;62:2–4.

136. Johns RB, Jemt T, Health MR: A multicenter study of overdentures supported by Branemark implants. *Int J Oral Maxillofac Implants* 1992;7:513–522.

137. Hutton JE, Heath MR, Chai JY, et al: Factors related to success and failure rates at 3-year follow-up in a multicenter study of overdentures supported by Branemark implants. *Int J Oral Maxillofac Implants* 1995;10:33–42.

138. Truhlar RS, Morris HF, Ochi S: Implant surface coating and bone quality-related survival outcomes through 36 months post-placement of root-form endosseous dental implants. *Ann Periodontol* 2000;5:109–118.

139. Degidi M, Piattelli A, Gehrke P, et al: Five-year outcome of 111 immediate nonfunctional single restorations. *J Oral Implantol* 2006;32:277–285.

140. Weng D, Jacobson Z, Tarnow D, et al: A prospective multicenter clinical trial of 3i machined-surface implants: results after 6 years of follow-up. *Int J Oral Maxillofac Implants* 2003;18:417–423.

141. Grunder U, Polizzi G, Goené R, et al: A 3-year prospective multicenter follow-up report on the immediate and delayed-immediate placement of implants. *Int J Oral Maxillofac Implants* 1999;14:210–216.

142. Higuchi KW, Folmer T, Kultje C: Implant survival rates in partially edentulous patients: a 3-year prospective multicenter study. *J Oral Maxillofac Surg* 1995;53:264–268.

143. van Steenberghe D, Lekholm U, Bolender C, et al: Applicability of osseointegrated oral implants in the rehabilitation of partial edentulism: a prospective multicenter study on 558 fixtures. *Int J Oral Maxillofac Implants* 1990;5:272–281.

144. Friberg B, Jemt T, Lekholm U: Early failures in 4,641 consecutively placed Brånemark dental implants: a study from stage 1 surgery to the connection of completed prostheses. *Int J Oral Maxillofac Implants* 1991;6:142–146.

145. Jemt T, Lekholm U: Implant treatment in edentulous maxillae: a 5-year follow-up report on patients with different degrees of

jaw resorption. *Int J Oral Maxillofac Implants* 1995;10: 303–311.

146. Glauser R, Ree A, Lundgren A, et al: Immediate occlusal loading of Branemark implants applied in various jawbone regions: a prospective, 1-year clinical study. *Clin Implant Dent Relat Res* 2001;3:204–213.

147. Bahat O: Treatment planning and placement of implants in the posterior maxillae: report of 732 consecutive Nobelpharma implants. *Int J Oral Maxillofac Impl* 1993;8:151–161.

148. Truhlar RS, Farish SE, Scheitler LE, et al: Bone quality and implant design-related outcomes through stage II surgical uncovering of Spectra-System root form implants. *J Oral Maxillofac Surg* 1997;55(Suppl 5):46–54.

149. Fugazzotto PA, Wheeler SL, Lindsay JA: Success and failure rates of cylinder implants in type IV bone. *J Periodontol* 1993;64:1085–1087.

150. Glauser R, Ruhstaller P, Windisch S, et al: Immediate occlusal loading of Branemark system TiUnite implants placed predominantly in soft bone: 4-year results of a prospective clinical study. *Clin Implant Dent Relat Res* 2005;7(Suppl 1): S52–S59.

151. Friberg B, Jisander S, Widmark G, et al: One-year prospective three-center study comparing the outcome of a "soft bone implant" (prototype Mk IV) and the standard Branemark implant. *Clin Implant Dent Relat Res* 2003;5:71–77.

152. Astrand P, Billstrom C, Feldmann H, et al: Tapered implants in jaws with soft bone quality: a clinical and radiographic 1-year study of the Branemark system mark IV fixture. *Clin Implant Dent Relat Res* 2003;5:213–218.

153. Steveling H, Roos J, Rasmusson L: Maxillary implants loaded at 3 months after insertion: results with Astra Tech implants after up to 5 years. *Clin Implant Dent Relat Res* 2001;3: 120–124.

154. Bahat O: Osseointegrated implants in the maxillary tuberosity: report on 45 consecutive patients. *Int J Oral Maxillofac Implants* 1992;7:459–467.

155. Glauser R, Lundgren AK, Gottlow J, et al: Immediate occlusal loading of Branemark TiUnite implants placed predominantly in soft bone: 1-year results of a prospective clinical study. *Clin Implant Dent Relat Res* 2003;5(Suppl 1):47–56.

156. Mericske-Stern R, Oetterli M, Kiener P, et al: A follow-up study of maxillary implants supporting an overdenture: clinical and radiographic results. *Int J Oral Maxillofac Implants* 2002;17: 678–686.

157. Ottoni JM, Oliveira ZF, Mansini R, et al: Correlation between placement torque and survival of single-tooth implants. *Int J Oral Maxillofac Implants* 2005;20:769–776.

158. Kline R, Hoar JE, Beck GH, et al: A prospective multicenter clinical investigation of a bone quality-based dental implant system. *Implant Dent* 2002;11:224–234.

159. Orenstein IH, Tarnow DP, Morris HF, et al: Three-year post-placement survival of implants mobile at placement. *Ann Periodontol* 2000;5:32–41.

160. Bahat O: Brånemark system implants in the posterior maxilla: clinical study of 660 implants followed for 5 to 12 years. *Int J Oral Maxillofac Implants* 2000;15:646–653.

161. Becker W, Becker BE, Alsuwyed A, et al: Long-term evaluation of 282 implants in maxillary and mandibular molar positions: a prospective study. *J Periodontol* 1999;70: 896–901.

162. Misch CE, Dietsh-Misch F, Hoar J, et al: A bone quality-based implant system: first year of prosthetic loading. *J Oral Implantol* 1999;25:185–197.

163. Tada S, Stegaroiu R, Kitamura E, et al: Influence of implant design and bone quality on stress/strain distribution in bone around implants: a 3-dimensional finite element analysis. *Int J Oral Maxillofac Implants* 2003;18:357–368.

164. Misch CE, Degidi M: Five-year prospective study of immediate/early loading of fixed prostheses in completely edentulous jaws with a bone quality-based implant system. *Clin Implant Dent Relat Res* 2003;5:17–28.

165. Herrmann I, Lekholm U, Holm S, et al: Evaluation of patient and implant characteristics as potential prognostic factors for oral implant failures. *Int J Oral Maxillofac Implants* 2005;20:220–230.

166. Rocci A, Martignoni M, Gottlow J: Immediate loading of Brånemark system TiUnite and machined-surface implants in the posterior mandible: a randomized open-ended clinical trial. *Clin Implant Dent Relat Res* 2003;5(Suppl 1):57–63.

167. Khang W, Feldman S, Hawley CE, et al: A multi-center study comparing dual acid-etched and machined-surfaced implants in various bone qualities. *J Periodontol* 2001;72:1384–1390.

168. Trisi P, Lazzara R, Rao W, et al: Bone-implant contact and bone quality: evaluation of expected and actual bone contact on machined and Osseotite implant surfaces. *Int J Periodontics Restorative Dent* 2002;22:535–545.

169. Iezzi G, Degidi M, Scarano A, et al: Bone response to submerged, unloaded implants inserted in poor bone sites: a histological and histomorphometrical study of 8 titanium implants retrieved from man. *J Oral Implantol* 2005;31: 225–233.

170. Feldman S, Boitel N, Weng D, et al: Five-year survival distributions of short-length (10 mm or less) machined-surfaced and Osseotite implants. *Clin Implant Dent Relat Res* 2004;6:16–23.

171. Roccuzzo M, Wilson T: A prospective study evaluating a protocol for 6 weeks' loading of SLA implants in the posterior maxilla: one year results. *Clin Oral Implants Res* 2002;13: 502–507.

172. Testori T, Del Fabbro M, Feldman S, et al: A multicenter prospective evaluation of 2-months loaded Osseotite implants placed in the posterior jaws: 3-year follow-up results. *Clin Oral Implants Res* 2002;13:154–161.

173. Cochran DL, Buser D, ten Bruggenkate CM, et al: The use of reduced healing times on ITI implants with a sandblasted and acid-etched (SLA) surface: early results from clinical trials on ITI SLA implants. *Clin Oral Implants Res* 2002;13:144–153.

174. Al-Nawas B, Hangen U, Duschner H, et al: Turned, machined versus double-etched dental implants in vivo. *Clin Implant Dent Relat Res* 2007;9:71–78.

175. Orsini G, Piattelli M, Scarano A, et al: Randomized, controlled histologic and histomorphometric evaluation of implants with

nanometer-scale calcium phosphate added to the dual acid-etched surface in the human posterior maxilla. *J Periodontol* 2007;78:209–218.

176. Morris HF, Ochi S, Orenstein IH, et al: Part V: factors influencing implant stability at placement and their influence on survival of Ankylos implants. *J Oral Implantol* 2004;30: 162–170.

177. Lazzara RJ, Testori T, Trisi P, et al: A human histologic analysis of Osseotite and machined surfaces using implants with 2 opposing surfaces. *Int J Periodontics Restorative Dent* 1999;19:117–129.

178. Strietzel FP, Nowak M, Kuchler I, et al: Peri-implant alveolar bone loss with respect to bone quality after use of the osteotome technique: results of a retrospective study. *Clin Oral Implants Res* 2002;13:508–513.

179. O'Sullivan D, Sennerby L, Jagger D, et al: A comparison of two methods of enhancing implant primary stability. *Clin Implant Dent Relat Res* 2004;6:48–57.

180. Wang TM, Leu LJ, Wang J, et al: Effects of prosthesis materials and prosthesis splinting on peri-implant bone stress around implants in poor-quality bone: a numeric analysis. *Int J Oral Maxillofac Implants* 2002;17:231–237.

181. Smedberg J-I, Lothigius E, Bodin I, et al: A clinical and radiological 2-year follow-up study of maxillary overdentures on osseointegrated implants. *Clin Oral Implants Res* 1993;4: 39–46.

182. Friberg B, Sennerby L, Gröndahl K, et al: On cutting torque measurements during implant placement. A 3-year clinical prospective study. *Clin Impl Dent Relat Res* 1999;1:75–83.

183. Piesold JU, Al-Nawas B, Grotz KA: Osteonecrosis of the jaws by long term therapy with biphosphonates. *Mund Kiefer Gesichtschir* 2006;10:287–300.

184. Scully C, Madrid C, Bagan J: Dental endosseous implants in patients on biphosphonate therapy. *Implant Dent* 2006;15: 212–218.

185. Marx RE, Sawatari Y, Fortin M, et al: Biphosphonate-induced exposed bone (osteonecrosis/osteopetrosis) of the jaws: risk factors, recognition, prevention, and treatment. *J Oral Maxillofac Surg* 2005;63:1567–1575.

186. Savoldelli C, Le Page F, Santini J, et al: Maxillar osteonecrosis associated with biphosphonate treatment and dental implants. *Rev Stomatol Chir Maxillofac* 2007;108:555–558.

187. Wang HL, Weber D, McCanley LK: Effect of long-term oral biphosphonates on implant wound healing: literature review and a case report. *J Periodontol* 2007;78:584–594.

188. Triplett RG, Mason ME, Alfonso WF, et al: Endosseous cylinder implants in severely atrophic mandibles. *Int J Oral Maxillofac Impl* 1991;6:264–269.

189. Lekholm U, van Steenberghe D, Hermann I, et al: Osseointegrated implants in the treatment of partially edentulous jaws: a prospective 5-year multicenter study. *Int J Oral Maxillofac Impl* 1994;9:627–635.

190. Graves SL, Jansen CE, Siddiqui AA, et al: Wide diameter implants: indications, considerations and preliminary results over a 20 year period. *Aust Prosthodont J* 1994;14: 173–180.

191. Bahat O, Handelsman M: Use of wide implants and double implants in the posterior jaw: a clinical report. *Int J Oral Maxillofac Implants* 1996;11:379–388.

192. Ivanoff CJ, Grondahl K, Sennerby L, et al: Influence of variations in implant diameters: a 3- to 5-years retrospective clinical report. *Int J Oral Maxillofac Impl* 1999;14:173–180.

193. Mordenfeld MH, Johansson A, Hedin M, et al: A retrospective clinical study of wide-diameter implants used in posterior edentulous areas. *Int J Oral Maxillofac Implants* 2004;19: 387–392.

194. Aparicio C, Orozco P: Use of 5-mm-diameter implants: Periotest values related to a clinical and radiographic evaluation. *Clin Oral Implants Res* 1998;9:398–406.

195. Summers RB: A new concept in maxillary implant surgery: the osteotome technique. *Compendium* 1994;15:152–158.

196. Schliepake H, Neukam FW, Wichmann M, et al: Langzeitergebnisse osteointegrierter Schraubenimplantate in Kombination mit Osteoplastik. *Z Zahnarztl Implantol* 1997;13: 73–78.

197. Tolman DE: Reconstructive procedures with endosseous implants in grafted bone: a review of the literature. *Int J Oral Maxillofac Implants* 1995;10:275–294.

198. Branemark P-I, Svensson B, van Steenberghe D: 10-year survival rates of fixed prosthesis on 4 and 6 implants ad modum Branemark in full edentulism. *Clin Oral Impl Res* 1995;6:227–231.

199. Branemark P-I: *Surgery and Fixture Installation. Zygomatic Fixture Clinical Procedures* (ed 1). Goteborg, Sweden, Nobel Biocare AB, 1998, p. 1.

200. Ivanoff CJ, Grondahl K, Bergstrom C, et al: Influence of bicortical or monocortical anchorage on maxillary implant stability: a 15-year retrospective study of Branemark system implants. *Int J Oral Maxillofac Impl* 2000;15:103–110.

27

UPDATED CLINICAL CONSIDERATIONS FOR DENTAL IMPLANT THERAPY IN IRRADIATED HEAD AND NECK CANCER PATIENTS

Takako Imai Tanaka, DDS, FDS RCSED,[1,2] Hsun-Liang Chan, DDS, MS,[2] David Ira Tindle, DDS, MS,[2] Mark MacEachern, MLIS,[3] and Tae-Ju Oh, DDS, MS[2]

[1]Department of Biomedical & Diagnostic Sciences, University of Detroit Mercy School of Dentistry, Detroit, MI
[2]Department of Periodontics and Oral Medicine, University of Michigan School of Dentistry, Ann Arbor, MI
[3]A. Alfred Taubman Health Sciences Library, University of Michigan, Ann Arbor, MI

The article is associated with the American College of Prosthodontists' journal-based continuing education program. It is accompanied by an online continuing education activity worth 1 credit. Please visit www.wileyhealthlearning.com/jopr to complete the activity and earn credit.

Keywords
Dental implant; head and neck cancer; irradiation; survival rate; oral rehabilitation.

Correspondence
Takako I. Tanaka, 2700 MLK Jr. Blvd., Detroit, MI 48208-2576. E-mail: tanakata@udmercy.edu

The authors deny any conflicts of interest.

Accepted November 11, 2012

Published in *Journal of Prosthodontics* August 2013; Vol. 22, Issue 6

doi: 10.1111/jopr.12028

ABSTRACT

An increasing number of reports indicate successful use of dental implants (DI) during oral rehabilitation for head and neck cancer patients undergoing tumor surgery and radiation therapy. Implant-supported dentures are a viable option when patients cannot use conventional dentures due to adverse effects of radiation therapy, including oral dryness or fragile mucosa, in addition to compromised anatomy; however, negative effects of radiation, including osteoradionecrosis, are well documented in the literature, and early loss of implants in irradiated bone has been reported. There is currently no consensus concerning DI safety or clinical guidelines for their use in irradiated head and neck cancer patients. It is important for healthcare professionals to be aware of the multidimensional risk factors for these patients when planning oral rehabilitation with DIs, and to provide optimal treatment options and maximize the overall treatment outcome. This paper reviews and updates the impact of radiotherapy on DI survival and discusses clinical considerations for DI therapy in irradiated head and neck cancer patients.

Cancer of the oral cavity and pharynx, the largest group of head and neck cancers, is the ninth most common cancer in males in the United States.[1] Approximately 40,000 people will be newly diagnosed with oral cancer with a 5-year survival rate of 57%.[2] Surgery is a well-established treatment and may include radiotherapy (RT) and/or chemotherapy.[3] Reconstruction of major surgical defects is required for a majority of the cases, followed by rehabilitation of missing teeth and restoring orofacial function.

Use of implants for prosthetic reconstruction has dramatically increased due to advancements in materials science and surgical techniques during the past three decades.[4] Implant-supported dentures seem to be a viable option, especially when RT's adverse effects, such as oral dryness or fragile mucosa, along with compromised anatomy, hamper the use of conventional removable dentures.[5]

An increased number of reports indicate successful implant-supported prostheses in irradiated cancer patients.[6–10] However, the negative effects of radiation are well documented,[11] and several studies in both animals and humans have shown an increased risk of early loss of dental implants (DI) in irradiated bone.[12–14] There is currently no consensus about the predictability, safety, or clinical guidelines for DI therapy in irradiated head and neck cancer patients. This paper reviews the impact of RT on DI therapy and discusses updated clinical considerations for DI therapy in those patients.

RT AND ITS ADVERSE EFFECTS

Cancer cells are in a continuous state of mitosis. Ionizing radiation produces energy that injures or destroys cells by damaging nuclear DNA or altering the molecular characteristics of individual cells.[2] Most patients with head and neck cancer receive between 50 and 70 Grays (Gy) as a curative dose. For concomitant use, 45 Gy are used preoperatively and 55 to 60 Gy postoperatively. These doses are typically fractionated over a period of 5 to 7 weeks, once a day, 5 days a week, with a daily dose of approximately 2 Gy.[2] Normally, each daily treatment lasts about 10 to 15 minutes. Fractionated radiation is used because in general, normal tissue repairs sub-lethal DNA damage better than tumor tissue, especially in the low-dose range.

Adverse effects of RT include mucositis, hyposalivation, loss of taste, radiation caries, trismus, and osteoradionecrosis (ORN) of the jaw. ORN, ischemic necrosis of bone, is one of the most serious complications.[11] Initial changes in bone caused by irradiation result from direct injury to the remodeling system (osteocytes, osteoblasts, and osteoclasts). In addition, vascular injury precedes hyperemia, followed by endarteritis, thrombosis, and a progressive occlusion and obliteration of small vessels. With time, the bone marrow

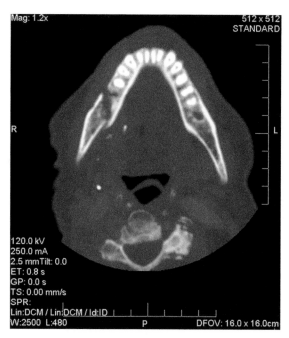

FIGURE 27.1   CT scan showing the fracture of the right mandible of a patient after tumor surgery, RT, and HBO.

exhibits marked acellularity and avascularity, with marked fibrosis and fatty degeneration.[14] ORN occurs in the mandible more often than the maxilla. Although 30% of cases may be asymptomatic, more patients with ORN present pain, fistula formation, and in more severe cases, spontaneous bone fracture (Fig 27.1). Recent systematic reviews found the risk of developing ORN in irradiated head and neck cancer patients as low as 2%; however, the risk can be higher after tooth extraction.[15,16] While peak time of spontaneous ORN was in the first 2 to 3 years after RT,[17] the risk of trauma-induced ORN might last indefinitely.[11] The risk and severity of ORN is known to be directly related not only to radiation dose and the volume of irradiated tissue, but also to the dental health of the patients.[15]

RT ON IMPLANT SURVIVAL

Many studies have shown that DI therapy in irradiated patients is not significantly less favorable than in the non-irradiated population (Table 27.1). These studies were identified via a PubMed search using Medical Subject Headings and keyword phrases for "dental implants," "dental prosthesis," "radiotherapy," "radiation effects," and other variations. The papers were limited to human studies, English language papers, and papers published since 2000. Clinical reports and studies with a sample size less than 10 were excluded. The identified studies reported implant survival rates or

TABLE 27.1 Summary of the Recent Literature on the Effect of RT on DI Survival

Authors (Year)	Study Type	Follow-up Period	Radiation Dosage	Timing of DI Placement	HBO	No. of Patients w RT	No. of Patients w/o RT	No. of DI w RT	No. of DI w/o RT	DI Survival/Success w RT	DI Survival/Success w/o RT	Remarks
Shaw et al (2005)[29]	Retrospective	0.3 to 14 years (median 3.5 years)	40 to 66 Gy (median 50 Gy)	Secondary (approximately 1 year after RT)	Yes (24/34 Pst)	34	43	172	192	Failure: 32% of patients, 18% of DI	Failure: 23% of patients, 13% of DI	Native/grafted bone
Schepers et al (2006)[3]	Retrospective	Up to 23 months	61 to 68 Gy as a boost dose on the primary tumor site and 10 to 68 Gy on the symphyseal area	Primary	?	21	27	61	78	OI success: 97% Prosthetic success: 75.4%	OI success: 100% Prosthetic success: 75.6%	Edentulous mandible only, native bone
Yerit et al (2006)[9]	Retrospective	0.3 to 13.6 years (mean 5.4 years)	50 Gy as a boost dose on the primary tumor site and 10 to 68 on the symphyseal area	Secondary (4 to 8 wks after RT)	No	71 (total)		154	84	SR: 93% (2 years) 90% (3 years) 84% (5 years) 72% (8 years)	SR: 99% (2 years) 99% (3 years) 99% (5 years) 95% (8 years)	Native/grafted bone, only mandibular-bar retained overdenture used
Nelson et al (2007)[28]	Retrospective	5 to 161 months (mean 10.3 years)	Up to 72 Gy	Secondary (a minimum of 6 months after RT)	?	29	64	124	311	SR: 84% (46 months) 54% (after 13.5 years)	SR: 92% (3.5 years) 84% (8.5 years) 69% (13 years)	The heavy nicotine users after RT excluded, antibiotics used for DI in irradiated patients
Schoen et al (2008)[47]	Prospective	12 months	60.1 ± 7.7 Gy	Primary	?	31	19	76	64	SR: 97%	SR: 97%	Edentulous jaws only
Cuesta-Gil et al (2009)[61]	Retrospective	6 months to 9 years	50 to 60 Gy	Primary (56.9%): secondary (43.1%, a minimum of 12 months after RT)	Yes (all)	79	42	395	301	OI failure: 27/395, prosthetic failure 48/395 implants	OI failure: 2/301, prosthetic failure 4/301 implants	Native/graft bone
Korfage et al (2010)[8]	Prospective	5 years	46 to 70 Gy, intraforaminal dose 12 to 70 Gy	Primary	?	32	18	123	72	SR: 89.4% (13 DI in 6 patients failure)	SR: 98.6% (1 DI failure)	Edentulous jaws only
Salinas et al (2010)[62]	Retrospective	4 to 108 months (mean 41.1)	>60 Gy	Secondary	Yes (all)	22	40	90	116	Success rate: 74.4%	Success rate: 93.1%	Mandible only, native/grafted (fibula flaps), adjunct chemotherapy (29.7%)
Buddula et al (2011)[12]	Retrospective	3 years	>50 Gy: 50.2 to 67.50 Gy (mean 60.7 Gy)	Secondary (median 3.4 years after RT)	?	48	n/a	271	n/a	SR: 98.9% (1 years) 89.9% (5 years) 72.3% (10 years)	n/a	Native/grafted bone

RT = radiation therapy; DI = dental implants; HBO = hyperbaric oxygen therapy; OI = osseointegration; SR = survival rate; Gy = gray.

success rates in patients with RT ranging from 74.4% to 98.9% with the majority reporting survival rates above 84%. Many additional studies also reported high function of implant-supported dentures in irradiated head and neck patients, with relatively high implant survival rates.[18–20] However, conflicting results exist. The major concerns for DI therapy in irradiated head and neck cancer patients are the potential for delayed healing and the later risk of ORN.[21,22] In a recent review of the literature evaluating RT effects on both dental and craniofacial implants in animal and human subjects, the relative risk of implant failure in irradiated bone was found to be 2 to 3 times greater than that of non-irradiated subjects.[23] Animal models have revealed compromised osseointegration of DI due to irradiation, such as impaired osteogenesis, bone strength reduction, and significant fibrosis of the periosteum, to be the common end-stage of tissue injury.[13,24,25] Some human studies show a lower survival rate of implants placed in irradiated bone compared to non-irradiated controls.[1,9,12] The differing methodologies among these studies, the varying definitions of implant survival and success, the improvements in implant surface features, and variations in treatment modalities may account for the controversies regarding DI predictability in these patients.[26–31] Many factors influencing treatment outcome have been suggested (Fig 27.2). In the following section, we will discuss the impact of RT on DI therapy.

IMPACT OF RT ON DI THERAPY

Radiation Dose and Implant Location

DI failures were seldom seen at cumulative doses less than 45 Gy[32] and more commonly seen at doses greater than 65 Gy.[33] ORN risk has been reported to be highest in the extraction of mandibular teeth within the radiation field with doses greater than 60 Gy.[7] Studies have shown that short survival of implants in irradiated patients was significant with total doses >50 to 55 Gy.[9,22,33] Many agree that DI survival in patients treated with cumulative RT doses lower than 50 Gy can be comparable to that in non-irradiated patients.[34–36]

Implants in the mandible have shown higher survival rates than those in the maxilla.[34,37] As mirrored by DI practice in the general population,[31] that is most likely due to high bone density of the mandible providing better initial primary implant stability. Visch et al, in their study with 130 consecutive cancer patients irradiated orally over a period of up to 14 years, found implant location in the maxilla or mandible (59% and 85%, respectively) as a dominant factor ($p = 0.001$) among other potential factors influencing implant survival.[22] Nelson et al reported similar results in the maxilla and mandible (70% and 92%, respectively) in their first 5 years of follow-up, though long-term survival rates (after 8 years) were found to be equivocal.[28] The region of the mandible

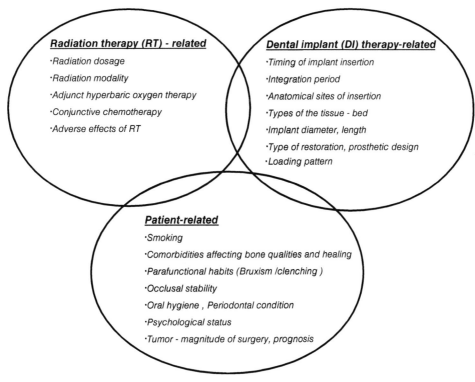

FIGURE 27.2   Potential factors impacting dental implant therapy in irradiated head and neck cancer patients.

anterior to the mental foramen is usually exposed to a lower dose than other sites during RT and seems to have better remodeling capability due to additional vascular supply from the facial artery.[38,39] It must be noted that the radiation dose per implant site ideally should be known to determine the impact of radiation dose on implant survival.[4] However, it is often not available in the literature.[23,40]

RT Modalities and Adjuvant Chemotherapy

Advancements in RT techniques have been developed to preserve function of normal tissue and enhance tumor control. Those include Intensity-Modulated Radiation Therapy (IMRT) and altered fractionation schedules (hyperfractionation and accelerated fractionation). IMRT is a computer-driven technology using rapid radiation beams of varying intensity to confine the dose to the target tissues.[41] IMRT in the head and neck region aims to preserve the parotid glands particularly, resulting in prevention of hyposalivation. Hyposalivation frequently results in dental caries and necessitates tooth extraction, which increases the risk of ORN.[16] Hyperfractionation delivers an increased number of fractions and total dose with a smaller dose per fraction. Accelerated fractionation provides radiation at a faster rate of accumulation than that of standard fractionation, and with a similar total dose to conventional RT.[40] A recent systematic review found that risk of ORN after tooth extraction in irradiated patients was reduced by accelerated fractionation with dose reduction but elevated by hyperfractionation.[16] However, studies focusing on the impact of RT modality on DI survival are scarce at this time.

Concomitant chemotherapy is often incorporated in cancer therapy to augment the anti-tumor effect of RT. Major side effects include acute mucositis and altered taste, which can be multiplied with RT; however, currently there is little evidence that chemotherapy influences DI therapy.[42] Nabil and Samman did not find significantly increased ORN risk in patients receiving chemoradiotherapy.[16]

Adjunctive Use of Hyperbaric Oxygen Therapy (HBO)

HBO has been used for a wide range of medical conditions such as syphilis, multiple sclerosis, and myocardial infarction. It raises levels and diffusion of oxygen in local tissue by inducing angiogenesis, increasing bone metabolism (enhancing osteoblast repopulation and fibroblast function), and stimulating collagen synthesis.[11] Therefore, it is expected that HBO increases the capacity to repair tissue damaged by RT.

The protocol of HBO used after RT in the head and neck region usually includes 20 to 30 sessions (lasting 90 minutes each) prior and 10 minutes after tooth extraction or implant placement, at a compression of 2.4 atmospheres absolute pressure with 100% oxygen.[43] Many support adjunctive use

of HBO to prevent and manage ORN, especially when the implant site is irradiated with more than 50 Gy and shows clinical signs of radiation damage.[6,15,35] Better wound healing on the implant site of the mandible was noted in irradiated patients who received HBO therapy during the 3 to 7 year follow-up period.[44] Granström et al[45] found significantly lower failure rates of craniofacial implants including DI in HBO-treated patients than those in the non-HBO-treated group (8.1% vs. 53.7%, respectively); however, opinions conflict on the prophylactic effect of HBO in reducing the risk of RT-induced ORN, and it has not been universally accepted in dentistry. Studies have shown that HBO could not enhance implant survival in irradiated mandibular bone.[29,46] Limited accessibility and its high costs in time and money might be concerns.[46] HBO requires approximately 1 month before tooth extraction, which may not always be practical for symptomatic cases. Potential complications such as middle ear barotraumas and myopia must also be taken into consideration, as well as contraindications including uncontrolled COPD.[46]

Timing of Implant Placement Related to RT

Optimal timing of DI insertion-related RT has been debated. Immediate implant insertion before RT, at the same time as the ablative tumor surgery, is referred to as primary placement, as opposed to secondary placement after RT. Primary placement of implants aims at achieving osseointegration prior to onset of the damaging effects of RT, and early oral rehabilitation by avoiding additional surgery.[3,47] Overall cost can be reduced; however, indications may be limited to low-grade tumors. Computer-guided implant placement has recently been introduced to improve identification of the ideal implant location during surgery.[48–50] Secondary placement of implants is probably more common in dental practice because primary placement is not always available to patients in the hospital setting. Delayed DI placement enables assessment of the postsurgical status of the patients (both functionally and psychologically), and more accurate cancer prognosis.[29] Patients will be given more time to choose prosthetic treatment options after their recovery from tumor therapy and prior to initiation of an extensive dental procedure.[24]

Recent publications have demonstrated encouraging results in primary placement of DI.[3,47] A human study shows better implant survival in primary placement than in secondary placement in edentulous mandibles of patients with oral squamous cell carcinoma.[3] However, a recent systematic review by Colella et al found a similar implant failure rate between the two groups (3.2% vs. 5.4%, respectively).[32] Choice of implant insertion timing (before RT vs. after RT) likely depends on the surgical team's personal preference.[11] No randomized controlled studies have been conducted regarding timing of implant therapy and implant success.

How long should we wait for implant placement after RT? The answer remains unclear at this time. Several studies showed that 6 months after RT, DI survival was not affected by placement timing.[9,22] However, to avoid early complications of tumor therapy, most clinicians agree to wait a minimum of 6 to 12 months.[24] Others have recommended waiting a little longer (12 to 18 months typically) to allow enough time for bone remodeling and muscle healing.[51,52] Tumor recurrence or developing a second malignancy in the adjacent region must be another important consideration.[34,53] The first 12 months after tumor therapy is generally considered to be the high risk period of recurrence. A longitudinal prospective study showed 44% of cancer patients who underwent mandibular resection had recurrence within 13 months of surgery.[34]

It must be noted that the risk of ORN may persist for years after RT in head and neck cancer patients.[4,14] Progressive loss of capillaries (therefore loss of tissue perfusion) without evidence of spontaneous revascularization over time was found in a study by Marx and Johnson, using serial biopsy specimens from more than 143 irradiated patient mandibles.[14] Granström et al reported progressive loss of DI due to failure of osseointegration up to 6 years after the placement.[54]

Oral Health and Psychological Status of Patients Related to RT

Although the direct impact of oral health status on DI survival is not clear in the literature, local effects of RT on periodontal tissue, and attachment loss particularly, have been reported in several studies.[55,56] Epstein et al observed tooth loss and progressive periodontal attachment loss in teeth within areas of high-dose radiation.[55] A study by Marques and Dib showed similar results and explained that inadequate homecare resulting from lack of motivation, RT-induced hyposalivation, and limited vertical opening might contribute to such significant periodontal destruction in irradiated head and neck cancer patients.[56] Poor oral health is known to increase ORN risk.[57,58] Katsura et al reported that oral conditions such as periodontal pocket depth >5 mm, dental plaque score >40%, and alveolar bone loss >60%, in the first or second year after RT, as well as smoking history after RT were significantly associated with ORN risk.[57]

Patients undergoing cancer therapies are often weak. RT can be detrimental to the patients' quality of life, compromising speech, swallowing, and sensory and masticatory function, in addition to compromised esthetics caused by major surgery.[11,29] After tumor therapies, patients often become apprehensive about further extensive dental treatment, which results in unloaded implants.[3,24] Compared to the high success rate of implant osseointegration, a lower success rate for prostheses has been reported.[24] In the study by Smolka et al, prosthetic success was reported as 42.9%, while implant success was 92% in 56 cancer patients who had mandibular free flap reconstruction.[59] Schepers et al found the ultimate rates of functional implant-supported dentures in the postoperative irradiated group versus surgery-only group were 75.4% versus 75.6%, respectively, compared to a 97% success rate of implant osseointegration during the 23-month follow-up.[3] In their study, 24.5% of the primary-placed implants never became functional because of cancer-related (tumor recurrence or metastasis) or psychological reasons.

DISCUSSION

Interpretation of published data needs special caution. Neither a high implant survival rate nor success of osseointegration assures functional DI or success of DI therapy in cancer patients; however, with careful case selection, DI therapy in oral rehabilitation in irradiated head and neck cancer patients can be successfully achieved. Before initiation of DI therapy, a patient's level of tolerance must be assured both physically and psychologically. Reasonable oncologic prognosis should be obtained from the physician. The planned implant site of the anterior mandible and a cumulative radiation dosage lower than 50 Gy may predict the outcome of DI therapy. If possible, consultation with the radiation oncologist is encouraged to obtain radiation dose distribution. A timespan of 12 months between the last RT and implant insertion seems reasonable from both the oncologic and dental prospective; however, later complications of RT, including ORN, are still not clear. In general, placement of a minimal number of implants is recommended.[2] It is the authors' opinion that options for primary placement of implants should be discussed prior to tumor surgery to avoid potential damage from RT for implant sites such as ORN. The impacts of adjunctive HBO, chemotherapy, or RT modality on implant survival remain uncertain.

Throughout the oral rehabilitation, it is important to maintain optimal periodontal health with appropriate management of any adverse effects of RT. General known risk factors of DI failure should be controlled to maximize the treatment outcome. Lack of communication and education among the patient and healthcare professionals have been raised as concerns.[2] New guidelines for prophylactic dental care prior to the head and neck cancer treatment that could damage the oral tissue in cancer patients are on the horizon.[11,60]

CONCLUSION

Multidimensional potential risk factors of DI failure must be considered when planning DI therapy in irradiated head and neck patients. Factors focusing on RT were discussed, and the negative impacts of RT on DI therapy are undeniable. The benefit of using implant-supported dentures over conventional dentures must outweigh the risks. Meticulous treatment planning along with careful preoperative oral examination and good coordination with oncologic specialists cannot be overemphasized. It is also important for the dental profession to keep abreast of the latest available RT technologies. Additional evidence-based clinical guidelines for implant use in head and neck patients undergoing RT are expected.

ACKNOWLEDGMENT

Dr. Robert Nisker is gratefully acknowledged for his contribution of the CT imaging.

REFERENCES

1. American Cancer Society: Cancer Treatment and Survivorship. 2012. Available at http://www.cancer.org/acs/groups/content/%40epidemiologysurveilance/documents/document/acspc-027766.pdf (accessed September 9, 2012).

2. Oral Cancer Foundation: Oral Cancer Facts. 2012. Available at http://www.oralcancerfoundation.org/facts/ (accessed September 9, 2012).

3. Schepers RH, Slagter AP, Kaanders JH, et al: Effect of postoperative radiotherapy on the functional result of implants placed during ablative surgery for oral cancer. *Int J Oral Maxillofac Surg* 2006;35:803–808.

4. Granström G: Osseointegration in irradiated cancer patients: an analysis with respect to implant failures. *J Oral Maxillofac Surg* 2005;63:579–585.

5. Dholam KP, Gurav SV: Dental implants in irradiated jaws: a literature review. *J Cancer Res Ther* 2012;8(Suppl 1): S85–S93.

6. Barrowman RA, Wilson PR, Wiesenfeld D: Oral rehabilitation with dental implants after cancer treatment. *Aust Dent J* 2011;56:160–165.

7. Jisander S, Grenthe B, Alberius P: Dental implant survival in the irradiated jaw: a preliminary report. *Int J Oral Maxillofac Implants* 1997;12:643–648.

8. Korfage A, Schoen PJ, Raghoebar GM, et al: Benefits of dental implants installed during ablative tumour surgery in oral cancer patients: a prospective 5-year clinical trial. *Clin Oral Implants Res* 2010;21:971–979.

9. Yerit KC, Posch M, Seemann M, et al: Implant survival in mandibles of irradiated oral cancer patients. *Clin Oral Implants Res* 2006;17:337–344.

10. Linsen SS, Martini M, Stark H: Long-term results of endosteal implants following radical oral cancer surgery with and without adjuvant radiation therapy. *Clin Implant Dent Relat Res* 2012;14:250–258.

11. Vissink A, Burlage FR, Spijkervet FK, et al: Prevention and treatment of the consequences of head and neck radiotherapy. *Crit Rev Oral Biol Med* 2003;14:213–225.

12. Buddula A, Assad DA, Salinas TJ, et al: Survival of dental implants in native and grafted bone in irradiated head and neck cancer patients: a retrospective analysis. *Indian J Dent Res* 2011;22:644–648.

13. Verdonck HW, Meijer GJ, Laurin T, et al: Implant stability during osseointegration in irradiated and non-irradiated minipig alveolar bone: an experimental study. *Clin Oral Implants Res* 2008;19:201–206.

14. Marx RE, Johnson RP: Studies in the radiobiology of osteoradionecrosis and their clinical significance. *Oral Surg Oral Med Oral Pathol* 1987;64:379–390.

15. Nabil S, Samman N: Risk factors for osteoradionecrosis after head and neck radiation: a systematic review. *Oral Surg Oral Med Oral Pathol Oral Radiol* 2012;113:54–69.

16. Nabil S, Samman N: Incidence and prevention of osteoradionecrosis after dental extraction in irradiated patients: a systematic review. *Int J Oral Maxillofac Surg* 2011;40: 229–243.

17. Thorn JJ, Hansen HS, Specht L, et al: Osteoradionecrosis of the jaws: clinical characteristics and relation to the field of irradiation. *J Oral Maxillofac Surg* 2000;58:1088–1093; discussion 1093–1095.

18. Fukuda M, Takahashi T, Nagai H, et al: Implant-supported edentulous maxillary obturators with milled bar attachments after maxillectomy. *J Oral Maxillofac Surg* 2004;62: 799–805.

19. Korfage A, Schoen PJ, Raghoebar GM, et al: Five-year follow-up of oral functioning and quality of life in patients with oral cancer with implant-retained mandibular overdentures. *Head Neck* 2011;33:831–839.

20. Taira Y, Sekine J, Sawase T, et al: Implant-retained overdenture following hemiglossectomy: a 10-year clinical case report. *J Oral Rehabil* 2006;33:313–315.

21. Harrison JS, Stratemann S, Redding SW: Dental implants for patients who have had radiation treatment for head and neck cancer. *Spec Care Dentist* 2003;23:223–229.

22. Visch LL, van Waas MA, Schmitz PI, et al: A clinical evaluation of implants in irradiated oral cancer patients. *J Dent Res* 2002;81:856–859.

23. Ihde S, Kopp S, Gundlach K, et al: Effects of radiation therapy on craniofacial and dental implants: a review of the literature. *Oral Surg Oral Med Oral Pathol Oral Radiol Endod* 2009;107:56–65.

24. Asikainen P, Klemetti E, Kotilainen R, et al: Osseointegration of dental implants in bone irradiated with 40, 50 or 60 Gy doses. An experimental study with beagle dogs. *Clin Oral Implants Res* 1998;9:20–25.

25. Renou SJ, Guglielmotti MB, de la Torre A, et al: Effect of total body irradiation on peri-implant tissue reaction: an experimental study. *Clin Oral Implants Res* 2001;12:468–472.

26. Carr AB: Oral cancer therapy may influence survival of dental implants. *J Evid Based Dent Pract* 2011;11:124–126.

27. Jokstad A: Can dental implants osseointegrate in oral cancer patients? *Evid Based Dent* 2011;12:82–83.

28. Nelson K, Heberer S, Glatzer C: Survival analysis and clinical evaluation of implant-retained prostheses in oral cancer resection patients over a mean follow-up period of 10 years. *J Prosthet Dent* 2007;98:405–410.

29. Shaw RJ, Sutton AF, Cawood JI, et al: Oral rehabilitation after treatment for head and neck malignancy. *Head Neck* 2005;27:459–470.

30. Anne-Gaelle B, Samuel S, Julie B, et al: Dental implant placement after mandibular reconstruction by microvascular free fibula flap: current knowledge and remaining questions. *Oral Oncol* 2011;47:1099–1104.

31. Strub JR, Jurdzik BA, Tuna T: Prognosis of immediately loaded implants and their restorations: a systematic literature review. *J Oral Rehabil* 2012;39:704–717.

32. Colella G, Cannavale R, Pentenero M, et al: Oral implants in radiated patients: a systematic review. *Int J Oral Maxillofac Implants* 2007;22:616–622.

33. Granstrom G: Placement of dental implants in irradiated bone: the case for using hyperbaric oxygen. *J Oral Maxillofac Surg* 2006;64:812–818.

34. Garrett N, Roumanas ED, Blackwell KE, et al: Efficacy of conventional and implant-supported mandibular resection prostheses: study overview and treatment outcomes. *J Prosthet Dent* 2006;96:13–24.

35. Larsen PE: Placement of dental implants in the irradiated mandible: a protocol involving adjunctive hyperbaric oxygen. *J Oral Maxillofac Surg* 1997;55:967–971.

36. Sammartino G, Marenzi G, Cioffi I, et al: Implant therapy in irradiated patients. *J Craniofac Surg* 2011;22:443–445.

37. Kovacs AF: Clinical analysis of implant losses in oral tumor and defect patients. *Clin Oral Implants Res* 2000;11:494–504.

38. de Oliveira JA, do Amaral Escada AL, Alves Rezende MC, et al: Analysis of the effects of irradiation in osseointegrated dental implants. *Clin Oral Implants Res* 2012;23:511–514.

39. Nishimura RD, Roumanas E, Beumer J, 3rd, et al: Restoration of irradiated patients using osseointegrated implants: current perspectives. *J Prosthet Dent* 1998;79:641–647.

40. Zackrisson B, Mercke C, Strander H, et al: A systematic overview of radiation therapy effects in head and neck cancer. *Acta Oncol* 2003;42:443–461.

41. Lee N, Puri DR, Blanco AI, et al: Intensity-modulated radiation therapy in head and neck cancers: an update. *Head Neck* 2007;29:387–400.

42. Scully C, Hobkirk J, Dios PD: Dental endosseous implants in the medically compromised patient. *J Oral Rehabil* 2007;34:590–599.

43. Marx RE, Johnson RP, Kline SN: Prevention of osteoradionecrosis: a randomized prospective clinical trial of hyperbaric oxygen versus penicillin. *J Am Dent Assoc* 1985;111:49–54.

44. Taylor TD, Worthington P: Osseointegrated implant rehabilitation of the previously irradiated mandible: results of a limited trial at 3 to 7 years. *J Prosthet Dent* 1993;69:60–69.

45. Granström G, Tjellstrom A, Branemark PI: Osseointegrated implants in irradiated bone: a case-controlled study using adjunctive hyperbaric oxygen therapy. *J Oral Maxillofac Surg* 1999;57:493–499.

46. Schoen PJ, Raghoebar GM, Bouma J, et al: Rehabilitation of oral function in head and neck cancer patients after radiotherapy with implant-retained dentures: effects of hyperbaric oxygen therapy. *Oral Oncol* 2007;43:379–388.

47. Schoen PJ, Raghoebar GM, Bouma J, et al: Prosthodontic rehabilitation of oral function in head-neck cancer patients with dental implants placed simultaneously during ablative tumour surgery: an assessment of treatment outcomes and quality of life. *Int J Oral Maxillofac Surg* 2008;37:8–16.

48. De Santis D, Malchiodi L, Cucchi A, et al: Computer-assisted surgery: double surgical guides for immediate loading of implants in maxillary postextractive sites. *J Craniofac Surg* 2010;21:1781–1785.

49. Fletcher-Stark ML, Rubenstein JE, Raigrodski AJ: The use of computer-aided manufacturing during the treatment of the edentulous mandible in an oral radiation therapy patient: clinical report. *J Prosthet Dent* 2011;105:154–157.

50. Horowitz A, Orentlicher G, Goldsmith D: Computerized implantology for the irradiated patient. *J Oral Maxillofac Surg* 2009;67:619–623.

51. Epstein JB, Wong FL, Stevenson-Moore P: Osteoradionecrosis: clinical experience and a proposal for classification. *J Oral Maxillofac Surg* 1987;45:104–110.

52. Meraw SJ, Reeve CM: Dental considerations and treatment of the oncology patient receiving radiation therapy. *J Am Dent Assoc* 1998;129:201–205.

53. De Ceulaer J, Magremanne M, van Veen A, et al: Squamous cell carcinoma recurrence around dental implants. *J Oral Maxillofac Surg* 2010;68:2507–2512.

54. Granström G, Tjellstrom A, Branemark PI, et al: Bone-anchored reconstruction of the irradiated head and neck cancer patient. *Otolaryngol Head Neck Surg* 1993;108:334–343.

55. Epstein JB, Lunn R, Le N, et al: Periodontal attachment loss in patients after head and neck radiation therapy. *Oral Surg Oral Med Oral Pathol Oral Radiol Endod* 1998;86:673–677.

56. Marques MA, Dib LL: Periodontal changes in patients undergoing radiotherapy. *J Periodontol* 2004;75:1178–1187.

57. Katsura K, Sasai K, Sato K, et al: Relationship between oral health status and development of osteoradionecrosis of the mandible: a retrospective longitudinal study. *Oral Surg Oral Med Oral Pathol Oral Radiol Endod* 2008;105:731–738.

58. Oelgiesser D, Levin L, Barak S, et al: Rehabilitation of an irradiated mandible after mandibular resection using implant/tooth-supported fixed prosthesis: a clinical report. *J Prosthet Dent* 2004;91:310–314.

59. Smolka K, Kraehenbuehl M, Eggensperger N, et al: Fibula free flap reconstruction of the mandible in cancer patients:

evaluation of a combined surgical and prosthodontic treatment concept. *Oral Oncol* 2008;44:571–581.

60. Patel Y, Bahlhorn H, Zafar S, et al: Survey of Michigan dentists and radiation oncologists on oral care of patients undergoing head and neck radiation therapy. *J Mich Dent Assoc* 2012;94:34–45.

61. Cuesta-Gil M, Ochandiano Caicoya S, Riba-Garcia F, et al: Oral rehabilitation with osseointegrated implants in oncologic patients. *J Oral Maxillofac Surg* 2009;67:2485–2496.

62. Salinas TJ, Desa VP, Katsnelson A, et al: Clinical evaluation of implants in radiated fibula flaps. *J Oral Maxillofac Surg* 2010;68:524–529.

28

IMPLANT TREATMENT RECORD FORM

TONY DAHER, DDS, MSED,[1] CHARLES J. GOODACRE, DDS, MSD,[2] AND STEVEN M. MORGANO, DMD[3]

[1]Associate Professor, Department of Restorative Dentistry, School of Dentistry, Loma Linda University, Loma Linda, CA
[2]Professor and Dean, School of Dentistry, Loma Linda University, Loma Linda, CA
[3]Professor and Director, Division of Postdoctoral Prosthodontics, Department of Restorative Sciences and Biomaterials, Goldman School of Dental Medicine, Boston University, Boston, MA

Keywords
Dental implant; implant record; implant form.

Correspondence
Dr. Tony Daher, 1413 Foothill Blvd. Ste A, La Verne, CA 91750. E-mail: tonydaher@verizon.net

Presented in part at the annual meeting of the Pacific Coast Society for Prosthodontics, San Francisco, CA, June 21–25, 2007.

Accepted April 25, 2008

Published in *Journal of Prosthodontics* June 2009; Vol. 18, Issue 4

doi: 10.1111/j.1532-849X.2008.00434.x

ABSTRACT

The identification of different dental implants and restorative components is difficult when dental records do not include an inventory of implant components. An implant record form is described. The form should be filled out and retained in the patient's chart for future use and implant maintenance visits.

The identification of different dental implant bodies and other implant components can be difficult. It is particularly challenging when patient treatment records are unavailable or when the records do not include an inventory of the implants and components used. The lack of information can be a very frustrating experience for both practitioners and their patients.

The mobility of individuals in today's society increases the need for a repository of pertinent information to be available for future dental care providers. In fact, even the practitioner who provided the initial implant treatment can find it difficult to subsequently recall details about the implants and components. The problem is compounded by the large number of implant systems currently available,

Journal of Prosthodontics on Dental Implants, First Edition. Edited by Avinash S. Bidra and Stephen M. Parel.
© 2015 American College of Prosthodontists. Published 2015 by John Wiley & Sons, Inc.

Patient Name:_____ Phone number:_____

Treating dentist _____ Phone:_____ Treating surgeon:_____
Phone:_____

Implant location (by tooth #)					
Company name					
Type					
Batch #					
Diameter					
Length					
Bone grafting date/site (if used)					
Graft type/ Donor site					
Placement date (Surgery)					
Restoration date (Prosthesis placed)					
Cement					
Screw head type					
Screw torque (Preload)					
Access screw location					
Type of abutment					
Abutment material					
Additional information					

FIGURE 28.1   Implant treatment record.

some of which have identical or similar designs. The extensive array of abutment types, abutment materials, and the number of customized parts that may have been used to restore dental implants makes it imperative to record important information for posterity.

There have been publications regarding the radiographic identification of implants[1,2] and also regarding the use of implant consultation forms to document presurgical and surgical information;[3] however, there have not been publications identifying the pertinent dental implant information that should be recorded in a patient's treatment record for future use. A specific form, an exhaustive list, that records pertinent information would be valuable for any future treating dentists. A copy of this form (Fig 28.1) can be given to patients for their records, as well as be retained in the practitioner's patient treatment file.

THE RECORD (FIG 28.1)

- "Location" is the tooth number(s) where the implant(s) was/were placed.
- "Company name" (i.e., Nobel Biocare, Zimmer Dental, Astra Tech, or Biomet 3i).
- "Type" is specific to the implant system used (i.e., Replace Select, Tapered Screw-Vent, MicroThread, OsseoSpeed, or Osseotite implant systems).
- "Batch #" records the batch number of the implants used.
- "Diameter" is specific to the size of the implant platform (i.e., 3.7 mm, 4.7 mm, or 5.0 mm).
- "Length" is the cervicoapical length of the implant (i.e., 8 mm, 10 mm, or 13 mm).
- "Bone grafting" specifies the date and site of the graft.
- "Graft type" is the trade name (i.e., Bio-Oss or Puros materials) or for autogenous grafts, the donor site (i.e., "from the chin").
- "Placement date" records the date of implant placement.

- "Restoration date" records the date of placement of the prosthesis.
- "Cement" specifies the type of cement for cemented restoration.
- "Screw head type" describes the type of screwdriver required for retrievability (i.e., hexagon head, star grip, or squared head).
- "Screw torque" specifies the amount of torque to tighten the screw.
- "Access screw location" specifies the location of the screw access hole, and is very useful if the abutment screw loosens with a cement-retained, implant-supported prosthesis.
- "Type of abutment" lists how the abutment was made (i.e., premade, custom cast, or computer-assisted design/computer-assisted machining).
- "Abutment material" lists what the implant abutment is made of (titanium, cast gold, zirconia).
- "Additional information" pertains to any additional information needed for the specific clinical situation.

ACKNOWLEDGMENT

The authors are grateful to Dr. Roy Yanase for editing the article and for his suggestions.

REFERENCES

1. Sahiwal IG, Woody RD, Benson BW, et al: Radiographic identification of nonthreaded endosseous dental implants. *J Prosthet Dent* 2002;87:552–562.
2. Sahiwal IG, Woody RD, Benson BW, et al: Radiographic identification of threaded endosseous dental implants. *J Prosthet Dent* 2002;87:563–577.
3. Rieder CE: An implant consultation form. *Calif Dent Assoc J* 1990;18:29–31.

INDEX

A

Abutment
  CAD/CAM designs, 15, 17, 22
  cast prosthetic abutments, 179
  collar heights, 15
  connection on stress distribution, 207
  design and esthetics, 47
  design, assessment criteria for, 11
  digital one-abutment/one-time concept, 21
  with internal connection and different angulations, 215
  selection, 19
  temporary, 48, 50
  titanium, 18
Acrylic resin, 29, 36, 37, 118, 119, 154, 194, 200, 202, 219
  retention, 162
Adhesive cement, 18, 44
All-on-Four™ concept, 115
  cumulative survival rate, 115
  panoramic radiograph, 161
Alloying elements, in dental noble alloys, 156
Alumina (Al₂O₃), 18, 219
  abutments, 17–19
American Dental Association (ADA) system, 5
American Psychiatric Association, 45
Angular cheilitis, 46
Anorexia nervosa (AN), 45
ANSYS Workbench 12.1 finite element software, 209
Antidepressants, 46
Applegate–Kennedy classification system, 4
Appropriate/inappropriate maxillary tooth positions, 154
Artificial teeth
  adequate support for, 160
  appropriate location, 162
    using laboratory c-silicon material, 178

extreme wear/abrasion of, 153
Atrophic maxilla, 103–105, 107, 109–111, 177, 180
  treatment of, 178

B

Bicon Dental Implant™ system, 53
Binge-eating disorder (BED), 45
Biological width, 28
Bone grafts, 8, 28, 37, 108, 110, 115, 132, 161, 178, 180
Bone preservation, 28, 167
800 Brånemark system implants
  following All-on-Four™ protocol, 115
  life table for
    axial implants, 117
    implants in female patients, 117
    implants in male patients, 117
    implants in mandibular arch, 116
    implants in maxillary arch, 116
    master life table of implants, 116
  materials and methods, 115–116
  number of failures
    based on bone quality, 117
    based on implant dimension, 117
    based on smoking status, 117
  panoramic radiograph
    following delivery of definitive prostheses for, 118
  postoperative panoramic
    radiograph following All-on-Four™ implant
      rehabilitation, 118
  preoperative panoramic
    radiograph of patient elected for, 118
  prosthesis survival rate, 119
  retrospective analysis, 115
  tilted implants, 117

Journal of Prosthodontics on Dental Implants, First Edition. Edited by Avinash S. Bidra and Stephen M. Parel.
© 2015 American College of Prosthodontists. Published 2015 by John Wiley & Sons, Inc.

Buccally positioned zygomatic implants
   cast prosthetic abutments, and prosthetic framework, 179
   challenge for restorative dentistry, 177
   clinical report, 178–180
   frameworks
      computer aided design/computer aided manufacturing
        (CAD/CAM) systems, 180
   frontal view of patient after rehabilitation, 180
   occlusal view of prosthesis, 179
   panoramic radiography showing the maxillary sinus
      pneumatization, 178
   professional training, 180
   prosthesis, occlusal view, 179
   rehabilitation, frontal view of, 180
   survival rate, 180
   use of overcast component, 181
   view of the implant inclinations, 179
   zygomatic fixation, 180
Bulimia nervosa (BN), 45

C
CAD/CAM implant framework, 153, 158
   JPEG images, 158
   titanium alloy, 158
CAD implant framework, with a modified I-bar design, 159
Cantilever length (CL), 94, 115, 155, 160, 173
   rationale for, 160
Caries, 41, 44, 46, 55, 255, 258
Cast base metal alloys, 157
Cast noble alloys, 94, 156
Cemented restoration, 41
Cemento-enamel junction (CEJ), 16
Cement-retained fixed prosthesis, 41
   caries removal and remargination and fabrication crown, 44
   cemented FPD separated from screw-retained implant
      abutments, 43
   clinical presentations, 42, 43
      Case I, 42, 43
      Case II, 43, 44
   crown separated from cast dowel-core substructure, 43
   retrieved PFM crown with custom cast dowel and core still
      cemented, 43
   screw access channels, to retrieve prosthesis and
      substructures, 42
Ceramo-metal, 59
Cobalt-chromium alloy, 179, 180
   prosthetic framework, 179
Cognitive-behavior therapy, 46
Commercial dental implants, 223
   ANOVA, cell adhesion rates, 230
   cell adhesion, 231, 232
      data, 231
      similar cell adhesion patterns, 227
   cell culture
      Astra and Straumann systems, 227, 228
      on implants, 224
   cell-surface interaction, 223
   clinical evidence of performance, 223
   distinct surface characteristics, 230
   EDS analysis of, 227
   evidence/criteria support, 223
   higher magnification
      cell culture, 229
      lateral view, 229
   implant surface/bone cells, interaction of, 231
   materials and methods, 224
      cell culture on implants, 224
      implants, 224
      optical profiler, 224
      primary osteoblastic cell isolation, 224
      quantitative analysis of cell culture, 224
      Raman microspectroscopy, 224
      SEM/EDS, surface morphology and elemental
        composition, 224, 226, 228, 229, 230
   optical profilometer
      3D roughness, 224
      roughness measurements from, 224–228
   osseointegration, concept of, 223
   osteoblastic cells, 231, 232
   Raman microspectroscopy analysis, 227, 228, 231, 232
   randomized controlled clinical trials (RCT), 223
   roughness
      comparison of, 225, 226
      measurements, 224
   Ryan-Einot-Gabriel-Welsch Multiple Range Test
      (REGWQ), 223
   SEM images of implants, 226
   surface
      properties, 223
      quality of implants, 229
      topography, 228
Computer aided design/computer aided manufacturing (CAD/
      CAM) technology, 22, 49, 167, 180, 199
   abutments, 15, 17
   fabricated restorations, 24
   mandibular implant, 153, 158
   milled and cast gold alloy, 156
   milled framework, 161, 162
      copy-milled, 203
      with L-beam design, 160
   Ti frameworks achieve implant, 158, 200, 201
   titanium framework, 94
   vs. cast frameworks, 159
Computer-guided implant treatment software, 46
Cone beam computed tomography (CBCT) files, 46
Conventional two-stage implant protocol, 36
   with delayed loading, 36
Copy milling, 158
Core-retained restoration, 41
Craniofacial implants (CFI's)
   copy-milled CAD/CAM framework, 203
   extraoral prostheses
      survival rates and associated clinical complications,
        202
   failure, common risk factors associated with, 203
CSRs. *See* Cumulative survival rates (CSRs)

Cumulative survival rates (CSRs), 59, 115, 116, 117, 132, 135, 158, 203
  prosthesis, 202

D

Dental implants, in osteoporotic patients, 238
  animal studies reviewed, 240–241
  dental implants and age, gender, and jawbone quality, 246
  human studies reviewed, 242–243
  materials and methods, 239
  practical measures, aimed at improvement of dental implant outcomes, 246–247
Dental implants, in restoration of partially and fully edentulous patients, 46
  clinical report, 46–49
  intraoral labial view of interim prostheses, 49
  maxillary anterior region, 46
  methods and technologies, 46
  periapical radiographs, 49
  pretreatment dental condition, 47
  temporary abutments, 48
  two four-unit zirconia FPDs cemented, 49
  zirconia abutments fabricated
    using CAD/CAM technology seated on implants, 49
Dental implant therapy, 167
  CT scan showing fracture of right mandible of a patient after, 255
  in irradiated head and neck cancer patients, 254
  potential factors impacting
    dental implant therapy in irradiated head and neck cancer patients, 257
  radiation dose and implant location, 257–258
  radiotherapy (RT)
    on DI survival, recent literature on effect of, 256
    on implant survival, 255, 257
    and its adverse effects, 255
Dental noble alloys
  composition and properties, 157
  roles of alloying elements, 156
Dental stone type IV, 178
Diamond Crown™, 53
Digitalization, 22
  direct, 22, 23
  indirect, 22
Double full-arch *vs.* single full-arch, implant-supported rehabilitations, 131–138
  biological complication incidence rate, 138
  final prosthetic protocol, 134
  immediate provisional prosthetic protocol, 134
  implant survival of completely edentulous rehabilitations using, 135, 136
  incidence of mechanical complications, 137
  limitations of study, 138
  marginal bone level, 134
    situated apically to implant platform, 137
  materials and methods, 133
  orthopantomography
    double full-arch All-on- 4 rehabilitation, 133
    mandibular single full-arch All-on-4 rehabilitation, 133

    of maxillary single full-arch All-on-4 rehabilitation, 133
  outcome measures, 134
  retrospective analysis of porcelain failures, 137
  sample size calculation, 133
  statistical analysis, 134
  surgical protocol, 134
  survival estimation, 136

E

Eating disorders not otherwise specified (ED-NOS), 45, 46
Edentulism, 78
  prevalence of, 167
Edentulous maxillary jaws, 115
Elastomer technology, 198
Elliptical designs, 159
Emergency profile
  customization, 16
  evaluation, 16–17
Endosseous craniofacial implants (CFI's), 198
Endosseous extraoral implants, 198
Esthetics, 17, 36, 38, 168, 186, 194, 216
  abutment design and, 47
  blueprint for, 88
  for certain jaw and lip, 89
  challenges, 16
  comfort, 115
  complications, 96
  demands with maxillary prostheses, 154, 155
  factors critical to prosthetic design selection, 90
  impacts buccal corridor, 88
  implant abutment, 17–19
  implant-supported restorations, 46
  by major surgery, 259
  outcome, 83
  and prosthetic complications, 12
  result of RPD improved by, 4
  screw-retained interim prostheses, 118
  variables, 174
Extraoral implants, for acquired nasal defect
  abutment impression copings, 200
  acrylic resin, framework fabricated, 200
  associated clinical complications and clinical survival rates, 202
  CAD/CAM framework, 201
  clinical report, 199
    implant placement, 200
    patient presentation, 199
    restorative treatment, 200–202
    treatment plan, 199
  common risk factors associated with craniofacial implant failure, 203
  endosseous craniofacial implants (CFI's), 198
  facial bones, 198
  failure with CFI implants, 202
  frameworks for fixed complete dentures, 199
  hygiene instructions and demonstrations, 201
  implant failure, common risk factors associated with, 203
  implant frameworks, 199, 201
  maxillofacial prosthetic rehabilitation, 198

Extraoral implants, for acquired nasal defect (*Continued*)
    osseointegrated implants, 198
  milling center, 200
  Minnesota Multiphasic Personality Inventory (MMPI), 198
  nasal and orbital implants, 202
  nasal prosthesis, 201
  preoperative frontal and lateral views, 199
  prosthesis cumulative survival rates (CSR's), 202
  prosthesis, magnetic housings, 201
  rhinectomy with left neck dissection, 199
  use of computer-assisted design and computer-assisted
      machining (CAD/CAM), 199
  wax prosthesis, lateral, frontal/left three-fourth views, 200

F
Facial prostheses, 187, 188, 190, 198
Family-based therapy, 46
Fibrous encapsulation, 36
Finite element analysis (FEA), 81, 110, 155, 208
Finite element methods (FEMs), 209
Fixed dental prostheses (FDPs), 22, 157, 158
Fixed partial denture (FPD), 42, 47, 54, 137, 155
Fluoride, 46
Fracture load, 215, 218, 219

G
Galileos imaging system, 168
Gingival
  biotypes, 17
  cervical crown junction of the MC design, 92
  crest, 15
  hyperplasia, 83
  index, 82
  margin, 15, 17, 53
  porcelain, 15
  sulcus, 53
  swelling, 37
  tissue thickness, 15
  zenith, 28
Gold alloy, 154–156, 199
  screws, 201
Graftless approach, 92
Grafts, 8, 11, 12, 15, 28, 37, 110, 115, 178
  assessment, 13
  autogenous onlay bone, 92
  composite, 177
  with pterygomaxillary implants, 92
  sinus, 90, 161, 177
GraphPad InStat version 3.01, 224

H
Healing
  abutments, 15, 25, 28, 31
  around titanium implants in osteoporotic bone, 239
  caps, 23, 25
  delay, 69, 71, 110, 118, 247, 257
  peri-implant mucosal, 30
  periods, 23, 24, 30, 36, 245

  for dental implants, 36
  phase, 46, 47, 222
  time, 29
  tissue gingival collar, 16
Hormone replacement therapy (HRT), 244
Hybrid implant prostheses, 153
  A/P spread and the "All-on-Four" protocol, 161
  CAD/CAM framework for fixing, 154
  cantilever
    extensions, 162
    length, rationale, 160
  clinical image of an acrylic resin, 154
  design considerations, 159–161
  fixed hybrid prostheses, original framework designs, 153–155
    complications, 156
    physical properties of metals, 156–159
  framework guidelines, 161–162
  historical perspective, 153–162
  metal implant frameworks, 153
  passively fitting implant frameworks, 155–156

I
ICK classification system, 5–8
  Kennedy Class I situations, 5
  Kennedy Class II situations, 6
  Kennedy Class III situations, 7
  Kennedy Class IV situations, 7
  for partially edentulous arches, 5
IFCD. *See* Implant, fixed complete denture (IFCD)
Iliac crest grafts, 177
Image Analysis System (AnalySIS), 224
Implant
  abutment, 17
    esthetics and function, 17
  angulation
    evaluation, 17
    issues, 17
  anterior-posterior (A-P) spread, 173
  craniofacial (*See* Craniofacial implants)
  dentistry, 11
  fixed complete denture (IFCD), 67, 68, 70, 71, 88–90, 94–96
  frameworks
    laser-welding of, 155
  hybrid prosthesis, 154
  ideal implant location to access hole, 17
  platform location and evaluation, 12–14
  pterygomaxillary, 92, 115, 119
  retained overdenture (IROD), 68–71
  retained prosthesis, 154
    laboratory palatal image of, 155
    mandibular, 154
  supported
    fixed complete prostheses, 155
    metal ceramic (MC) reconstructions, 68
    overdenture, 68, 69
  surgery (*See* Implant surgery)
  titanium, 28
  treatment record form, 263–265

Implant possibilities, on atrophic maxilla
    anatomic considerations
        extrinsic morphology, 104, 109
        intrinsic morphology, 108–109
    biomechanics in atrophic maxilla, 110–111
    materials and methods, 104
    relevant studies
        on biomechanical aspects for implant possibilities, 103–104,
            107, 108
        on intrinsic and extrinsic anatomical aspects, 105, 106
Implant restorations, for mandibular edentulous patient
    differential treatment planning, 67
        considerations for implant treatment, 68
        evidence-based criteria for, 67–72
        immediate loading protocols, 69–71
        implant fixed complete denture, 70
        implant overdenture, 68–69
        implant restoration of edentulous mandible, 68
            rationale for placing implants, 68
        metal ceramic fixed dental prosthetic design, 71
Implant restorations, for maxillary edentulous patient
    differential treatment planning, 87
        algorithm for decision making in treatment planning, 96
    display of residual alveolar ridge without any prosthesis,
        90
    Dolder bar anchorage system, 91
    evidence-based criteria, 87–96
    exaggerated smile of patient with maxillary fixed complete
        denture, 90
    facebow registration using Kois Facial Analyzer, 91
    facial profile
        with flangeless denture, 89
        with no prosthesis in place, 89
    frontal view of vertical extent of residual ridge resorption, 89
    general considerations, for implant therapy, 88
    gingival-cervical crown junction of the MC design, 92
    gold occlusal design, on posterior teeth to thwart attrition, 92
    implant fixed complete denture, 92, 94
        framework design, 94
        immediate loading protocol, 95
        maintenance, 94–95, 95–96
        metal ceramic design, 95
        number of implants, 94
    implant overdenture, 93
        anchorage design/maintenance, 93
        immediate load protocols, 93–94
        number of implants, 93
    indications for implant restoration, of edentulous maxilla, 88–89
    Locator abutments, evenly distributed for maxillary
        overdenture, 91
    maxillary and mandibular dentures, on resilient casts, 91
    measurement of space allowance, before prosthetic design, 91
    milled bar mesostructure for overdenture, 92
    mounting of maxillary denture, with laboratory putty in, 91
    Sackett's hierarchy of evidence, 88
    sagittal view of horizontal defect, of premaxilla region, 89
    screw-retained metal ceramic (MC) design, 92
    selection of fixed or removable implant prosthetic design, 89–93

    suprastructure
        milled bar overdenture with swivel latches engaged on, 92
        overdenture in place over Locator abutments, 91
        in place over Dolder bar, 91
Implant-supported facial prostheses, by maxillofacial unit, 185
    age distribution, population of, 188
    degree of comfort, 189
    discoloration of, 190
    longevity of prosthesis, 188
    longevity, patient expectation, 190
    materials/methods, 188
    nasal defect and dental implant position
        lateral view demonstrating, 186
    nasal defect, lateral view, 186
    orbital defect, 187
    overall opinion, 189, 190
    patients' perception of quality, 189
    prosthesis
        life span, 189
        longevity of, 187, 188
        proportion of, 188–189
    quality of edge, 189
    restorative dentists, 187
    stomatognathic and associated facial structures, 186
Implant surgery, 23
    antibiotics, 23
    CAD design, 23
    control X-ray, 23
    implant placement, 23
    restoration options, 23
    scan data
        exported in STL format and, 23
        imported into a CAD-Software, 23
    scanning, 23
    screw-retained crown fabricated in, 24
    second-stage surgery, 24
        placement of screw-retained final crown, 24
        raising mucosal flap and undermining buccal soft tissue, 24
    situation during implant placement, 23
    wound healing and sutures removal, 23
Implant-surrounding bone, stress distribution
    abutment/implant interface, 208
    adequate implant system, 208
    bone/implant contact, 211
    bone/implant interface, 208
    CTI database, 208
    3D CAD software, 208
    internal hexagon (IH)/Morse taper (MT), 208
        buccal and lingual models, 210, 211
        maximum displacement stress, 210
            image analysis of, 210
        stresses in trabecular bone implants, 210
        stresses on cortical bone, 210
        Von Mises stress, 211
    long-term survival of dental implants placed, 208
    materials and methods
        anatomical structure, mechanical proprieties, 209
        implant manufacturer, 208

Implant-surrounding bone, stress distribution (*Continued*)
    model reconstruction, 209
    Von Mises criterion, 209
    peri-implant bone tissues
        transmission of occlusal load, 208
    tension distribution, 211
    vestibulo-lingual direction, 211
    Von Mises stress analysis, 212
Incomplete cement, removal, 53
Integrated Abutment Crown™, 53
Internal engaging/nonengaging connection evaluation, 14
Internal hexagon (IH), 208
    buccal and lingual models, 210, 211
    maximum displacement stress, 210
        image analysis of, 210
    stresses in trabecular bone implants, 210
    stresses on cortical bone, 210
    Von Mises stress, 211
Intraoral scanning device, 22
IROD. *See* Implant, retained overdenture (IROD)
Irreversible hydrocolloid material, 178

K
Kennedy method of classification, 4
    guidelines, 4
Keratinized tissues, 16
Kolmogorov-Smirnov test, 217, 218

L
Laboratory occlusal image, of a resin pattern, 159
L-beam design, 153, 160
    CAD/CAM milled framework, 160
Le Fort I osteotomy, 177
Lesions, 46, 105, 179
    nasal, 199
Lithium disilicate, 23–25, 118

M
Mandibular
    implant CAD/CAM framework
        for a fixed hybrid implant prosthesis, 153
    implant-retained framework designed as an I-bar, 153
    prosthesis
        fixed hybrid, 153, 154
        mandibular implants, planned position of, 168
        mock-up of, 169
        scan and digital design of, 169
Mandibular implant overdenture treatment, 77–84
    combination syndrome associated with dental implants, 82
    consensus of opinion *vs.* controversy, 83
        areas of controversy, 84
        areas of general consensus, 84
    conventional denture treatment, 78
    dental implants
        with bar attachment fixation in anterior mandible, 81
        with bar attachment in anterior mandible, 80
        located within anterior mandibular alveolar bone, 80
        utilization, 78–79

denture base fracture
    associated with mandibular implant overdenture treatment, 83
    diminished supporting tissue volume, negative influence, 78
    edentulism, 78
    implant overdenture treatment, 79
    independent dental implants with O-ring attachments in anterior mandible, 80
    interconnected *vs.* independent implants, 80–82
    natural teeth *vs.* dental implants, 79
        sparse and controversial, 79
    number of implants required, 80
    patient satisfaction, 83
    peri-implant response, 82
    preservation of bone, 79–80
    totally implant-supported prosthesis in anterior mandible, 79
    treatment complications, 82–83
Marginal bone loss (MBL), 28
    associated with immediately loaded implants inserted into, 30
    delayed loading protocol (two stages), 29
    difference in values between mesial and distal surfaces, 32
    at different time intervals, 32
    digital intraoral radiographs of implants placed into, 31
    evaluation in extraction sites, 30
    formation and maturation of soft tissue around implants, 32
    immediate loading protocol (one stage), 29
    materials and methods, 28
    measurement technique, 30
    nonsignificant error margin, 30
    null hypothesis, 28
    patient selection criteria, 28–29
    prosthetic techniques, around titanium implants, 28
    radiological criteria to assess, 28
    statistical analysis, 29, 30
    surgical and prosthetic factors, influencing, 28
    surgical phase, 29
    two-phase surgical procedures associated with, 30
    vascular ischemia associated with, 31
Maxillary
    anterior region, 46
    bone, tumor resection surgery
        treatment of, 178
    complete dentures, 155
    sinus grafts, 177
    sinus pneumatization
        initial panoramic radiography, 178
Maxillary tumor, 193
Maxillomandibular relationships
    abutment level impression, 168
MBL. *See* Marginal bone loss (MBL)
MDIs. *See* Mini dental implants (MDIs)
Micro-CT techniques, 110
Milled green-state zirconia prosthesis, 169
Milled titanium alloy framework, 159
Milled zirconium frameworks, 157
Mini dental implants (MDIs)
    challenge to treating prosthodontist, 192
    clinical report, 193–195
    finger driver, 193

heat-processed acrylic resin, 194
immediate implants
   postoperative intraoral photograph, 194
interim obturator with resilient liner/incorporated O-ring
     housings, 194
ligated surgical obturator, 193
master cast, secondary impression, 195
maxillary tumor, preoperative photograph of, 193
O-ring housings, 194
postoperative panorex, 194
pressure-indicating paste, 195
surgical obturator, 193
transitional/modular implants, 195
Minnesota Multiphasic Personality Inventory (MMPI), 198
Missing teeth, repalcement, 36
cementation of acrylic resin crown, 37
clinical treatment, 37
comparison study of two groups of patients, 38
complications and failures, 37
contours of restoration, 37
immediate provisionalization protocols, treatment option, 39
implant distribution frequency, 38
implant failure rate by type, 39
implant sites, 37
implant survival rates
   by location and bone quality, 39
   by location and implant length, 38
integrity of acrylic resin margins, 37
materials and methods, 36
Nobel Biocare implants, 37
patients, 36
surgical procedure, 36
teeth in a day prosthetic procedures, 36–37
Monolithic zirconia fixed dental prosthesis (MZ-FDP), 167
analytic methods, 169–170
assessment/conventional denture fabrication, 168
biologic and prosthetic outcomes, 170–171
complications, 170–171
fracture, 173
implant survival in edentulous mandible, 171–174
inclusion/exclusion criteria, 168
master cast, 168
materials and methods, 168–170
mean OHIP-49 extent scores, 171, 172
mean OHIP-49 severity scores, 171, 172
milled green-state zirconia prosthesis, 169
mock-up of mandibular prosthesis, 169
observation period, 170
   complications by participant, 170
   complications by type/timing, 171
OHIP-49 questionnaire, 169–170
   severity score, 171
OHIP-49 subscale analysis, 173
participant characteristics
   and OHIP-49 severity and extent scores at enrollment, 171
planned position of mandibular implants, 168
scan and digital design of mandibular prosthesis, 169
sintered and polished definitive zirconia prosthesis, 170

stained, presintered zirconia prosthesis, 169
surgical procedures, 168
zirconia prosthesis fabrication, 168–169
Morse taper (MT), 208
buccal and lingual models, 210, 211
maximum displacement stress, 210
   image analysis of, 210
stresses in trabecular bone implants, 210
stresses on cortical bone, 210
Von Mises stress, 211
Mortality rates, 46
MT. *See* Morse taper (MT)
Mucosal barrier, 28
Muscle
attachments, 69, 78
grafts, 107
healing, 259
movements, 119
MZ-FDP. *See* Monolithic zirconia fixed dental prosthesis (MZ-
    FDP)

N
Nasal defect, 186, 199, 202
lateral view, 186
Nickel-chromium alloys, 180
Nobel Biocare implant, 225, 226
Noble metal alloy, 44, 153, 156

O
One-piece casting procedures, for homogeneous frameworks, 158
Oral/facial symmetries, 154
Oral health quality of life (OHQoL), 167
Oral implant, 132
Osseointegrated dental implants. *See also various dental implants*
characteristics of data collected, 123
description of anticipated and unanticipated prosthetic and
    biologic events, 123
events, 129
   addressed for, 127
   summary of anticipated and unanticipated events and visits to
     address, 126
   summary of patient experiences with, 127
implant failures, 127
long-term practice outcome data, 127–128
most common prosthetic and biologic events, 125–127
outcomes
   comparison, 128
   research, 128
overview
   of events, 124–125
   of prosthesis survival, 124
population characteristics, 128
practice application, 129
practice-based evidence, and management of edentulous jaw
    using, 121
   materials and methods, 122–123
prosthesis-specific survival, 129
summary

Osseointegrated dental implants (*Continued*)
    of patient-centered questions, 128
    of patient specific features, 124
Osseointegration, 30, 36, 39, 88, 116, 132, 141, 148, 155, 198,
       199, 202, 222, 228, 230, 231, 239–241, 244, 245, 247,
       257–259
Osteoporosis, 238
  animal studies deficiencies, 244–245
  biphosphonate therapy, 246
  definition of, 238
  dental implants and, 238
  epidemiology of, 238
  human studies deficiencies, 245–246
  pathophysiology of, 238
  risk factors, 239
  steroid-induced, 244
  systemic complications of, 238
  WHO criteria, 244
    defined, 244
    diagnosis, 244
Oxidized-titanium-surfaced implants, 36

P
Palladium/silver alloys, 157
Partial edentulism, 4
  rationale of classification, 4
Peri-implant mucosa, 22
  architecture, 28
Peri-implant pathology
  attributable risk fraction, 148
  components of an implant-prosthetic rehabilitation, 141
  controlling risk factors for the incidence of, 147
  crude odds ratio (OR) with confidence intervals, 148
  frequencies and percentages of variables related to
      characteristics of reconstruction, 144–146
  implant:crown ratio (ICR), 142
  implant-supported prostheses
    screwed/cemented, 142
  implants with hydroxyapatite surface, 141
  influence of rehabilitation, characteristics in incidence of, 141
  machined surfaces constituted risk factor, 146
  materials and methods, 142–143
  material used, in prosthesis influenced risk status, 146
  measuring critical bending moment, 146
  mechanical complications, 142
  pathogenesis, described as, 141
  presence of cantilevers, in a fixed prosthesis, 142
  prosthetic screw loosening, 142
  restorative material, used in prosthesis, 142
  results from bivariate analysis for variables in, 147
  statistical analysis, 143
Phonares I denture teeth, 168
Plaster model, 22
Platform switch evaluation, 14–15
Polished definitive zirconia prosthesis, 170
Poly(vinyl siloxane) impression material, 178
Porcelain
  fracture, 96, 137

fused-to-gold implant-supported crown, 37
fused-to-metal fixed partial denture, 47
gingival, 15, 17
ideal thickness, 11
incisal chipping, 30
to mask the defect, 15
structural integrity and establish unstable occlusal contact, 42
tendency to change to a green color with, 157
veneer fractures, 157, 158
Presintered zirconia prosthesis, 169
Prosthesis
  esthetic and functional examination, 179
  occlusal view, 179
  waxed on master cast, 178
Prosthetic complications, 156
Prosthetic preangulated abutments, 17
Prosthodontic Diagnostic Index (PDI), 8
Provisionalization, 36, 37, 39

Q
Quality of life (QoL), 67, 69, 71, 72, 88, 89, 174

R
Randomized controlled clinical trials (RCT), 88, 104, 138, 222, 223
Removable partial denture (RPD), 4, 193
  design, 154
  metal frameworks, 162
Restorative space
  cementable restoration, 11
  choice of fixed restoration, 11
  classification, 11
  evaluation, 11
  ideal space for a fixed prosthesis, 11
  interocclusal distances exceeding, 12
Rhinoceros 4.0 NURBS Modeling, 208

S
Scanning, 18, 23
  CAD/CAM frameworks, 162
  images, filter size, 224
  intraoral device, 22, 23
  template, 200
Screwless and cementless technique, 52–61
  clinical and radiographic
    view of an IAC on a maxillary right second premolar, 60
  complications and failures, 55
    loosening of IACs, 61
    loosening of nine maxillary anterior IACs, 61
    plaque accumulation, 61
    postinsertion, 61
  data management and statistics, 55
  descriptive statistics and univariate analysis for risk factors,
    56–58
  descriptive statistics for patient questionnaire, 58
  insertion of IAC, 53
  Kaplan–Meier survival IACs, 58
  materials and methods, 54
  multivariate marginal cox regression models for risk factors, 59

patient questionnaire, 55
periapical radiographs, 54, 60
soft tissue parameters, 55
study variables, 54
    anatomic-tooth specific variables, 54
    health status variables, 54
    implant-specific variables, 54
    prosthetic-soft tissue variables, 54
    reconstructive variables, 54
survival estimate for IACs, 55, 61
Shear bond strengths (SBS), 162
Silver palladium alloys, 155
Single-tooth implants, 25, 36, 37, 39
failure rates in immediate provisionalization of, 39
screwless and cementless technique for restoration of, 52–61
Sintered definitive zirconia prosthesis, 170
Stained zirconia prosthesis, 169
Standard tessellation language (STL) format, 23
Stereolithographic models, 46
Subgingival margins, 53
Substance abuse, 46

T
Tilted implants, 92, 115
Tissue
collar height evaluation, 15–16
diminished supporting tissue volume, 78
evaluation, soft and hard, 12
inflammation, 82
keratinized, 93
mucosal, hyperplasia of, 82
peri-implant, 28, 138
  infections, 208
prosthetic-soft tissue variables, 54
prosthetic-tissue junction, 89
soft and hard tissue evaluation, 12, 22
Titanium alloy, 53, 94, 158, 161, 162, 180, 195, 199, 200, 226

U
Ultrasonic vibration device, 42

V
Vickers hardness, 156
Vistafix System, 200
Von Mises criterion, of maximal distortion, 209

W
Wax prosthesis, 200

X
Xerostomia, 46

Y
Yttria tetragonal zirconia polycrystal (Y-TZP), 157

Z
Zirconia, 15, 18, 23, 25
abutments, 16, 17, 19, 49, 158, 217, 219
  fabricated using CAD/CAM technology, 49
ceramics, 158
definitive zirconia prosthesis, 174
fractured distal extension segment of zirconia prosthesis
  through screw access hole, 173
frameworks, milled, 157
monolithic, 167, 168
oxide materials, flexural strength, 157
prosthesis
  cementable single unit, 174
  chipping complication, 172
  fractured distal extension segment of, 173
restorations, implant supported, 158
stained, presintered zirconia prosthesis, 169
yttria-stabilized, 18, 216
Zirconia custom abutments, with internal connection,
    216
artificial dynamic thermal, aging, 218, 219
ceramic abutment material, 216
cubic acrylic jigs, implant replicas placed, 217
failure risk, 218
fracture load, 218
fracture load means, 218
fracture pattern of, 218
group distribution, 217
implant/abutment connection, types, 218
Instron machine, 217
lever arm vector and fracture behavior, 218
materials and methods, 216
  experimental design, 216–217
  one-piece zirconia custom abutments, mean fracture load
    of, 218
  sample size/power calculation, 216
  specimen preparation, 217
  statistical analysis, 217–218
one-piece abutments, 216
one-piece zirconia custom abutments, 218
regular cross-fit zirconia custom abutments, 217
stress-strain diagram, 217
zirconia custom abutments, 217
Zygomatic fixation technique, 178
Zygomatic implants, 92, 96, 110, 111, 177, 178
implant inclinations, 179
impression copings, 178
panoramic radiography, 178